D1805271

Surgical Pathology Dissection

Second Edition

Springer
*New York
Berlin
Heidelberg
Hong Kong
London
Milan
Paris
Tokyo*

Surgical Pathology Dissection
An Illustrated Guide

Second Edition

William H. Westra, M.D.
Department of Pathology
The Johns Hopkins University
School of Medicine
Baltimore, Maryland

Ralph H. Hruban, M.D.
Department of Pathology
The Johns Hopkins University
School of Medicine
Baltimore, Maryland

Timothy H. Phelps, M.S.
Department of Art as Applied to Medicine
The Johns Hopkins University
School of Medicine
Baltimore, Maryland

Christina Isacson, M.D.
Department of Pathology
Virginia Mason Medical Center
Seattle, Washington

With Forewords by Frederic B. Askin, M.D.

With 58 Illustrations

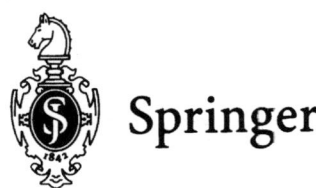 Springer

William H. Westra, M.D.
Department of Pathology
The Johns Hopkins Hospital
The Weinberg Cancer Building, Room 2242
401 North Broadway
Baltimore, MD 21231-2410, USA

Ralph H. Hruban, M.D.
Department of Pathology
The Johns Hopkins Hospital
The Weinberg Cancer Building, Room 2242
401 North Broadway
Baltimore, MD 21231-2410, USA

Timothy H. Phelps, M.S.
Department of Art as Applied
 to Medicine
The Johns Hopkins University
 School of Medicine
1830 East Monument Street,
 Suite 7000
Baltimore, MD 21205-2100, USA

Christina Isacson, M.D.
Department of Pathology
Virginia Mason Medical Center
1100 Ninth Avenue, C6-Path
Seattle, WA 98101, USA

Cover illustration: Extrahepatic biliary tract resection for carcinoma of the common bile duct. Illustration by Timothy H. Phelps.

Library of Congress Cataloging-in-Publication Data
Surgical pathology dissection: an illustrated guide/[edited by] William H. Westra . . . [et al.].—2nd ed.
   p.; cm.
  Includes bibliographical references and index.
  ISBN 0-387-95559-3 (s/c: alk. paper)
   1. Pathology, Surgical—Laboratory manuals. 2. Human dissection—
Laboratory manuals.   I. Westra, William H.
   [DNLM: 1. Pathology, Surgical—Laboratory Manuals.
 2. Dissection—Laboratory Manuals.   WO 142 S9615   2002]
 RD57. S87. 2002
 617'.07—dc21   2002029448

ISBN 0-387-95559-3   Printed on acid-free paper.

© 2003, 1996 Springer-Verlag New York, Inc.
All rights reserved. This work may not be translated or copied in whole or in part without the written permission of the publisher (Springer-Verlag New York, Inc., 175 Fifth Avenue, New York, NY 10010, USA), except for brief excerpts in connection with reviews or scholarly analysis. Use in connection with any form of information storage and retrieval, electronic adaptation, computer software, or by similar or dissimilar methodology now known or hereafter developed is forbidden.
The use in this publication of trade names, trademarks, service marks, and similar terms, even if they are not identified as such, is not to be taken as an expression of opinion as to whether or not they are subject to proprietary rights.
While the advice and information in this book are believed to be true and accurate at the date of going to press, neither the authors nor the editors nor the publisher can accept any legal responsibility for any errors or omissions that may be made. The publisher makes no warranty, express or implied, with respect to the material contained herein.

Printed in the United States of America.

9 8 7 6 5 4 3 2 1   SPIN 10888565

www.springer-ny.com

Springer-Verlag New York Berlin Heidelberg
A member of BertelsmannSpringer Science+Business Media GmbH

To the Breakfast Club. Fond memories of hooping it up.

To the team: Sharon, Caryn, Janine, and Willem.
William H. Westra

To my wonderful wife, Claire, and our three terrific children, Zoe, Emily, and Carolyn.
Ralph H. Hruban

To my wife, Lyn, for her ever-present love and support; my two children, Katie and Kevin, who bring me great and constant joy; my art instructors of the past for all they have shared with me; and, particularly and most importantly, my Father; and in loving memory of my Mother.
Timothy H. Phelps

To my sisters, Charlotte and Patty.
Christina Isacson

Foreword to the Second Edition

It is a pleasure, an honor, and a distinct privilege to write the foreword for the second edition of *Surgical Pathology Dissection: An Illustrated Guide.* I am delighted to see that my predictions were accurate in regard to this effective and useful book. It has become an extremely popular dissection manual with regard to both its text and illustrative material. In fact, the manual and its medical illustrator, Timothy H. Phelps, received the Illustrated Book Award from the Association of Medical Illustrators in 1996. Pathologist reviewers have uniformly characterized the text as valuable and inclusive while still leaving room for individual variation in specimen handling.

Just as our other clinical colleagues continually endeavor to improve patient care by adding new diagnostic tests and techniques, it is incumbent on anatomic pathologists to do the same. The authors' goal in the development of the second edition of this manual was not to replace the first edition but, rather, to build on its strength. In this second edition, one finds the addition of new coauthors with recognized expertise in their respective fields of interest. These coauthors have provided chapters on contemporary topics not covered in the first edition and new illustrations (the specifics are listed in the Preface). In addition, a number of the original illustrations, such as the breast specimen dissection, have been significantly revised and improved. In an attempt to provide more uniform description and tumor staging, the existing chapters have been updated to conform with the recently published College of American Pathologists (CAP) and Association of Directors of Anatomic and Surgical Pathology (ADASP) guidelines.

The basic goals for the first edition have been retained: to provide an accurate, concept-oriented, easy-to-use manual that provides a logical, concise approach to the most commonly encountered specimens. Although new authors and new material have been added, the basic solid framework of the manual persists. I am confident that the second edition provides significant improvements and that this manual will continue to be a mainstay in the anatomic pathology armamentarium.

Frederic B. Askin, M.D.
Professor of Pathology
The Johns Hopkins University
School of Medicine
and
Director of Surgical Pathology
The Johns Hopkins Hospital
Baltimore, MD 21231-2410, USA

Foreword to the First Edition

The modern surgical pathology cutting room is replete with tools of the electronic age. Computers, automatic cassette labelers, bar coding, and even electronic voice-recognition systems are available to help the surgical pathologist be an effective, efficient, and highly productive cog in the machinery of healthcare delivery. In spite of this automated armamentarium, much of our ability to render diagnoses rests with the surgical pathology "cutters." These personnel need to be trained to handle surgical specimens consistently and appropriately, with the goal of providing optimal diagnostic information and adequate pathologic correlation with clinical and radiologic findings.

This dissection manual is an outgrowth of what Waldemar Schmidt has called the "oral tradition" of surgical pathology. Traditionally, the senior pathologist passed down to the trainee an individual accumulation of expertise on the handling of specimens. This transfer of information was often random and based solely on the specific case at hand. Now, despite the importance of training personnel, the exigencies of modern practice limit the amount of time available for individual training, and so most laboratories have developed their own local manual. Unfortunately, many of these manuals are incomplete or not user-friendly.

Drs. Hruban, Westra, and Isacson have prepared this manual with the help of a distinguished and talented medical artist. Timothy H. Phelps's pen and ink drawings bring a unique vitality and multidimensional effect to the reader throughout the manual as dissection techniques are explained and illustrated. The editors and contributors have effectively shared their talents and experience by providing general principles that can be employed to resolve even the most complex problems in dissection and effective tissue sampling. The methods are broadly applicable and unusually easy to follow.

This text should be at hand in all surgical pathology laboratories, where it will be useful to a wide variety of personnel including staff pathologists, residents, pathologist's assistants, histotechnologists, and other laboratory personnel. It is highly likely that many surgeons would also benefit from use of this manual, through which they can gain an understanding of how specimens are dissected and can become familiar with the way in which margin and tumor sampling are carried out.

This is a very practical manual. The authors discuss the clinically important features of various types of specimens and lesions in each organ system. They instruct the prosector in every instance as to what information is needed to provide the clearest clinical picture. I suspect that this work will be most valuable to the surgical pathology cutter late in the evening or on weekends, when the redoubtable oral historian of surgical pathology is not available. This manual should serve as a cornerstone on which to build a stable but malleable standard of excellence in the surgical pathology cutting room.

Frederic B. Askin, M.D.
Professor of Pathology
The Johns Hopkins University
School of Medicine
and
Director of Surgical Pathology
The Johns Hopkins Hospital
Baltimore, MD 21231-2410, USA

Preface

Our goal in writing the first edition of *Surgical Pathology Dissection: An Illustrated Guide* was to create a user-friendly, hands-on guide for the dissection of surgical pathology specimens. To do this, we brought a team of surgical pathologists with a broad range of expertise together with Timothy H. Phelps, one of the leading medical illustrators in the United States. In so doing, we believe we created a manual that provides a logical, concise approach to the most commonly encountered specimens. In the years since the first edition was published, *Surgical Pathology Dissection: An Illustrated Guide* has emerged as the standard in the field, and in 1996, Timothy H. Phelps was awarded the Illustrated Book Award from the Association of Medical Illustrators for his artwork in the book.

We have made a number of significant improvements in the second edition of *Surgical Pathology Dissection: An Illustrated Guide*. First, new coauthors were asked to join the existing team to add a fresh perspective to key chapters. For example, Elizabeth Montgomery, Robb E. Wilentz, Michael Torbenson, Susan Abraham, E. Rene Rodriguez, and Pedram Argani have helped update key chapters on the digestive system, heart, and breast. Second, new chapters, including chapters on transplantation and sentinel lymph nodes, have been added, reflecting emerging trends in surgical pathology practice. Importantly, these new chapters retain the user-friendly style characteristic of the first edition. Third, new illustrations, including those for dissection of an explanted heart, craniofacial bones, and sentinel lymph nodes, have been added. In addition, a number of the original illustrations, such as for the dissection of breast specimens, have been significantly revised and improved. Fourth, updates to existing chapters, particularly where they were needed to conform to the more recently published College of American Pathologists (CAP) and Association of Directors of Anatomic and Surgical Pathology (ADASP) guidelines, have been made. These changes were made with the goal of keeping *Surgical Pathology Dissection: An Illustrated Guide* user-friendly and up to date. Each chapter therefore continues to include descriptions and illustrations of the mechanics involved when handling each specimen as well as a conceptual framework for questions to keep in mind during the dissection. At the end of each chapter, the section entitled "Important Issues to Address in Your Pathology Report" helps guide the user to the key information needed to stage most tumors accurately.

Finally, to reflect the equal contributions of the two first authors, Drs. Westra and Hruban have switched places in authorship, and Dr. Westra is now the first author on the second edition.

We believe the second edition is a significant improvement over the first edition, and we continue to hope that this illustrated guide will make the dissection of any specimen an important and enjoyable endeavor.

William H. Westra, M.D.
Ralph H. Hruban, M.D.
Timothy H. Phelps, M.S.
Christina Isacson, M.D.

Acknowledgments

The authors thank Amanda Lietman and Sandy Markowitz for their superb assistance in preparing, proofreading, and editing this manual and for their patience and understanding. It is impossible to praise their talents and efforts enough. The authors also thank Drs. Frederic B. Askin and Grover M. Hutchins for their constructive criticism of the book and Drs. Michael Borowitz, Joseph Califano, David Eisele, Jonathan Epstein, Kristin Fiebelkorn, Stanley R. Hamilton, Zdenek Hruban, Wayne Koch, Ralph Kuncl, Robert Kurman, and Charles Yeo for sharing their expertise. The authors also thank Claire E. Hruban.

William H. Westra, M.D.
Ralph H. Hruban, M.D.
Timothy H. Phelps, M.S.
Christina Isacson, M.D.

Contents

Foreword to the Second Edition vii
Foreword to the First Edition ix
Preface xi
Acknowledgments xiii
Contributors xix

I. General Approach and Techniques

Chapter 1 General Approach to Surgical Pathology Specimens 2

Chapter 2 Laboratory Techniques 14
William M. Fox III and Robert H. Rosa, Jr.

Chapter 3 Tissue Collection for Molecular Genetic Analysis 22

Chapter 4 Photography 26
Norman J. Barker

II. Lymph Nodes for Metastatic Tumors

Chapter 5 Lymph Nodes 34

III. The Head and Neck

Chapter 6 Larynx 38

Chapter 7 Major Salivary Glands 43

Chapter 8 Complex Specimens 44

Chapter 9 Maxilla 48
James J. Sciubba

Chapter 10 Radical Neck Dissection 54

IV. The Digestive System

Chapter 11 Esophagus 58
Elizabeth Montgomery

Chapter 12 Stomach 62
Elizabeth Montgomery

Chapter 13	Non-Neoplastic Intestinal Disease	66
	Robb E. Wilentz	
Chapter 14	Neoplastic Intestinal Disease	70
	Elizabeth Montgomery	
Chapter 15	Appendix	74
	Elizabeth Montgomery	
Chapter 16	Liver	76
	Michael S. Torbenson	
Chapter 17	Gallbladder and Extrahepatic Biliary System	82
	Susan Abraham	
Chapter 18	Pancreas	88

V. The Cardiovascular/Respiratory System

Chapter 19	Heart, Heart Valves, and Vessels	94
	E. Rene Rodriguez	
Chapter 20	Lungs	102
Chapter 21	Transplantation	110

VI. Bone, Soft Tissue, and Skin

Chapter 22	Bone	114
	Edward F. McCarthy, Jr.	
Chapter 23	Soft Tissue, Nerves, and Muscle	120
	Elizabeth Montgomery	
Chapter 24	Skin	124
	Thomas D. Horn	

VII. The Breast

Chapter 25	Breast	132
	Pedram Argani	

VIII. The Female Genital System

Chapter 26	Vulva	142
Chapter 27	Uterus, Cervix, and Vagina	146
Chapter 28	Ovary and Fallopian Tube	160
Chapter 29	Products of Conception and Placentas	166

IX. The Urinary Tract and Male Genital System

Chapter 30	Penis	172
Chapter 31	Prostate	176
Chapter 32	Testis	180
Chapter 33	Kidney	184
Chapter 34	Bladder	188

X. The Ocular System

Chapter 35	Eye	194
	Robert H. Rosa, Jr., and W. Richard Green	

XI. The Endocrine System

Chapter 36	Thyroid	202
Chapter 37	Parathyroid Glands	206
Chapter 38	Adrenal Glands	208

XII. Pediatric Tumors

Chapter 39	Pediatric Tumors	212
	Elizabeth J. Perlman	

XIII. The Central Nervous System

Chapter 40	Brain and Spinal Cord	218
	Peter C. Burger	

XIV. The Hematopoietic and Lymphatic System

Chapter 41	Lymph Nodes	224
Chapter 42	Spleen	228
Chapter 43	Thymus	231
Chapter 44	Bone Marrow	232

XV. Odds and Ends

Chapter 45	Common Uncomplicated Specimens	236

Closing Comments	239
References	240
Suggested Web Sites and Suggested Readings	242
Index	253

Contributors

Susan Abraham, M.D.
Assistant Professor of Pathology, Division of Gastrointestinal/Liver Pathology, The Johns Hopkins School of Medicine, Baltimore, MD 21287-6971, USA

Pedram Argani, M.D.
Assistant Professor of Pathology, The Johns Hopkins University School of Medicine, Baltimore, MD 21231-2410, USA

Frederic B. Askin, M.D.
Professor of Pathology, The Johns Hopkins University School of Medicine; and Director of Surgical Pathology, The Johns Hopkins Hospital, Baltimore, MD 21231-2410, USA

Norman J. Barker, M.S., R.B.P.
Assistant Professor of Pathology and Art as Applied to Medicine and Director of Pathology Photography, The Johns Hopkins University School of Medicine, Baltimore, MD 21287-6971, USA

Peter C. Burger, M.D.
Professor of Pathology, Oncology, and Neurosurgery, The Johns Hopkins University School of Medicine, Baltimore, MD 21287-6971, USA

William M. Fox III, B.S., M.S., P.A.-C.
Mercy Medical Center, Baltimore, MD 20201, USA

W. Richard Green, M.D.
International Order of Odd Fellows Professor of Ophthalmology, and Professor of Pathology, the Wilmer Ophthalmological Institute, The Johns Hopkins University School of Medicine, Baltimore, MD 21287-6971, USA

Thomas D. Horn, M.D.
Professor of Dermatology and Pathology, and Chairman, Department of Dermatology, University of Arkansas for Medical Sciences, Little Rock, AR 72205, USA

Ralph H. Hruban, M.D.
Professor of Pathology and Oncology, The Johns Hopkins University School of Medicine; and Director, Division of Gastrointestinal/Liver Pathology, The Johns Hopkins Hospital, Baltimore, MD 21231-2410, USA

Christina Isacson, M.D.
Pathologist and Deputy Chief of Pathology, Virginia Mason Medical Center, Seattle, WA 98101-0900, USA

Edward F. McCarthy, Jr., M.D.
Professor of Pathology and Orthopedic Surgery, The Johns Hopkins University School of Medicine; and Director, Bone Histomorphometry Laboratory, The Johns Hopkins Hospital, Baltimore, MD 21231-2410, USA

Elizabeth Montgomery, M.D.
Associate Professor of Pathology, Division of Gastrointestinal/Liver Pathology, The Johns Hopkins School of Medicine, Baltimore, MD 21205-2410, USA

Elizabeth J. Perlman, M.D.
Professor of Pathology, Northwestern University; and Head, Department of Pathology, Children's Memorial Hospital, Chicago, IL 60614, USA

Timothy H. Phelps, M.S., FAMI, C.M.I.
Associate Professor of Art as Applied to Medicine, The Johns Hopkins University School of Medicine, Baltimore, MD 21205, USA

E. Rene Rodriguez, M.D.
Associate Professor of Pathology, The Johns Hopkins School of Medicine; and Director, Clinical Services Cardiovascular Pathology, The Johns Hopkins Hospital, Baltimore, MD 21205-2410, USA

Robert H. Rosa, Jr., M.D.
Associate Professor, Departments of Ophthalmology and Pathology, Scott and White Clinic, Texas A&M University System Health Science Center, Temple, TX 76508, USA

James J. Sciubba, D.M.D., Ph.D.
Professor of Otolaryngology, Head and Neck Surgery, Pathology, and Dermatology, The Johns Hopkins University School of Medicine, Baltimore, MD 21287-6971, USA

Michael S. Torbenson, M.D.
Instructor of Pathology, Division of Gastrointestinal/Liver Pathology, The Johns Hopkins School of Medicine, Baltimore, MD 21205-2410, USA

William H. Westra, M.D.
Associate Professor of Pathology and Otolaryngology, Head and Neck Surgery, The Johns Hopkins University School of Medicine, Baltimore, MD 21231-2410, USA

Robb E. Wilentz, M.D.
Assistant Professor of Pathology, Division of Gastrointestinal/Liver Pathology, The Johns Hopkins School of Medicine, Baltimore, MD 21205-2410, USA

I General Approach and Techniques

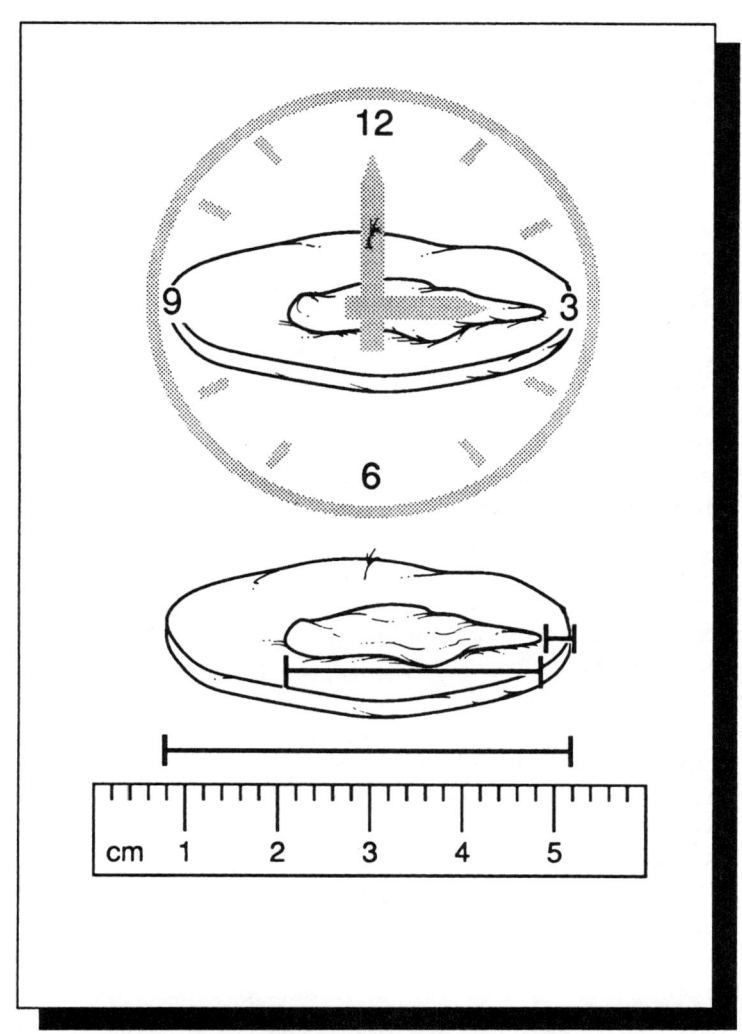

General Approach to Surgical Pathology Specimens

Safety in the Surgical Pathology Laboratory

The key to safety in the surgical pathology laboratory is to recognize that this area is a dangerous place. A variety of noxious chemicals are routinely used in the surgical pathology laboratory, and tissues infected with the human immunodeficiency virus (HIV), hepatitis viruses, mycobacteria, and other agents enter through its doors on a daily basis. Not only are these infectious agents present in the laboratory, but their transmission is also facilitated by the frequent handling of bloody tissues and the routine use of surgical blades, knives, saws, and other sharp instruments. Clearly, the surgical pathology laboratory is no place to "let down one's guard" by becoming careless or distracted. Rather, safety in the work area should become an ingrained habit, and universal precautions should be exercised with all specimens.

Protective Gear

The prosector should regard all tissues as potentially infectious, not just those tissues removed from patients known to have an infectious disease. For the protection of oneself and for the safety of others, the prosector should wear protective gear in the cutting area at all times. Protective gear prevents contact of potentially infectious materials with the skin and mucous membranes, and it diminishes the transfer of infectious material outside of the surgical pathology laboratory. At the very least, protective gear should include surgical scrubs, waterproof shoe coverings, a surgical gown and/or waterproof forearm wraps, gloves, a cap, a mask, and eye protection. A waterproof apron should also be worn to prevent the absorption of fluids onto the clothing and skin. Hands should be protected by well-fitting surgical gloves. To prevent seepage of fluids, two pairs of gloves are preferred to one pair, and these gloves should be changed frequently. Keep in mind that even two pairs of gloves will not protect against punctures and cuts. Fine mesh metallic or synthetic gloves that are cut-resistant are recommended in those instances where one is unfamiliar with the use of a sharp instrument or when one is dissecting a specimen with sharp edges (e.g., a bone resection). Soiled or bloody garments and coverings should not be worn outside of the cutting area.

Disposal of Instruments and Trash, and Storage of Specimens

In order to avoid inadvertent wounds, there should be no more than one blade in the dissection field at any one time. Needles, razor blades, scalpel blades, and other sharp disposable objects should be promptly discarded into appropriate containers following their use. Trash items soiled with blood or other potentially infectious materials should be discarded into designated biohazard containers located in the cutting area. Upon completion of the dissection, the specimen should be stored in a container with adequate formalin. Specimen containers should be wiped clean of any potentially infectious materials, securely closed to prevent leakage, accurately labeled, and stored in a designated storage area.

In cases of known viral hepatitis, HIV infection, or tuberculosis, the cutting area should be washed clean and wiped with a disinfectant such as dilute bleach, and a biohazard label should be affixed to the specimen container.

Radioactive Specimens

With the increasing use of radioactive materials as a means to identify sentinel lymph nodes, the proper handling of radioactive materials has become an increasing concern in the surgical pathology laboratory. Although the risk of significant radiation exposure associated with these sentinel lymph nodes is believed to be very low, each institution should nonetheless develop written procedures for handling all radioactive specimens. These procedures should be developed in conjunction with the institution's radiation safety officer and should encompass issues related to the labeling, transportation, processing, storage, and disposal of radioactive specimens. The radiation safety officer is also responsible for training pathology personnel regarding safety issues. Do not be shy about contacting your institution's radiation safety office if you have questions about general policy issues or specific concerns regarding a radioactive specimen.

Fundamentals of Dissection

At first glance the challenges facing the surgical pathology cutter appear almost insurmountable. The types of specimens that come across the cutting table seem endlessly diverse, and the complexity of these specimens may at times be perplexing. To top it off, each specimen, whether a simple needle biopsy or a convoluted composite resection, must be handled with equal care and precision. How then does one confidently and effectively function in the surgical pathology laboratory, given the bewildering diversity and complexity of specimens that enter its doors? Where does one even begin?

For any specimen, the best place to begin is at the end. Even before making the first cut, take time to visualize the end result of your work, the surgical pathology report. Consider the issues that need to be addressed in that report, and then plan a dissection of the specimen that will help address these important issues. While it is true that no two specimens are exactly alike, you will find that the questions they pose are remarkably similar. Even the most complex of specimens can be reduced to three fundamental issues: *What structures are present? What is the nature of the pathologic process? How extensive is that process?* If you are not familiar with the important issues for a given organ, the Association of Directors of Anatomic and Surgical Pathology have an excellent website that summarizes the important diagnostic and prognostic issues for many of the major tumor types (www.panix.com/~adasp/). Regardless of the complexity or novelty of the specimen, these issues can be efficiently addressed by a systematic four-step approach. By mastering these four fundamental steps of surgical dissection, the surgical pathology cutter will be well equipped to tackle even the most intimidating of specimens with confidence.

Step 1. Specimen Orientation

If the surgical pathology report is the end result of the dissection, specimen orientation might be regarded as a road map by which to reach that ultimate destination. With orientation, an otherwise confusing conglomerate of tissue is placed in its proper clinical and anatomic context and appreciated as a structural unit. Then a proper course of dissection can be chartered. Without orientation, specimen dissection can proceed speedily but may never reach its desired aims.

The Requisition Form

Orientation is usually thought of in terms of the structural anatomy of the specimen. While these anatomic considerations certainly are important, a specimen must also be understood in terms of its clinical context. No specimen should be dissected in a "clinical vacuum"; rather, a strategy for the dissection of any specimen should be directed by the clinical history. For example, a uterus removed for leiomyomas is handled very differently from one removed for cervical cancer. Fortunately, clinical orientation usually does not require a full review of the patient's medical chart. Instead, a pertinent clinical history can often be succinctly communicated through a requisition form (Appendix 1-A). The requisition form should accompany every surgical specimen. It identifies the patient and the type of specimen, provides relevant clinical history, and alerts the prosector to specific biohazards. Referring physicians are responsible for providing this clinical information. Sometimes the information on the requisition form may not be complete, or a case may be so complex that additional clinical information is required. These situations may necessitate a review of the medical chart, evaluation of imaging studies, and/or direct communication with the requesting clinician. Do not be shy or timid; if in doubt, call the clinician.

Anatomic Orientation

The anatomic orientation is best appreciated at the outset of the dissection while the specimen is still intact. The further the dissection progresses, the more difficult it can become to reconstruct and orient the specimen. Even when the specimen is entirely intact, orientation is not always a simple task. Unlike the surgeon viewing the specimen as it is situated in the patient, the prosector frequently cannot fully appreciate the anatomic context of the isolated specimen lying on the cutting table. Nonetheless, two steps can be taken to overcome this obstacle and confidently orient the specimen: *appreciation of anatomic landmarks* and *communication with the surgeon*.

Anatomic landmarks can be thought of as consistent features (a shape, a contour, a structure, etc.) that serve to indicate a specific structure or designate a position. For example, the uterus can be correctly oriented by the relative positions of its peritoneal reflections, and the orientation of the eye may be guided by the insertion of a specific extraocular muscle. Before proceeding with any dissection, the prosector should be familiar with the anatomy of a specimen and should be able to recognize and interpret its unique anatomic landmarks. Toward this end, an anatomy atlas should be within easy reach of the cutting table.

Sometimes, even with the guidance of an anatomy atlas, the prosector may not be able to orient the specimen. Either the specimen is too complex, or it simply does not possess any useful anatomic landmarks. In these instances, communication with the surgeon takes on a very important role. This communication may take one of several forms. Sometimes a surgeon will use tags, sutures, and/or an accompanying diagram to designate important structures or locations on a specimen. At other times, specimen orientation may require direct communication with the surgeon.

Step 2. Dissecting the Specimen

The Cutting Station

The cutting station should be clean and orderly. Most routine dissections require a ruler, a scale, a scalpel with disposable blades, scissors, forceps, a probe, and a long sectioning knife. At the beginning of each day, the prosector should make certain that these tools are well maintained, clean, and within easy reach. Between dissections, these instruments and the cutting table itself should be rinsed clean of fluids and tissue fragments. This practice will help eliminate contamination of a specimen with tissue fragments from a prior dissection. Similarly, sectioning blades should be rinsed regularly during a dissection so that fragments of a friable tumor are not inadvertently transferred throughout the specimen or to other cases. Nothing is worse than not being sure if a minute fragment of cancer on a slide was a "pickup" from another case.

No more than a single specimen should be on the cutting table at any one time. Although it may seem time efficient to work on multiple specimens simultaneously, this dangerous practice openly invites the loss and mislabeling of specimens. For example, a small biopsy specimen is easily overlooked and discarded when overshadowed by a large and messy specimen on the same cutting table, while specimens of similar size and shape may easily be confused and mislabeled.

Handling of Tissues

While all tissues are to be handled cautiously and gently, small specimens in particular are susceptible to ill-treatment. Small and delicate tissue fragments may be crushed during transfer to a tissue cassette, they may desiccate if not placed in fixative in a timely manner, and they even may be lost during processing if they are not easily seen.

These problems can be minimized by adhering to a few simple guidelines:

1. Small specimens should never be forcibly squeezed between the ends of a forceps or the tips of the fingers. Instead, small specimens should be gently lifted from the specimen container using the end of a wooden applicator stick or pickups. Alternatively, small specimens can be filtered directly into a tissue bag, avoiding instrumentation altogether.
2. Small specimens should be quickly placed in fixative. Ideally, most small specimens (i.e., less than 1 cm) should reach the surgical pathology laboratory already in fixative. This requires that physician offices, biopsy suites, and operating rooms be supplied with appropriate fixatives, and that all personnel involved be instructed as to their proper use. Sometimes delays in fixation are necessary, as when a frozen section is required or when special tissue processing is indicated. In these instances, the tissue should be kept damp in saline-soaked gauze. Never leave small tissue fragments exposed to the air on the cutting table, and never place these small fragments directly on a dry paper towel. These practices are sure to hasten tissue desiccation.
3. For extremely small specimens, the journey from specimen container to histologic slide is a treacherous one, and they may be lost at any point along the way. For this reason, it is a wise practice to identify these small tissue fragments first and then mark the fragments so that they can be found more easily by the histotechnologist. Before the specimen container is even opened, check its contents for the size and number of tissue fragments, and record these in the gross description. If no tissue is seen or if inconsistencies with the requisition form are noted, carefully open the specimen container and thoroughly examine its surfaces (including the undersurface of the lid) for adherent tissue fragments. If no tissue is found or if discrepancies persist, the submitting physician should be notified immediately, and the outcome of this investigation should be documented in the surgical pathology report.

Once all of the tissue is identified in the specimen container, efforts should be taken to ensure that it safely reaches the histology laboratory and that it is easily identified for embedding and sectioning. Minute tissue fragments should be wrapped in porous paper or layered between porous foam pads before they are placed in the tissue cassette. Before these fragments are submitted to the histology laboratory, they can be marked with eosin or mercurochrome so that they are easier for the histotechnologist to see.

Inking the Specimen

Various inks and colored powders can be used to mark critical points on the specimen. These dyes and powders may help orient both the gross specimen and the histologic section. For example, colored tattoo powder sprinkled on the outer surface of a cystic mass can be used to distinguish between the outer and inner aspects of the cavity. Similarly, India ink can be painted on the surgical margins so that they can be easily recognized at the time of histologic examination. Indeed, many times the critical distinction of whether a neoplasm extends to the surgical margin depends entirely on the absence or presence of ink.

Given the important implications of an inked surface, these inks should be carefully and judiciously applied to the gross specimen. Keep in mind that just as the effective use of inks can facilitate the histologic interpretation, the careless and improper use of these inks can befuddle the microscopic findings. Consider, for example, the implications of sloppily applied ink that runs across a surface where it does not belong. The following guidelines outline the proper application of inks:

- If possible, apply ink before sectioning the specimen.
- Do not use excessive ink.
- Dry the surface of the specimen with paper towels before applying ink. When applied to a dry surface, ink is more likely to stick to the desired surface and less likely to run onto other areas of the specimen.
- Allow the ink to dry before further processing the specimen. Do not cut across wet ink, as the knife is likely to carry the ink onto the cut surface.

Opening and Sectioning the Specimen

The manner of opening and dissecting specimens is variable, depending on the type of specimen and the nature of the lesion. Bone marrow biopsies may simply be placed directly into a tissue cassette without any further manipulation, while the dissection of complex bone resections may require a multistep process involving special chemical reagents, imaging machines, and bone saws. Although this manual provides specific dissection guidelines for most of the specimens you will encounter, a few general guidelines underlie many of the instructions.

First, localize the lesion before sectioning the specimen. One effective way to localize the lesion is simply to palpate the specimen. For example, a small peripheral lung tumor may be readily appreciated simply by palpating the lung parenchyma, and a colorectal tumor can usually be detected by probing the lumen of the specimen with a gloved finger. Sometimes further measures are needed to localize the lesion. Review of specimen radiographs, for example, may be necessary to uncover the size and location of a lesion when it involves a bone. Once the lesion is localized, the specimen can be sectioned in the plane that best demonstrates the pathology.

Second, open the specimen in such a way as to expose the lesion while maintaining its relationships to surrounding structures. In general, the walls of hollow structures (e.g., large bronchi, stomach, intestines) should be opened along the side opposite the lesion to maintain the structural integrity of the lesion and to preserve important anatomic relationships. For tumors involving solid organs, the specimen should be cut along the longest axis of the tumor to demonstrate the tumor's greatest surface area.

Third, remember to dissect and examine the entire specimen. Often, the dissection is so focused on a localized lesion that the rest of the specimen is not examined. Incomplete dissections represent lost opportunities to fully disclose the extent of a lesion and to uncover unsuspected pathologic processes.

Fixing the Specimen

Before tissue is processed in the histology laboratory, it should be well fixed. Some institutions prefer to fix the specimen before it is dissected and sampled, while other institutions would rather you dissect and sample the specimen in the fresh state. Each method has its advantages and disadvantages. Specimen fixation greatly facilitates tissue sectioning. For example, tissue fixation permits thin sectioning of fatty tissues, and it helps to preserve the structural detail of thin-walled cysts, mucosa-lined organs, and friable tumors. One major disadvantage of specimen fixation is simply that it takes time. Fixation of larger specimens may require submersion in formalin for a full day or longer. Delays caused by fixation can be eliminated by dissecting and sampling the specimen while it is fresh. Although this practice may compromise the quality of the histologic sections, it can significantly reduce case turnaround time. Another major disadvantage of specimen fixation is that certain diagnostic studies require fresh, unfixed tissues. This demand for unfixed tissues is rapidly expanding owing to recent advances in genomic assays that require undegraded DNA and/or RNA (see Chapter 3). Most of the dissection descriptions in this manual include a step for fixation. Simply skip this step if your institution does not fix specimens before dissection or if fresh tissue needs to be collected for appropriate studies.

Even when one chooses to fix a specimen, a limited dissection of the fresh specimen is usually necessary. Fixative will not diffuse into the center of an unopened specimen, especially if the specimen is large and fatty. To overcome this, hollow organs and large cysts should be opened and solid tissues should be sectioned. Furthermore, a limited dissection is usually needed to expose a lesion if fresh tissue is required for frozen section evaluation, ancillary diagnostic studies (e.g., cytogenetic studies, flow cytometry), research purposes, or storage in a tissue bank. These important decisions regarding the distribution of tissue must be made while the specimen is fresh, not after the specimen has been submerged in fixative. A detailed description of the various fixatives available and their uses is given in Chapter 2.

Storing the Specimen

The tissue remaining after a specimen has been thoroughly dissected and sampled should not be discarded. Instead, it should be stored in such a way as to ensure easy retrieval and reconstruction of the specimen. Tissues for storage should be placed in a well-sealed container that holds enough fixative to cover the specimen. For a given case, separate parts should be stored in separate containers. Each container should be clearly labeled with the surgical pathology number, the part number, the patient's name, the patient's medical record number, and a biohazard warning when indicated. Specimens that may be of special interest, either from a teaching, diagnostic, or medicolegal perspective, should be so designated and stored in a permanent storage area. Medical devices likewise should be placed in a properly labeled container and segregated into an area where they can be stored for long periods of time and easily retrieved. Unlike routine tissue specimens, storage of these prosthetic devices does not require fixation.

When preparing a specimen for storage, anticipate the need to return to the specimen at a later time, either to review the gross findings or to submit more sections for histology. Although the specimen may be quite fragmented and distorted following its dissection, efforts should be made to reconstruct the specimen before placing it on a storage shelf. There are many examples of how this can be done. Lymph nodes and their associated soft tissues can be separately wrapped and labeled according to their respective regional levels. Residual slices of a serially sectioned organ can be fastened together in their original positions. Important landmarks can be designated with tags or safety pins. These simple methods of reconstructing the specimen can become invaluable later, when, for example, you have to return to a colectomy to find more lymph nodes, to a prostatectomy to submit additional slices of prostate tissue, or to a mastectomy to sample a specific quadrant of the breast.

Step 3. The Gross Description

Correlation between the macroscopic and microscopic findings is important when evaluating a specimen and rendering a diagnosis. Just as glass slides represent a permanent record of the histologic findings, the gross description represents a permanent record of the specimen's macroscopic features. The goal of the gross description is threefold. First, it serves as a descriptive report that enables the reader to reconstruct the specimen mentally and envision the location, extent, and appearance of the pathologic process. Second, it serves as a slide index, enabling the pathologist to correlate each slide to a precise location on the specimen. Third, it accounts for the distribution of the tissue, documenting how a specimen has been apportioned for various diagnostic and research purposes.

To help reconstruct an image of a specimen, the gross description must be logical, factual, and succinct. A logical description is one that follows an orderly sequence. The first sentence should identify the patient and the specimen. It should tell the reader who the patient is, what the specimen is, and what structures are present. The description should then move from one individual component of the specimen to another in a methodical progression. Proceed from overall to specific, from abnormal to normal, and from relevant to ancillary. The best way to avoid a description that is fragmented and chaotic is to dictate after the specimen has been dissected and examined. This approach allows one to gather all of the information, then integrate the gross findings into a narrative that is comprehensive and complete.

A factual description is one that records the objective characteristics of the specimen. With few exceptions, these characteristics include the size, weight, color, shape, and consistency of the specimen and any specific lesions. Among these, size is particularly important. For example, in resections of neoplasms, the size of the neoplasm is critical in staging the tumor, and the distance from the edge of the tumor to the surgical margin may help to determine the adequacy of excision and the need for adjuvant therapy. For excisions of parathyroid glands, the important distinction between a normal and proliferative gland is made on the basis of the gland's weight.

Quite commonly, the gross description is so diluted by trivial details and technical minutiae that the important macroscopic features are not easily recognized by the reader. A concise dictation is one that ignores this minutiae and records only information that serves to achieve the three goals of the gross description. A leaner description can often be achieved by cutting the fat from two areas of the gross description. First, eliminate verbose descriptions of normal anatomy. Descriptions of normal structures should be restricted to pertinent negative findings and to terse statements about size, color, consistency, and shape that help reconstruct the appearance of the specimen. Second, do not describe the mechanics of the dissection. These technical details are already laid out in the dissection manual and do not belong in the gross dictation unless they clarify the histologic findings or unless your dissection deviates from routine methods (e.g., inflation of a lung with formalin).

Another important function of the gross description is its role as a slide index (Appendix 1-B). The slide index places each histologic slide in its appropriate anatomic context. Consider, for example, the importance of knowing whether a section of a neoplasm was sampled from the center of a tumor or from the margin of surgical resection. Only the prosector knows for sure where and how the specimen was sampled, and it is the prosector's responsibility to communicate this information in the gross description. This information should be summarized at the end of the gross description in the form of a slide index. The slide index should state the number of pieces submitted in each tissue block, the designations used to identify each tissue block, and the precise meanings of these designations. Tissue designation should strive for simplicity, rationality, and standardization. The designations themselves should use as few letters or numbers as possible, but the meanings of these designations should be specific. For example, two sections of tumor could be designated "TA" and "TB," respectively. Remember that slides are frequently sent to other hospitals for consultation, and so these designations also need to be clear to someone not familiar with your institutional idiosyncrasies.

The gross description should also document the distribution of tissue for diagnostic and/or research purposes. Sometimes tissue may be sent for ancillary diagnostic studies including electron microscopy, cytogenetics, and flow cytometry. In some instances fresh tissue may be frozen and stored in a tissue bank so that it can be retrieved at a later time, or tissue may be requested by various laboratories for research purposes. Not only is it important to supervise (under the guidance of a pathologist) the distribution of these tissues, but it is also important to document in the gross description where the tissue has been sent and for what purposes.

Other methods may be used to supplement the description of the macroscopic findings. Among them, photography (see Chapter 4) plays an especially versatile role. Indeed, recent advances in computer technology have expanded the role of photography as an adjunct to the gross dictation. Digital images of the gross specimen can be stored as electronic files, which can be readily retrieved for publication or research purposes or simply to clarify the gross description. Liberal photography is a practice that is to be encouraged as an effective supplement to the gross description.

Finally, remember that the gross description is a legal document, so the typed gross description should be proofread as carefully as the final diagnosis.

Step 4. Specimen Sampling

Mindless sampling of a specimen introduces errors at two different extremes. At one extreme, tissue sampling is inadequate, either because the number of sections is too few or the quality of sections is too poor. In these instances, important issues cannot be adequately addressed in the surgical pathology report. Forgetting to assess a surgical margin, failing to determine the extent of local tumor infiltration, and neglecting to check for metastases to regional lymph nodes are common examples of inadequate sampling. At the other extreme, tissue sampling can be excessive. An inordinate number of tissue sections may exact a costly toll on the resources of the surgical pathology laboratory.

The key to an approach that is both economical and thorough is *selective sampling*. Selective sampling is a strategic approach which attempts to maximize the information that can be obtained from a given tissue section. As opposed to random and indiscriminant sampling of a specimen, tissue sampling that is selective increases the information that can be obtained histologically, and it requires fewer sections to do so. Appendix 1-C lists some fundamental guidelines for selective tissue sampling.

Sampling a Tumor

The goals of tumor sampling go beyond the question of "What is it?" Tumor sampling is concerned not just with the type of a tumor but also with its histologic grade and the degree to which it has extended into surrounding structures. A tumor should be sampled with the objective of addressing all three of these issues.

In general, most sections of a tumor should be obtained from its periphery. This peripheral zone is often the best preserved region of a tumor, while the central zone is frequently so necrotic that it yields no useful histologic information. In addition, the tumor's periphery demonstrates the interface of the tumor with adjacent tissues. This interface zone may provide evidence regarding where a tumor has arisen (e.g., colorectal carcinoma arising in a pre-existing villous adenoma);

Fundamentals of Specimen Dissection

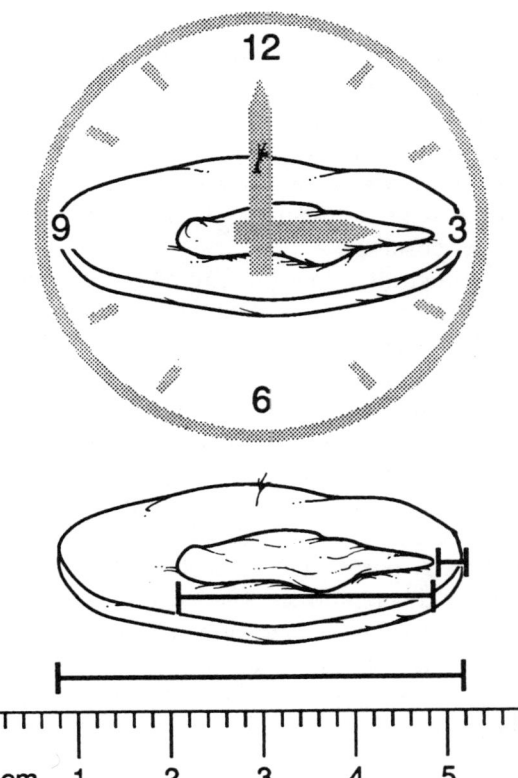

1. Orient
Use anatomic landmarks and/or surgical designations to help orient the specimen. In the illustration, the surgeon has placed a suture at the 12-o'clock position of the skin ellipse.

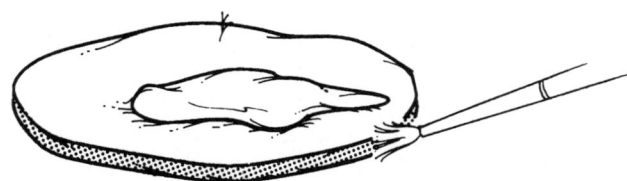

2. Measure
Size is one of the most important parameters to document in the gross dictation. Include not only the overall dimensions of the specimen but also the size of the lesion and its distance from the surgical margin.

3. Ink
Application of ink to the cut surface of the specimen is a good way to mark the resection margin.

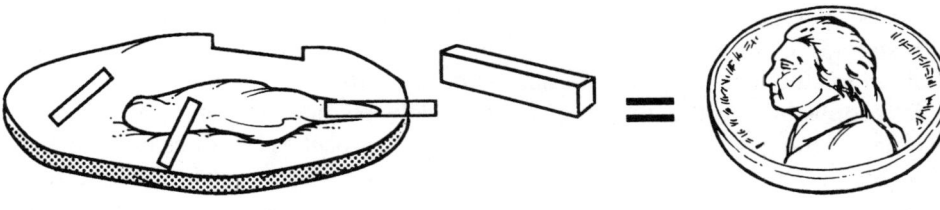

4. Sample
Adequately sample the specimen. Include sections of the lesion, normal tissue, and the margins. Sections should be no bigger than the diameter and thickness of a nickel.

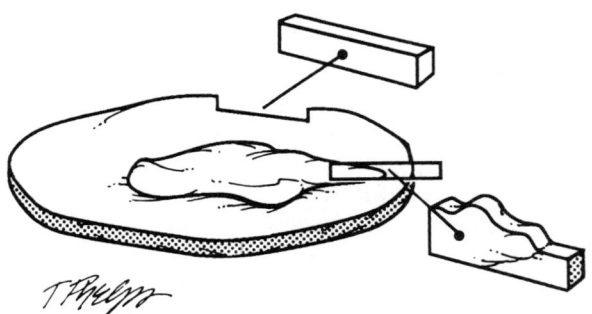

5. Assess Margins
A perpendicular section is a good way to evaluate the margin when it is closely approached by a lesion. This section shows the distance of the lesion to the edge of the specimen. A parallel section evaluates a larger surface area of the margin, and it may be used to evaluate a margin that is not closely approached by the lesion.

important clues about the biologic behavior of the tumor (e.g., transcapsular invasion of a follicular thyroid carcinoma); and information regarding the degree of local tumor invasion (e.g., depth of invasion of a cancer into the wall of the colon).

Questions frequently arise regarding the number of sections that should be taken of a tumor. Unfortunately, there is no single answer, since the appropriate number of sections depends on the type of specimen. For example, a single section from a solitary liver nodule may be sufficient to confirm that it is a metastasis, but such limited sectioning of a solitary thyroid nodule may not allow distinction between a follicular adenoma and a follicular carcinoma. Despite this tremendous variability between specimens, a few general considerations should guide the sampling of a tumor. First, when trying to assess the histologic type and grade of a neoplasm, be sure to sample all areas of the tumor that, on gross inspection, appear different. Even strict adherence to rigid rules such as "one section per 1 cm of tumor" may not be adequate if the sections are not selectively taken from areas of the tumor that appear grossly distinct. Second, sections of large cysts should be taken from areas where the cyst wall appears thickened or where the cyst lining has a complex appearance (e.g., shaggy, papillary excrescences). Sections from these areas are most likely to reveal the proliferative areas of the cyst lining and to demonstrate tumor infiltration of the cyst wall. Third, when concern exists about malignant transformation within a benign lesion or premalignant process, the lesion should be extensively if not entirely submitted for histologic evaluation. A number of examples fall under this category, including mucinous cystic neoplasms of the ovary and pancreas, adenomas of the gastrointestinal tract, Barrett's esophagus with dysplasia, *in situ* transitional carcinoma of the urinary bladder, and many others.

Sampling a Margin

The margin is the edge or the boundary of the specimen. It represents the plane where the surgeon has sectioned across tissues to remove the specimen from the patient. The surgical margin may be free of disease; that is, a rim of uninvolved tissues may surround a pathologic lesion that has been completely resected. Alternatively, the lesion could extend to the edge of the specimen, implying that the lesion has not been completely removed. Clearly, the status of a surgical margin is an important indicator of the potential for the disease to recur and of the need for further therapy. Therefore, the assessment of these margins, both grossly and microscopically, is of considerable importance.

As illustrated, margins can be sampled in one of two ways: They can be taken as either as perpendicular section or a parallel section. A perpendicular section is one taken at a right angle to the edge of the specimen. In this type of section, the true margin is present at one of the two ends of the section. The advantage of a perpendicular section is that it can be used to demonstrate the relationship of the edge of the tumor to the margin. A perpendicular section allows the important distinction between a lesion that truly extends to the margin and a lesion that very closely approaches but does not involve the margin. Since only a small surface area of the margin is represented in a perpendicular section, the margin must be carefully inspected and then selectively sampled from those areas where it is most closely approached by the tumor.

A shave section is one taken parallel to the edge of the specimen. Because the entire shave section spans the margin, a relatively large surface area at the margin can be evaluated with a single section. A shave section is ideal for obtaining complete cross sections of small luminal or cylindrical structures. Unlike the perpendicular section, the shave section does not effectively demonstrate the relationship between the margin and the edge of the tumor. Its major drawback is that it cannot be used to distinguish between a lesion that truly extends to the margin and one that very closely approaches but does not actually involve the margin. For this reason, shave sections should be reserved for those instances when the margin appears widely free of tumor or when dealing with small luminal or cylindrical structures that are not easily sampled using perpendicular sections.

To help the pathologist interpret the histologic findings, the slide index portion of the gross description should clearly document how the margin was sampled. The presence of tumor in a margin section may have entirely different implications, depending on whether the margin was sampled using a perpendicular or parallel section.

Sampling Lymph Nodes

A specimen dissection is not complete until the lymph nodes, when present, have been found and sampled. Sampling of lymph nodes is especially important for resections of neoplasms where critical staging information may depend on the number and location of lymph nodes involved by metastatic tumor.

Although the lymph node status is clearly important in staging neoplasms, finding these lymph nodes can be a tedious and frustrating job. They may be small, inconspicuous, and entirely overshadowed by the fibroadipose tissues in which they are embedded. Skill at finding lymph nodes develops over time, but a few guidelines may enhance the efficiency of your search. First, it is generally best to orient the specimen, designate the various regional lymph node levels, and submit margins of the soft tissues before a lymph node dissection is undertaken. Keep in mind that lymph node dissections require significant distortion and manipulation of the soft tissues such that the specimen may not be easily reconstructed following a thorough search for lymph nodes. Second, many prefer to look for lymph nodes in the fresh specimen. Lymph nodes are often best appreciated by touch, and smaller lymph nodes may elude detection when the surrounding soft tissues have been hardened by fixation.

Lymph nodes larger than 5 mm should be serially sectioned at 2- to 3-mm intervals. A common error is to submit multiple slices from more than one lymph node in the same tissue cassette for histologic evaluation. This may cause considerable confusion regarding the number of involved lymph nodes if more than one tissue fragment contains metastatic tumor. To avoid this confusion, a given cassette should contain slices from only one lymph node. A more detailed description of the processing of lymph nodes for the evaluation of metastatic disease is provided in Chapter 5.

Sampling Normal Tissues

Even tissues that do not appear to be involved by a pathologic process should be sampled for histologic evaluation. Histologic evaluation can uncover diseases that may not have been appreciated on gross inspection. These microscopic alterations may be entirely unrelated to the primary lesion, or they may be closely associated findings that provide important insight into the origin of the primary lesion. It is also important to sample normal tissues to document the structures that were surgically removed. For example, a section taken from the adrenal gland in a radical nephrectomy specimen clearly documents that this organ was removed, identified, and examined.

The Surgical Pathology Report

The surgical pathology report is a comprehensive statement that integrates the macroscopic and microscopic findings. It represents the summation of efforts on the part of the prosector, the histotechnologist, and the pathologist. Forms are now available that have standardized the reporting of the pathologic findings in a comprehensive way. For the prosector facing a complex and intimidating specimen, the time to contemplate the content of the surgical pathology report is not after the dissection is completed but before the first cut is even made. With this in mind, this manual describes the dissections of various specimens, including a tabulation of important issues to address in the surgical pathology report. These lists are provided so relevant clinical issues can be kept in mind as specimens are dissected, described, and sampled.

Appendix 1-A. Information to Be Included in the Specimen Requisition Form

Patient Identification	Type of Specimen	Clinical History	Additional Notations
Full name	Date of specimen collection	Pertinent clinical history	Special requests
Identifying number	Site of specimen	Differential diagnosis	Biohazard alerts
Date of birth	Type of procedure	Operative findings	Name/phone number of physicians to contact

Appendix 1-B. Example: Slide Index for a Modified Radical Mastectomy

Designation	Meaning	No. of Pieces of Tissue
FSC	Frozen section control	1
TA	Tumor—(A = first tissue block)	1
TB	Tumor—(B = second tissue block)	1
UIA	Upper inner quadrant	1
UIB		1
UOA	Upper outer quadrant	1
UOB		1
LIA	Lower inner quadrant	1
LIB		1
LOA	Lower outer quadrant	1
LOB		1
N	Nipple	2
S	Skin	1
LNIA	Level I lymph nodes	3
LNIB		2
LNIIA	Level II lymph nodes	2
LNIIB		4
LNIIIA	Level III lymph nodes	3
LNIIIB		4

Total blocks: 19

Total pieces of tissue: 32

Appendix 1-C. Selective Specimen Sampling

Tumor Sampling

- Sections from the periphery of a tumor are usually more informative than are sections from the center of a tumor.
- For heterogeneous tumors, sample all components of the tumor.
- For cystic lesions, sample areas of the cyst wall that are thickened or lined by a complex surface.
- If there is concern about a hidden focus of malignant transformation within a benign neoplasm or premalignant process (e.g., infiltrating carcinoma arising in a pre-existing villous adenoma), the lesion should be extensively, or even entirely, sampled for histologic evaluation.

Margin Sampling

- Always sample the specimen margins, even from lesions that are clinically thought to be benign (e.g., gastric ulcers).
- Perpendicular sections show the relationship of the lesion to the margin. Perpendicular sections are usually preferred to parallel sections, especially when the margin is closely approached by the tumor.
- Shave (i.e., parallel) sections are sometimes best when the margin appears widely free of tumor or for samples of a cylindrical or tubular structure (e.g., optic nerve or ureter margins).

Lymph Node Sampling for Tumor Staging

- Orient the specimen, submit soft tissue margins, and designate regional lymph node levels before dissecting the soft tissues for lymph nodes.
- Lymph nodes are easiest to find in unfixed tissues where they can be more readily appreciated by palpation.
- Lymph nodes larger than 5 mm should be sectioned to facilitate tissue fixation.
- Never submit multiple sections from more than one lymph node in a single tissue cassette.

Normal Tissue Sampling

- At least one representative section should be taken from each grossly normal structural component of the specimen.

2 Laboratory Techniques

William M. Fox III, B.S., M.S., P.A.-C.
Robert H. Rosa, Jr., M.D.

General Comments

The modern surgical pathology laboratory is equipped to perform a staggering number of routine and special diagnostic procedures. Most are carried out by the laboratory technologist; however, gross room personnel should be familiar with the basic concepts and initial steps of these procedures. Failure to handle tissue appropriately may preclude the performance of needed diagnostic studies and ultimately delay or even prevent the establishment of a diagnosis. This chapter provides a basic introduction to the more common techniques employed in tissue fixation, staining, decalcification, and intraoperative consultation.

Fixation

Adequate fixation by an appropriate fixative is central to any histologic preparation. Tissue that is inadequately or inappropriately fixed will lead to difficulties in microtomy, staining, and performing ancillary tests. These problems may not be correctable at a later stage.

Unfortunately, there is no "all-purpose" fixative. No single fixative is good for all specimens. It is therefore essential that surgical pathology personnel be familiar with a variety of fixatives and their uses. Although the exact mechanism of action of many fixatives is unknown, fixatives can broadly be classified into four groups based on their mechanism of action. The aldehydes, such as formaldehyde and glutaraldehyde, act by cross-linking proteins, particularly lysine residues. Oxidizing agents, such as osmium tetroxide, potassium permanganate, and potassium dichromate, also probably cross-link proteins, although their precise mechanism of action is unknown. Acetic acid, methyl alcohol, and ethyl alcohol are all protein-denaturing agents. The fourth and final group of fixatives acts by forming insoluble metallic precipitates, and these agents include mercuric chloride and picric acid. The choice of the appropriate fixative is based on the type of tissue being fixed and on projected needs for ancillary tests such as special stains, immunohistochemistry, *in situ* hybridization, and electron microscopy. Table 2-1 lists some common fixatives, their basic uses, and their advantages and disadvantages.

Ten percent neutral buffered formalin (4% formaldehyde) is the standard fixative used in most laboratories. Formalin tends to remove water-soluble substances such as glycogen, and it is therefore generally not suitable for the fixation of tissues for electron microscopy. Ten percent neutral buffered formalin penetrates and fixes tissues at a rate of approximately 2 to 3 mm/24 h at room temperature.

Glutaraldehyde, a common fixative for electron microscopy, is one of the slowest penetrating fixatives. Tissue for electron microscopy should be cut into 1-mm cubes and immediately placed in refrigerated glutaraldehyde. Glutaraldehyde (4%) must be kept refrigerated before use.

Ethyl alcohol (70% to 100%) is seldom used as a primary fixative. It may be useful in fixing tissue for preserving glycogen and for some histochemical studies, but it has several disadvantages. Ethyl alcohol penetrates tissues very slowly, and because it denatures proteins by abstracting water from the tissue, it can cause excessive hardening, tissue shrinkage, and cell distortion. Alcohol can also dissolve fats and should not

TABLE 2-1. Common fixatives.

Fixatives and their major components	Tissue	Special stains (+ = stain can be used with fixative) (− = stain should not be used with fixative)	Advantages (+) and disadvantages (−)
10% Neutral buffered formalin (4% Formaldehyde, 7.2 pH phosphate buffer, methanol)	All	+ Warthin-Starry (spirochetes) + Oil red O (fat) + Grimelius (neuroendocrine granules)	+ Routine fixative + Preservation, general staining + Immunohistochemistry + Molecular analyses + Long-term storage
2% Glutaraldehyde (50% Glutaraldehyde, 0.2 M cacodylate buffer)	All	− PAS (false positivity)	+ Electron microscopy + Preservation of collagen − Routine fixative − Slow penetration − Must be refrigerated
B5 (Mercuric chloride, sodium acetate, 37% formalin)	Lymph node Spleen Bone marrow		+ Cytoplasmic, nuclear staining − Routine fixative − Must be prepared fresh − Requires iodine treatment to remove mercury before routine staining − Timed exposure needed because overfixation causes hardening
Zenker's (Mercuric chloride, potassium dichromate, sodium sulfate, glacial acetic acid)	All	+ Sheehan (chromaffin) + Mallory's PTAH (collagen and muscle) + Viral inclusions (Negri bodies) + Feulgen (DNA) + Trichromes (collagen and muscle) + Verhoeff-van Gieson (elastic fibers)	+ Routine fixative + Preserves mitochondria − Must be washed overnight to remove excess chromate − Requires iodine treatment to remove mercury before routine staining − Must be prepared fresh − Molecular analyses − No metal instruments − Immunohistochemistry
Zenker's formol (Helly's fluid) (Mercuric chloride, potassium dichromate, sodium sulfate, 37% formaldehyde)	Bone marrow Spleen All blood-containing organs		+ Routine fixative + Preserves mitochondria + Preserves red blood cells − Must be washed overnight to remove chromate − Requires iodine treatment to remove mercury before routine staining − Molecular analyses − Immunohistochemistry
Bouin's (Picric acid, formalin, glacial acetic acid)	Testicular biopsies	+ Masson trichrome (collagen and muscle)	+ Routine fixative − Lyses red blood cells − Removes ferric iron − Dissolves some proteins − Molecular analyses − Immunohistochemistry − Carbohydrates

TABLE 2-1. Continued.

Fixatives and their major components	Tissue	Special stains (+ = stain can be used with fixative) (− = stain should not be used with fixative)	Advantages (+) and disadvantages (−)
Ethyl alcohol	All	+ Congo red (amyloid) + Von Kossa's (calcium) + Weigert's stain for fibrin + Mallory's stain for iron + Gomori's methenamine silver stain for urate crystals − Ziehl-Neelsen (AFB)	+ Enzyme histochemistry + Molecular analyses + Impression smears + Blood smears + Preserves glycogen + Preserves crystals: uric acid, sodium urate − Causes excessive hardening − Routine fixative − Dissolves lipids
Acetone 0–4°C	All	− Ziehl-Neelsen (AFB)	+ Enzyme histochemistry − Routine fixative − For best results, must be refrigerated − Dissolves lipids
Carnoy's (Glacial acetic acid, absolute ethanol, chloroform)	All	+ Methyl green pyronin (DNA and RNA) + Congo red (amyloid) + Giemsa (mast cells) − Ziehl-Neelsen (AFB)	+ Cytologic fixative + Rapid penetration + Nuclear detail + Fixes RNA + Preserves glycogen − Dissolves cytoplasmic elements − Hemolyzes red blood cells

be used when lipid studies or stains for myelin are being considered. Carnoy's is a fixative that combines ethanol, chloroform, and glacial acetic acid. It quickly fixes tissues and it is a good fixative for glycogen, plasma cells, and nucleic acids. Because of its quick action, some laboratories use Carnoy's to fix biopsies that require urgent processing.

The mercury-based fixatives (e.g., B5) provide excellent nuclear detail and are useful in evaluating lymphomas. Mercury-based fixatives precipitate proteins without firmly binding to them. These fixatives generally must be prepared fresh; once fixed, the tissues require special processing in the histology laboratory (iodine treatment to remove the mercury). Overfixation with B5 can cause excessive hardening of the tissue.

Bouin's, a picric acid-based fixative, is the fixative of choice for testicular biopsies. Picric acid reacts with basic proteins and forms crystalline picrates with amino acids. Therefore, tissues fixed with picric acid-based fixatives retain little affinity for basic dyes, and the picric acid must be recovered from the tissue before staining. Picric acid penetrates tissues well and fixes them rapidly, but it also causes cells to shrink. Picric acid causes DNA methylation; hence, many polymerase chain reaction (PCR)-based molecular diagnostic tests cannot be performed on tissues fixed with picric acid.

An appropriate fixation technique is just as important as choosing the correct fixative. Appropriate fixation requires adequate tissue exposure and a duration of fixation sufficient to allow full penetration of the fixative. For most tissues, a volume of fresh fixative 15 times the volume of tissue is needed to fix the tissue adequately within 12 to 18 hours. The rate of fixation varies depending on the type of fixative, the type of tissue, and the thickness of the tissue sections. Adipose tissue (due to its hydrophobic nature) and fibrous tissue (due to its density) may require longer periods of fixation when hydrophilic fixatives are employed.

There can be no more important tenet of fixation than to do it early. The process of autolysis begins immediately, and even the best fixative can only arrest, not reverse, this process. Small amounts of tissue may arrive in fixative or saline, whereas larger tissues usually arrive fresh. Large specimens generally do not fix well unless first prepared. Even then, specimens often require a limited dissection to maximize the surface area exposed to the fixative, thereby ensuring adequate fixation. Tissue with a hollow viscous or lumina should be opened and solid tissue partially serially sectioned at 5- to 10-mm intervals. To maintain proper orientation, these partially sectioned tissues can be pinned onto a wax block and floated in a fixation tank. Paper towels can be inserted between the sections. The towels act as a wick, drawing more fixative to the sections, thereby facilitating rapid fixation. In general, tissue submitted for processing should never exceed a thickness of 4 mm, and tissues comprised of adipose or dense fibrous tissue should be no more than 3 mm. Optimally, you should routinely aim to submit your tissue sections as 2 mm slices. There should be at least a 3-mm space between the cassette and tissue on all sides. Cramming oversized tissue to make it fit into a cassette often results in inferior slide preparation, time consuming reprocessing, and ultimately a delay in diagnosis.

Special Stains

A variety of special stains are employed in the surgical pathology laboratory. Most of these are performed by specially trained laboratory personnel, and a detailed description of all of these stains is beyond the scope of this manual. The surgical pathologist and pathologist's assistant, however, should be able to perform a few basic stains: hematoxylin and eosin (H&E), oil red O (ORO), periodic acid-Schiff (PAS), Gram Weigert's (GW), Ziehl-Neelsen, and Papanicolaou (PAP) stains.

While the details of each stain vary from laboratory to laboratory, examples of "cookbook-style" instructions for the performance of each of these six stains on frozen tissue sections follow.

Stain: Hematoxylin and Eosin (H&E)
Approximate time: 3 minutes
Technique: 4 to 6 µm frozen section, touch prep, smear, crush prep
Any slides
Fixative: Absolute alcohol
Procedure:
1. Absolute alcohol, 60 seconds
2. Rinse in tap water (one change); dip until clear
3. Hematoxylin (Harris), 60 seconds
4. Rinse in tap water (three changes); dip until clear
5. Blue in Scott's water, 15 seconds
6. Rinse in tap water (two changes); dip until clear
7. Eosin-phloxine, 5 seconds
8. 50% Alcohol, five dips
9. 70% Alcohol, five dips
10. 95% Alcohol, five dips
11. Absolute alcohol, five dips (two changes)
12. Xylene (two changes); dip until clear
13. Mount and coverslip with resinous media
Results: Nuclei: blue to purple
Cytoplasm: pink to red

Stain: Oil Red O (ORO)
Approximate time: 10 minutes
Technique: 6 to 8 µm frozen section, touch prep, smear, crush prep
Poly-L-lysine or sialinated slides
Fixative: 10% Neutral buffered formalin
Procedure:
1. 10% Neutral buffered formalin, 60 seconds
2. Wash in tap water and blot dry
3. Oil red O, 5 minutes
4. Wash in tap water
5. Hematoxylin (Harris), 60 seconds
6. Rinse in tap water (two changes)
7. Blue in Scott's water, 15 seconds
8. Rinse in tap water (two changes)
9. Mount and coverslip with *aqueous* media
Results: Fat: orange to bright red
Nuclei: blue
Cytoplasm: transparent

Stain: Periodic Acid-Schiff (PAS)
Approximate time: 35 minutes
Technique: 4 to 6 µm frozen section,
Poly-L-lysine or sialinated slides

Fixative:	Absolute alcohol
Procedure	1. Absolute alcohol, 60 seconds
	2. Rinse in distilled water (one change)
	3. 0.5% Periodic acid solution, 5 minutes
	4. Rinse in distilled water (three changes)
	5. Schiff reagent, 15 minutes
	6. Wash in running tap water, 2 to 5 minutes or until pink color develops
	7. Hematoxylin (Harris), 60 seconds
	8. Wash in tap water, 2 minutes
	9. 50% Alcohol, five dips
	10. 70% Alcohol, five dips
	11. 95% Alcohol, five dips (two changes)
	12. Absolute alcohol, five dips (two changes)
	13. Xylene (two changes); dip until clear
	14. Mount and coverslip with resinous media
Results:	Fungi: red to rose
	Glycoproteins, mucopolysaccharides: red to rose
	Nuclei: blue
	Cytoplasm: light pink

Stain:	**Gram Weigert's (GW)**
	Approximate time: 10 minutes
Technique:	4 to 6 μm frozen section, touch prep, smear, crush prep
	Poly-L-lysine or sialinated slides
Fixative:	Absolute alcohol
Procedure:	1. Absolute alcohol, 60 seconds
	2. Eosin, 60 seconds
	3. Rinse in tap water (one change)
	4. Sterling's gentian violet, 60 seconds
	5. Rinse in tap water (one change)
	6. Gram's iodine, 2 minutes
	7. Blot slides
	8. Differentiate with aniline/xylene mixture (two to three changes) until the black color is lost.
	9. Xylene (two changes); dip until clear
	10. Mount and coverslip with resinous media
Results:	Gram-positive bacteria and *Pneumocystis carinii*: purple to blue
	Nuclei: blue
	Cytoplasm: light pink

Stain:	**Modified Ziehl-Neelsen** (Acid Fast)
	Approximate time: 60 minutes
Technique:	4 to 6 μm frozen section, Poly-L-lysine or sialinated slides
Fixative:	10% Neutral buffered formalin
Procedure:	1. Absolute alcohol, 60 seconds
	2. Rinse in tap water
	3. Carbol-fuchsin, 45 minutes
	4. Wash in tap water
	5. 1% Acid alcohol (one to two quick dips)
	6. Wash in tap water
	7. Methylene blue, 10 to 20 seconds
	8. 50% Alcohol, five dips
	9. 70% Alcohol, five dips
	10. 90% Alcohol, five dips (two changes)
	11. Absolute alcohol, five dips (two changes)
	12. Xylene (two changes); dip until clear
	13. Mount and cover slip with resinous media
Results:	Acid-fast bacilli: bright red
	Background: light blue

Stain:	**Papanicolaou (PAP)**
	Approximate time: 60 minutes
Technique:	Touch prep, crush prep, smear, fine needle aspiration
	Poly-L-lysine or sialinated slides
Fixative:	95% Alcohol
Procedure:	1. 95% Alcohol, 15 minutes
	2. 75% Alcohol, five dips
	3. 50% Alcohol, five dips
	4. Distilled water, five dips
	5. Hematoxylin, two to three minutes

6. Wash in tap water
7. 0.25% HCl, one to two quick dips
8. Wash in tap water
9. 30% Alcohol, five dips
10. 75% Alcohol, five dips
11. 95% Alcohol, five dips
12. Orange G, 2 minutes
13. 95% Alcohol, five dips (three changes)
14. Eosin-azure 50, 2 minutes
15. 95% Alcohol, five dips (two changes)
16. Xylene, five dips (three changes)
17. Mount and cover with resinous material

Results: Nuclei: blue
Cytoplasm: pink, gray, to green

Immunohistochemical Stains

Immunohistochemical studies employ an unlabeled antibody to a specific tissue antigen followed by treatment in one or more steps with an enzyme-labeled antibody. These studies are extremely versatile and can be used to detect an ever-expanding number of antigens. Depending on the specific antigens, they can be performed on fresh-frozen or formalin-fixed, paraffin-embedded tissues. The effectiveness of immunohistochemistry depends on the integrity, stability, and availability of the target antigen. Three steps can improve the results of your immunohistochemical staining. First, sample a viable and representative area of the process to be studied. Immunohistochemical stains of necrotic material are practically worthless. Second, choose the appropriate method of stabilizing the tissue. While formalin is generally a good fixative for most immunohistochemical stains, some stains work best in other fixatives, and other stains work only on fresh-frozen tissue. Finally, do not overfix the tissue. Overfixation may result in the loss of antigenicity. In general, tissue fixation for longer than 24 hours compromises immunohistochemical analysis.

Decalcification

A wide variety of calcified specimens are received in the surgical pathology laboratory. While some of these should be cut with specialized, expensive equipment, the vast majority of calcified specimens can be handled by a routine histology laboratory if they are appropriately decalcified. Decalcification is the process whereby calcium salts are removed from bone and other calcified tissues. Three general methods are employed to decalcify tissues. These include acid hydrolysis, organic chelation, and electrolysis (see Table 2-2). The important points to remember about decalcifying specimens follow:

1. The tissue must be fixed before decalcification. In most cases, fixing a specimen for at least 24 hours in 10% neutral buffered formalin is adequate. If you use a different fixative, make sure that the fixative employed is compatible with the method of decalcification chosen.
2. Decalcification should be carried out at room temperature and with constant magnetic stirring. While heat accelerates decalcification, it also induces numerous artifacts and thus should be avoided.
3. Do not decalcify longer than necessary, as excessive decalcification will introduce artifacts. To avoid overdecalcification, delicate tissues should be examined every hour and larger tissues examined as established by laboratory protocol.
4. Residual acid will destroy nuclear detail. Therefore, acid decalcification solutions must be removed from bone specimens before they are processed by washing them in water for at least 24 hours.
5. The volume of the decalcification solution should be 10 to 15 times that of the tissue being decalcified. These solutions should also be changed on a regular basis.

Intraoperative Consultation

Important decisions in the operating room are frequently based on intraoperative consultation with a pathologist. These intraoperative consultations often require the rapid microscopic examination of fresh tissue. This examination can be accomplished either by the preparation of cytologic slides or by the preparation of histologic slides using the frozen section technique.

Cytologic slides can be prepared from fresh specimens by one of three methods. Impression smears are produced by touching a microscopic

TABLE 2-2. Acid decalcification methods.

Decalcification method	Tissue	Comment	Advantages (+) and disadvantages (−)
Acid hydrolysis, 3% HCl	Routine decalcification of cortical bone, large thick bone, ossified cancellous bone	Compatible with most routine and special staining methods May interfere with immunoperoxidase and other special studies Method of choice for large specimens	± Immunohistochemistry − Swells cells − Overdecalcification results in extreme eosinophilia
Acid hydrolysis, 5% HNO_3	Routine decalcification of cortical bone, large thick bone, ossified cancellous bone	Compatible with most routine and special staining methods but yields substandard results	− Damages nuclear detail − Immunohistochemistry − Swells cells
Acid hydrolysis, 5% formic acid	Light decalcification of delicate tissue, bone marrow, bones of inner ear	Compatible with most routine and special staining methods Method of choice for small specimens	+ Immunohistochemistry + Good preservation of nuclear detail

slide to the cut face of the tissue. This procedure is also known as a touch preparation. The slide can be air dried or immediately fixed in alcohol for subsequent staining. The crush preparation is performed by taking a small (1-mm cube) piece of tissue and crushing it between two glass slides. The crush preparation can be fixed or air dried, then stained. Extremely hard tissues can be *scraped* with a sharp blade and the scrapings drawn across another slide in much the same way that a blood smear is prepared. Each of these techniques can be used on different tissues with varying degrees of success in terms of preparation artifacts and quantity of cells obtained. For example, crush preparations work best on very soft tissues, while scrapings are needed on very firm tissues.

The frozen section is another procedure frequently used in intraoperative consultations. The details of preparing a frozen section vary greatly from one laboratory to another; however, one should become familiar with a few general concepts.

The first step is to select and prepare a piece of the specimen to freeze. Select a section that demonstrates the interface of the lesion with normal tissue, and try to avoid fatty or calcified tissues. The section should not be greater than 2×2 cm, and wet tissue should be gently blotted dry to avoid the formation of ice crystals. Very small pieces are easily lost in opaque embedding medium, so they should be stained with a drop of eosin or India ink before sectioning.

The second step is to freeze the tissue. Tissues are usually frozen on a tissue chuck in freezing medium by immersion in liquid nitrogen. This technique will lead to the formation of ice crystals, which can distort the histology. Some laboratories therefore prefer to use either refrigerated units with isopentane or cryostats equipped with specialized heat extractors.

Once the specimen is frozen, it is ready for sectioning. A variety of sectioning artifacts can be reduced with a few simple tricks. For example, sections that have been overly frozen will crumble when sectioned. In these cases, simply warm up the block by pressing a gloved thumb firmly onto its surface. (Be careful not to cut your finger on the cryostat blade.) Inadequate freezing, on the other hand, will cause the sections to stick and bind. In these cases, the specimen can be frozen to the appropriate temperature using a cooling spray, such as Histofreeze. Lines and knife marks can be avoided by using a clean and extremely sharp blade. Finally, loosely set screws can contribute to vibration artifacts, so if the sections look like corduroy pants, tighten all of the screws holding the block.

Once the section has been cut, it should be placed on a glass slide, fixed, and stained. A variety of stains are employed in different laboratories (see earlier for the H&E technique); but whichever stains are used, remember to take your time and follow the staining protocol. Too frequently, staining procedures are rushed, and the slides to be stained barely touch the staining solution. The resultant slides can be impossible to interpret or, ironically, may take longer to interpret than a slide stained correctly. Also, when one rushes, one often transfers solutions from one Coplin jar to the next. As a result, solutions are contaminated, and the quality of subsequent frozen sections is diminished. This problem can be reduced simply by touching the edge of the slide to the edge of the jar before transferring the slide to a new solution. Another problem encountered during staining is that tissue can fall off of the slide. If this happens, try using sialinated or other specially treated slides. The ultimate goal in preparation of a frozen section is to render a timely and accurate intraoperative diagnosis. Remember to save the piece of tissue that was frozen so that it can serve as a frozen section control for diagnostic and quality control purposes.

3 Tissue Collection for Molecular Genetic Analysis

Completion of the Human Genome Project will soon result in the identification of more than tens of thousands of new genes. Insight into the function and complex interaction of these genes is of more than just academic interest. Indeed, an understanding of the molecular genetic underpinning of human disease will fundamentally change the practice of surgical pathology.

In the past, a major role of the prosector was to submit well-fixed tissue sections for traditional light microscopic examination. Toward this end, the routine handling of specimens generally involved refrigeration for variable periods of time, fixation in formalin or other denaturing solutions, sampling for microscopic evaluation, and ultimate disposal of excess tissues. The role of the prosector is clearly evolving. These changes will first affect research hospitals, but the pace of change is so great that soon everyone practicing surgical pathology will have to be familiar with tissue collection for molecular genetic analysis. In this new era of functional genomics, there is a new emphasis on rapid collection of fresh, unfixed tissues to optimize preservation of undegraded DNA and RNA for genomic studies. Toward this end, handling of specimens now emphasizes prompt dissection, avoidance of formalin and denaturing solutions, multiplex processing for diverse diagnostic assays, and long-term storage of excess fresh tissues. A flow diagram for the increasingly complex and ever-evolving nature of tissue distribution is shown in Figure 3–1.

The bane of genomic studies is the degradation of RNA and DNA, and thus the major aim when securing tissue is to do so as quickly as possible. Degradation of DNA and RNA begins at the moment the blood supply to a tissue has been interrupted. Therefore, rapid tissue collection involves a coordinated network that begins with punctual delivery of specimens from the operating room to the pathology laboratory and ends with prompt processing of the specimen in the surgical pathology suite. The time allowed from surgical resection to specimen processing depends on a host of factors, but as a rule of thumb: *the faster the better*. In busy surgical pathology laboratories, rapid tissue collection requires prioritization of specimens potentially requiring molecular genetic evaluation over specimens that do not. Hence, be on the lookout for hematopoietic tumors and primitive tumors (i.e., "small round blue cell tumors") of children and young adults, as the molecular genetic profile of these tumors already plays a central role in tumor characterization and patient treatment. Chromosome analysis, molecular cytogenetics, and molecular assays are becoming increasingly useful in the diagnosis of other tumors as well. Table 3–1 provides a partial list of heterogeneous mesenchymal lesions where the identification of certain specific chromosomal translocations now permits more thorough and accurate classification. If any one of these lesions is considered in the differential diagnosis, the specimen should be targeted for rapid tissue collection.

The optimal way to process tissues for molecular genetic studies obviously depends on the nature and methodology of the analysis. Flow cytometry, cytogenetics, and other studies that entail the growth of living cell cultures require fresh sterile tissue samples. These samples should be collected as 0.5- to 1.0-cm cubes of tissue. A balanced physiologic solution such as Roswell Park Memorial Institute (RPMI) medium serves as an excellent medium for short-term storage and

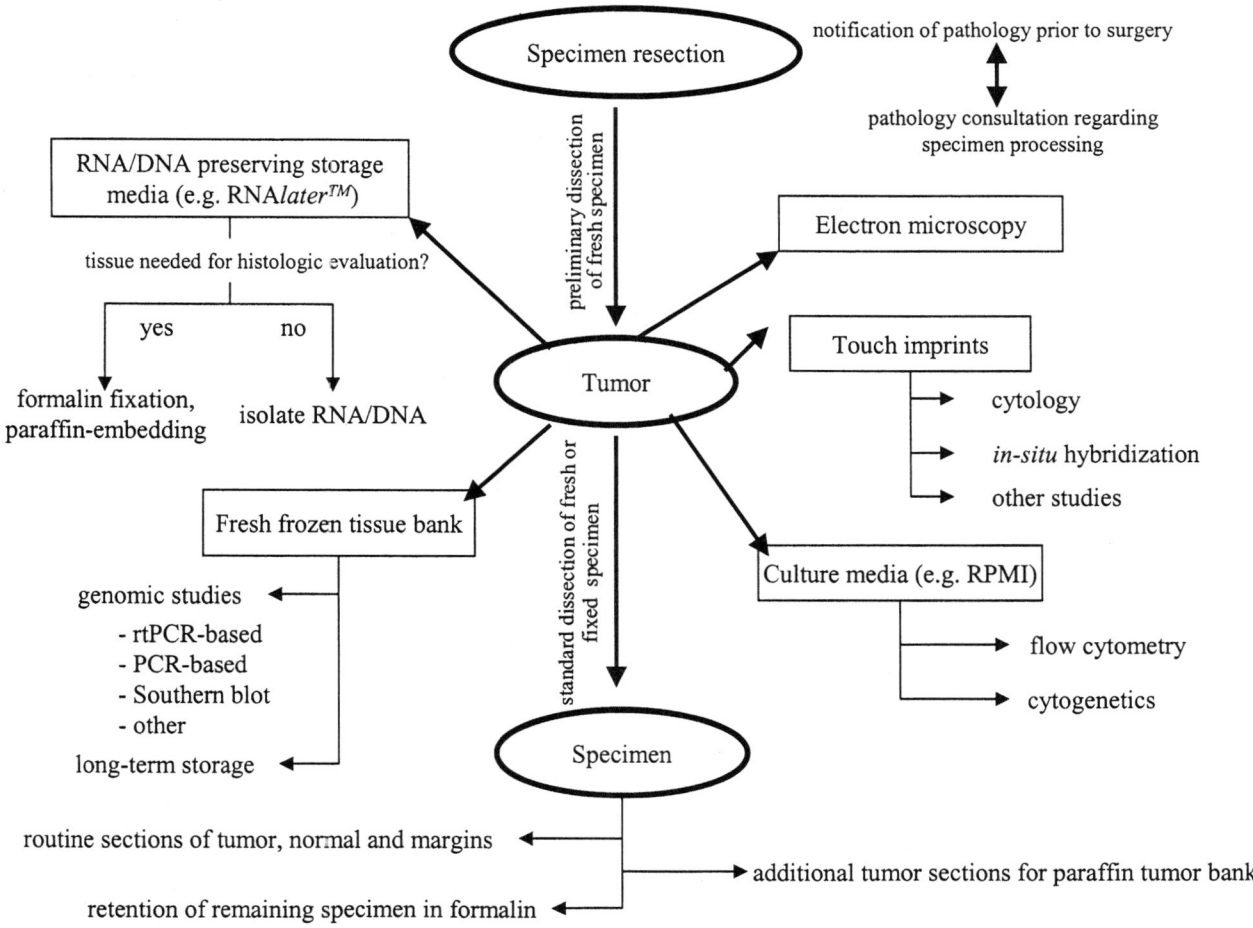

Fig. 3-1. Flow diagram of tissue distribution. (Modified from Florell SR, Coffin CM, Holden JA, et al. Preservation of RNA for functional genomic studies: a multidisciplinary tumor bank protocol. Mod Pathol 2001; 14: 116–128,[1] with permission.)

TABLE 3–1. Tumor-specific chromosomal translocations helpful in classifying mesenchymal lesions.

Tumor type	Chromosomal translocation
Alveolar soft part sarcoma	der(17)t(X;17)(p11.2;q25)
Myxoid/round cell liposarcoma	t(12;16)(q13;p11)
Extraskeletal myxoid chondrosarcoma	t(9;22)(q22;q12)
Dermatofibrosarcoma proteberans	t(17;22)(q22;q13)
Giant cell fibroblastoma	t(17;22)(q22;q13)
Infantile fibrosarcoma	t(12;15)(p13;q25)
Synovial sarcoma	t(X;18)(p11.2;q11.2)
Clear cell sarcoma of tendon sheath	t(12;22)(q13;q12)

transportation. Although various methods are being developed to optimize DNA and RNA extraction from formalin-fixed tissues, polymerase chain reaction (PCR)-based techniques looking for DNA and RNA alterations are best performed on fresh, unfixed tissues. This tissue can be snap-frozen in liquid nitrogen and stored for long periods at −80°C. Advances are being made in the development of more versatile tissue media (e.g., RNA*later*™) that preserve the integrity of DNA and RNA for molecular analysis and at the same time maintain the histologic and immunohistochemical properties of the tissue. Remember that PCR-based techniques are highly sensitive for detecting rare abnormal cells among large numbers of normal cells. Careful attention to cleanliness, such as the use of fresh cutting utensils and changing gloves between specimens, is therefore critical if one is to avoid the effects of specimen contamination.

Given the breakneck pace at which genomic studies are finding increasing diagnostic and therapeutic applications, it is often prudent to store excess fresh tissue in a repository should it be needed for future analysis. This need to collect, store, process, and distribute well-characterized human tissues for diagnostic and investigative purposes has resulted in the emergence of *tissue banks*. Unlike traditional archival banks where the tissues are stored as formalin-fixed and paraffin-embedded blocks, the tissues in tissue banks are generally stored at −80°C in an unprocessed state or as pellets of extracted DNA or RNA.

Not only may these banked fresh frozen tissues be utilized for present and future diagnostic studies, they are of considerable value as resources for molecular genetic translational research. A few guidelines should be kept in mind when collecting and distributing tissues for investigative purposes. First, the pathology laboratory should not distribute tissue for research purposes without prior documentation of approval from the local Institutional Review Board (IRB). IRBs have been established to define the obligations of researchers and to ensure that the use of human tissues conform to federal regulations. Second, patient care must always come first. There may be instances when it is simply not possible to submit tissues for investigative studies without compromising your ability to optimize patient care. In the case of limited specimens (e.g., biopsies), there may not be enough tissue to support microscopic examination and research studies; and for anatomically complex specimens, where it is vital to maintain the integrity of the specimen for proper orientation and evaluation of margins, it may not be prudent to violate the specimen to obtain fresh tissue when formalin fixation is necessary. What ever the scenario, whenever patient care collides with basic science requirements, patient care must win.

Molecular genetic analysis of human tissues is a constantly changing field. New and exciting techniques are being developed every day. Surgical pathology prosectors familiar with the latest developments in molecular diagnoses are best prepared to handle resected and biopsied tissues appropriately.

4 Photography

Norman J. Barker, M.S., R.B.P.

Quality gross specimen photographs are an essential part of surgical pathology. Aesthetically pleasing 35-mm color slides, black-and-white prints, and digital images are used not only to document the diagnosis but also for conferences, presentations, teaching, and publications. Unfortunately, photographs are often not taken; or if they are taken, they are not useful because of underexposure, overexposure, inappropriate lighting, poor selection of background, or blood-stained or blood-smeared backgrounds. Fortunately, with care and a standardized system, you can produce consistent high-quality photographs. This chapter first describes how to set up a standard photographic system and then describes how to photograph specimens and trouble shoot a variety of problems.

Setting Up a Photographic System

Photographic Stand

A variety of camera stands are on the market. Pick one with a sturdy column. Sturdy columns eliminate camera vibration, which causes photographs to be out of focus. Probably the most versatile and easy to use system on the market is the Polaroid MP4, which consists of a heavy-duty stand, a 4 × 5-inch camera, and permanently mounted but adjustable lighting (Fig. 4-A). It also has an adapter for a 35-mm camera. With this system, Polaroid 4 × 5-inch black-and-white negative film can be used to produce an instant print and negative. The print serves as an instant record, documenting the size and condition of the specimen, and notes can be made directly on the print, providing a visual correlate of the gross description. The negative can be filed and prints for publication made from it at a future date.

Lens Selection

Most major camera manufacturers offer a choice of two types of macro lenses. The 60-mm macro lens is sufficient for 95% of routine work in the surgical pathology laboratory. The 105-mm macro lens allows for more working distance between the specimen and the front of the lens. This feature is helpful when doing close-up work. Both of these macro lenses are extremely useful because they can focus down to a point where the image on the negative is the same size as the specimen, and they will cover specimens ranging in size from a large colon down to small polyps. One of the scales that is not present on most ordinary lenses, but that is printed on macro lenses, is the reproduction ratio. You should be familiar with this scale because, as discussed later, it can be used to determine the appropriate exposure for a specimen (Fig. 4-B).

Background Selection

Before lighting the subject, background selection must be considered. The correct background will enhance and highlight the subject to be photographed. A background table can be easily made or commercially purchased. The latter is a good choice but is only good for medium to small specimens. The Aristo Box DA-17 (Fig. 4-C) has a cool rectangular, fluorescent light inside. The

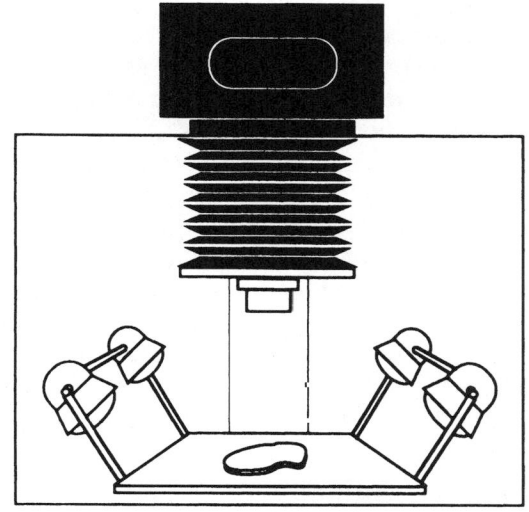

Fig. 4-A. The Polaroid MP4 system.

Film T-64 60-mm macro lens		
f-Stop	Time (s)	Reproduction Ratio
22 ½	¼	1 : 10
22	¼	1 : 7
16 ½	¼	1 : 3
16	¼	1 : 1

Fig. 4-B. Example of a gross stand exposure chart. Create a chart such as this one to calculate the f-stop when doing close-up work. The reproduction ratio value is printed on most lenses.

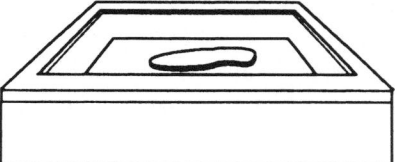

Fig. 4-C. Aristo DA-17 light box.

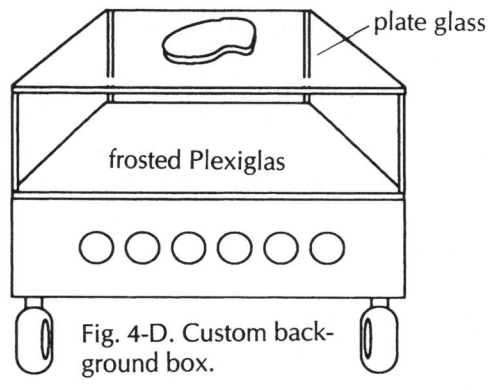

Fig. 4-D. Custom background box.

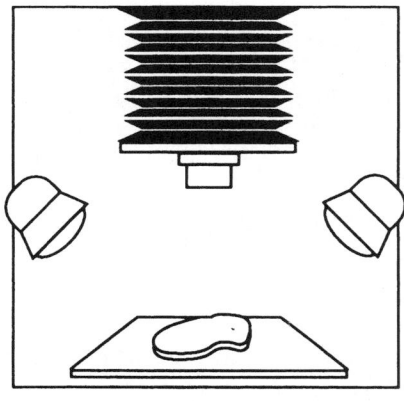

Fig. 4-E. Standard flat copy lighting.

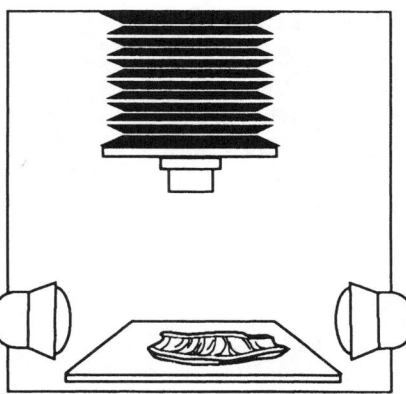

Fig. 4-F. Side lighting—texture.

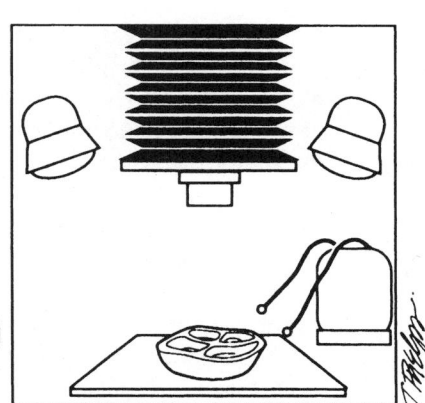

Fig. 4-G. Fiber-optic lighting—cavity.

box gives a flat shadowless illumination or, if turned upside down, a black background.

A more versatile system (Fig. 4-D) can be custom-made to fit space requirements. A custom background box should have even fluorescent lighting below a glass surface on which specimens can be placed. Immediately on top of the fluorescent lights is a place for opal glass or Plexiglas, which diffuses the light for an even background. Colored gels can then be placed on top of the Plexiglas for a variety of background selections. There is then a space of about 6 to 8 inches between the background and the specimen glass. This system eliminates shadows on the background.

If colored gels are used for backgrounds, great care must be taken. An ill-chosen background color can affect the color of the specimen in the photograph. For many specimens, red, yellow, and green are colors to avoid. Shooting an actual test photograph is the only way to tell for sure. One very simple type of background is a piece of black velvet available in fabric shops. This material will absorb all light that falls on it, yielding a pure black background. Therefore no shadows from the specimen will be seen. A solid black background also has the advantage of hiding liquids that have seeped out from a specimen. This makes a cleaner presentation in the final photograph.

Lighting

Important features of a specimen may be hidden when the lighting is too dim or obscured when the lighting is too bright. Appropriate lighting, on the other hand, will actually enhance the photographic demonstration of these findings. One of the many advantages of the Polaroid MP4 stand is the fact that the lights may be easily moved to highlight the features of a particular specimen. Lights placed in the standard 45° position (standard copy lighting) provide an even, flat illumination for the majority of specimens (Fig. 4-E).

The standard 45° positioning of the light source may not be optimal for every specimen. For example, when three-dimensional information is most important, the lights should be positioned at a lower angle (Fig. 4-F). This will provide shadows that will help suggest a relief or distinguish a form from its background. This positioning of the light source can help show texture as well. Another technique is to unplug the lights on one side so that a stronger contrast can be seen. The main thing to keep in mind is that lighting should not obscure information.

A good addition to a lighting system is a fiber-optic light source (Fig. 4-G). Manipulable fiber optic wands provide an excellent source of illumination when close-ups are required. They are particularly useful in illuminating cavities and crevices. When used in combination with other light sources, fiber-optic lights are also effective in "filling in" otherwise darkened areas. Keep in mind that when lighting changes are made, some changes in exposure may also be necessary.

Thirty-Five–Millimeter Slides

Not only can 35-mm slides be used for projection at conferences, they can be used for publication as well. The slides also can be scanned into a computer, and letters, numbers, or arrows may be added. Other slides can be scanned and combined together, such as a gross and microscopic view on one slide. A 35-mm slide may be converted to a black-and-white print for publication.

Color slides are best obtained with a 35-mm single-lens-reflex camera with through-the-lens light metering. The best results are achieved with fine-grain films. A film should be selected for accurate color rendition, and it should match the Kelvin temperature of the lights used. Most gross specimen photography is done with tungsten halogen lamps (3200 K) as opposed to an electronic flash (5500 K). Unlike the transient illumination of the electronic flash, tungsten lamps provide constant illumination so that the lighting can be critically evaluated before the photograph is taken. Kodak Ektachrome tungsten EPY-64 is a good choice of film. This film is balanced for tungsten lamps, it has a high resolution, tends to match the true specimen colors, and is a user-processed film. (User-processed film can be processed at most hospital in-house photographic departments, usually on a same-day basis.) Films such as Kodachrome, on the other hand, tend to enhance red and yellow colors and must be sent to outside laboratories for processing.

Standardized Exposure Determination

The amount of light that reaches the film or digital camera can be controlled in two ways. One is to change the aperture. The *aperture* refers to the diameter of the lens diaphragm, and this can be adjusted by changing the f-stop. Each f-stop setting changes the amount of light passing through the lens by a factor of 2. The smaller the f-stop number, the larger the aperture and the more open the lens. For example, an f-stop of 2 will let more light into the camera than an f-stop of 22. The aperture also controls the *depth of field*, which refers to the zone of sharpness in front of and behind the point of focus. With large apertures (smaller f-stop numbers), everything outside the plane of focus abruptly becomes blurred. At very small apertures (such as an f-stop of 22), objects remain in focus over a greater depth of field. Therefore, optimal clarity is best achieved using a smaller aperture (higher f-stop).

The amount of light hitting the film is also controlled by the shutter speed. The *shutter speed* refers to the length of time that the lens is open. Each shutter speed, like the f-stop, doubles or halves the exposure at the next setting. Standard speeds on modern shutters are 1, ½, ¼, ⅛, 1/15, 1/30, 1/60, 1/125 second, etc. Keep in mind that both the aperture and shutter control the amount of light falling on the film.

You need to identify the best f-stops and shutter speeds for your particular system by running a series of exposure tests for each different specimen magnification. To do this, you need a light meter. An incident light meter works best because it measures the light falling on the specimen. The reflected light meters that are found in most cameras can be "fooled" and give incorrect readings because of the light coming from the background. For example, reflected light meters may read too much of the background and not enough of the specimen when a lightly colored specimen on a black background is being photographed. Once the exposure is approximated with the hand-held incident light meter, a series of test exposures should be made at different magnifications (reproduction ratios). Most manufactured lenses have reproduction ratios listed on the lens barrel for each magnification. In making this test run, choose a standard exposure such as ¼ second, and then vary the aperture of the camera by one half of an f-stop at each magnification. This exposure time will enable you to use small apertures, which result in a better depth of field and translate into better specimen focus. The best aperture then can be determined for a specific image magnification, and a chart can be made listing the correct aperture that matches each magnification (Fig. 4-B). While this system is easy to use, it may be necessary to modify the exposure for very dark blood-red specimens or very light white specimens.

Scale

While many find scales and labels unnecessary distracters in an otherwise aesthetic photograph, at least one of the specimen photographs should include a scale along with the specimen identification number. A scale helps the viewer orient the specimen and provides a benchmark for the perception of size, while specimen labeling ensures that the photographs will not be lost or misidentified later. Commercially prepared plastic rulers are available that can be made into various sizes to accommodate different specimens. Small adhesive labels with the specimen identification number can be attached directly to the ruler. When placing the scale in a photograph, be sure to place it in the anatomical inferior position. The scale should be positioned at the level of the specimen so that it is in plane of focus.

Digital Photography

When it comes to photographing gross specimens, digital images offer several advantages over conventional 35-mm photography. First and foremost is the ease with which an image, once captured in digital format, can be edited, organized, catalogued, and stored. Second, a digital system permits immediate review of the image captured. Most digital cameras have a video "out" port that allows for the image to be captured and displayed on a video monitor in real time. Some digital cameras are also equipped with small screens for reviewing the image captured. Third, digital imaging is cost-effective. For laboratories that routinely use photography as a component of their gross dissections, digital image photography can reduce film and processing costs.

Digital imaging technology is advancing at breakneck speed. Each month seems to bring an updated digital camera that is less costly and of higher quality than the previous model. There are literally hundreds of digital cameras now on the market, and choosing the best one is a formidable task. When selecting a digital camera, one of the most important features to keep in mind is the resolution of the image sensor. Resolution has to do with the ability to appreciate fine detail in an image. Digital photographs are made up of thousands to millions of picture elements known as pixels, and the quality of an image depends, in part, on the number of pixels used to create the image. High pixel numbers enhance detail, sharpen edges, and provide a more meaningful record of the specimen. Conversely, low pixel numbers obscure fine detail and result in images that have less value for teaching, publication, and documentation of the gross findings. Keep in mind that a high-resolution digital camera is not a substitute for good judgment and technique. No matter how good the camera, informative images still require careful attention to specimen orientation, lighting, and exposure.

Some Pointers on Photographing Specimens

General Principles

A few simple steps will improve the aesthetic quality of your photographs. First, photograph the cut surface of the specimen. A photograph of the external surface of a specimen is seldom informative. Section the specimen using a fluid sweeping motion to create a cut surface that is smooth and unruffled. Take the photograph before gouging out tissue for frozen section evaluation or tumor collection; or if these studies are urgently needed, take the tissue from an area that will not be shown in the photograph. Gently rinse blood and fluid from the surface of the specimen, and then blot the surface of the specimen dry so that fluid does not seep across the field of view.

Second, decide whether the pathology is best demonstrated in the specimen before or after it is fixed. Color is best seen when the specimen is photographed fresh, while fine structural details are sometimes better appreciated in fixed specimens, which reflect less light.

Third, position the specimen so that (1) the area of interest is centered in the field of view; (2) its long axis is oriented along the long axis of the frame; and (3) the specimen fills at least 75% of the frame. For bivalved specimens, there is no need to photograph both halves of the specimen. Instead, fill the frame with a closer view of just one of the two halves. To point out a focal area of interest, use a clean and unassuming probe or pointer (not a finger).

Fourth, make sure the background is clean and free of distracters. Remember that your work is not over once the photograph is taken. Remove the specimen, and clean the background so that it is ready for the next user.

Dark Specimens

Many fresh specimens and bloody specimens tend to produce dark images on film. As a general rule, you can compensate by opening the lens by one f-stop (decrease the f-stop number). This will lighten the specimen in the final photograph.

Light Specimens

Photographs of fixed specimens can sometimes be bleached white with little or no color information. Try taking one photograph at the normal exposure. Then take several more photographs while increasing the f-stop number in half increments (e.g., f-stop 16, 16½, 22, etc.) This intentional closing of the lens and consequent underexposure should provide more detail in the very light areas.

Large Specimens

Large specimens generally require at least two sets of photographs: one of the entire specimen and the other a close-up of the area of interest. The close-up photograph will demonstrate the finer details of a lesion, while the overall view will show the relationship of the lesion to the rest of the specimen.

Small Specimens

Most normal lenses will not focus when moved very close (i.e., within 2 feet) to the specimen. A special macro lens is needed for very small specimens or for close-up photographs to show fine detail. The 105-mm macro lens is especially suitable for these purposes. It can focus to a point where the image on the negative is the same size as the specimen, while maintaining a comfortable working distance between the front of the lens and the specimen. Remember that focus is critical in close-up work. Even small specimens can have depth, so avoid focusing only on the top of the specimen by focusing on a point about one third of the way down from the top of the specimen. Also, use a small camera aperture (an f-stop of 22) for increased depth of field.

Oddly Shaped Specimens

Oddly shaped specimens are a nuisance to photograph when they cannot be maintained in the correct position. A simple solution is modeling clay, which can be used to prop up the specimen. Mold the clay into shape, and use it as a base to hold the specimen. Before taking the picture, be sure to look through the viewfinder to make sure that the clay will not show up in the final photograph. Small fishhooks with nylon cord and an attached weight can be used to hold areas open. For example, this technique can be useful when photographing the interior of heart valves.

Cavities

Under standard lighting conditions, the walls of a cavity cast shadows that obscure the base of the cavity. To circumvent this problem, place the lights as high as possible, so that they illuminate the depths of the cavity. This type of vertical illumination will help reduce shadows as well as light the entire cavity. A separate fiber-optic light source can also be of great help. Make sure that you are focused on the area of interest because depth of field can be a problem.

Three-Dimensional Structures

Side lighting is the best lighting to demonstrate surface detail or to show the three-dimensional quality of a tumor. The lower the angle of the light, the more surface relief will be seen. Shadows give the form shape, depth, and contrast. Be careful not to set the lights too low, as this can create harsh shadows that obscure detail.

Troubleshooting

Reflection

If you are using a piece of glass to support the specimen, watch out for reflections. A valuable photograph can be ruined when overhead (ceiling) lights, the photographer's hand, or the photographer's face is seen reflected in the background. Always use a cable release (the extender cable that allows the photographer to trigger the shutter from a distance), not only to keep the camera still but also to avoid reflections in the glass. Fixed specimens reflect much less light than fresh specimens. If the specimen is fresh, reflected light can be reduced by drying the surface of the specimen with a paper towel. Before tripping the shutter, look through the viewfinder and study the field. Make sure that the lighting and arrangement best demonstrate the pathology of interest.

Exposure

Once an exposure test has been made and an exposure chart posted, the camera should consistently produce uniform high-quality exposures. A photograph that is too light is likely due to overexposure. The simple solution is to close the aperture. (For example, an f-stop setting of 11 can be changed to a setting of 16 or 22.) If the photograph is too dark, simply open the aperture so that the film receives more light. With a little practice and a standard system, you should be well on the way to top-quality specimen photographs.

Maintenance of the Photography System

Not surprisingly, a system designed for use by many users is particularly susceptible to abuse and neglect. Proper maintenance of a photography system is a daily task that is less likely to be neglected if assigned to one person. This person should be responsible for: maintaining clean lenses and viewfinders as well as a fresh supply of film; checking that the cameras are loaded with film; and checking that the film is delivered for processing in a timely fashion. There is nothing worse than spending valuable time in photographing an important specimen and afterward finding out that there was no film in the camera!

Things to Remember when Photographing a Specimen

- Always make sure the background is clean. A spray bottle and towels should be part of the photography setup.
- Orient the specimen. Mark the specimen with a proper identification tag, and include a scale in the plane of focus.
- Always use a cable release to eliminate unwanted camera vibration and reflection.
- Double-check the focus and exposure settings.
- Verify that the lighting shows what you want. Take great care to avoid shadows that obscure features of particular interest.

Commercial Products/ Equipment Vendors

1. Aristo DA-17 Light Box: Aristo Grids Lamp Products, 65 Harbor Rd., P.O. Box 769, Port Washington, NY 11050.
2. Polaroid MP4 Camera: Polaroid Corp., 575 Technology Square, Cambridge, MA 02139.
3. Nikon Inc., 1300 Walt Whitman Dr., Melville, NY 11747-3064 (www.NIKONUSA.com).
4. 150-mm Rulers (Cat. No. 09-016): Fisher Scientific Co., 711 Forbes Ave., Pittsburgh, PA 25219.
5. Photodyne Technologies, Inc., 19441-134 Business Center Dr., Northridge, CA 91324 (www.Photodyne.com).

II Lymph Nodes for Metastatic Tumors

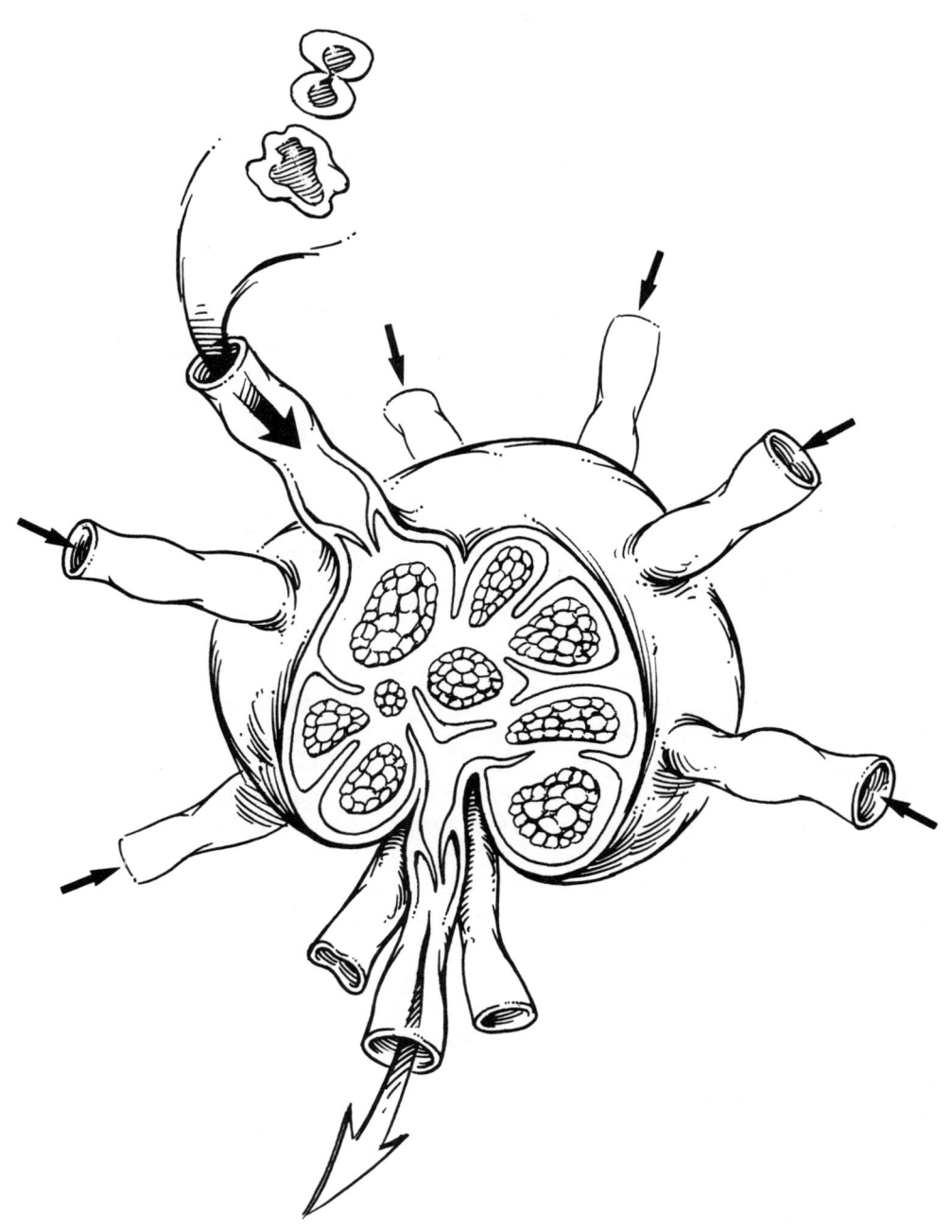

5 Lymph Nodes

Metastatic spread to lymph nodes carries profound treatment and prognostic implications for patients with carcinomas, melanomas, or any other malignant neoplasm with metastatic potential. Accordingly, assessment of lymph node specimens is every bit as important as evaluating a neoplasm at its primary site.

Lymph Node Dissections

A general approach to sampling lymph nodes is described in Chapter 1, and the organ-specific approach to the dissection of regional lymph nodes is detailed in each organ-specific chapter. In this chapter we review a few general guidelines that can be broadly applied when it comes to evaluating lymph nodes for metastatic disease.

Lymph nodes are easiest to appreciate in the fresh state before subtle distinctions in tissue density are obscured by tissue fixation. Submersion of specimens in certain clearing agents may be helpful in eliminating the bulk of adipose tissue, but this is an unnecessary and time-consuming step that does not improve on meticulous examination of the fresh tissues. When appropriate, the anatomic levels of the lymph nodes should be maintained and separately reported in the surgical pathology report (e.g., colectomy specimens and neck dissection specimens). In cases where important anatomic landmarks do not accompany the specimen, it may not be possible to identify levels without the help of the submitting surgeon.

Although tedious, the objective of any lymph node dissection for metastatic disease is nothing less than detection and processing of every lymph node contained in the specimen. There is practically no role for representative nodal sampling when searching for metastatic spread. Each lymph node identified should be submitted for microscopic examination. If tumor is grossly visible, a section that includes the tumor suffices. If tumor is not grossly visible, the lymph node should be sectioned in 3- to 4-mm slices and all of the sections submitted for microscopic evaluation. You can slice the lymph node along its long or short axis, but longitudinal sections are generally preferable, as this minimizes the number of slices. No single cassette should contain slices from more than one lymph node unless colored inks are used to distinguish different lymph nodes. For these nonsentinel lymph node dissections, one hematoxylin and eosin (H&E)-stained section per tissue block is adequate.

Sentinel Lymph Node Biopsy

As noted above, the standard pathologic practice for the evaluation of nonsentinel lymph nodes is to examine microscopically one section from each lymph node using the simple H&E technique. Although this approach may be practical for evaluating large numbers of lymph nodes, most pathologists would concede that such limited analysis consistently underestimates the true incidence of occult nodal metastases. Recent improvements in our clinical ability to identify the lymph nodes most likely to harbor metastases have facilitated the accurate staging of cancers. The sentinel lymph node strategy is particularly appealing because the surgical removal of just one or several selected lymph nodes permits a more comprehensive pathologic search for small and localized metastatic deposits.

Methods for detecting tumor cells in sentinel lymph nodes have become increasingly sophisticated and sensitive, ranging from routine histologic examination of serial sections to reverse transcriptase-polymerase chain reaction-based methods for detecting a single tumor cell among a sea of lymphocytes. Outside of routine H&E staining, however, most detection methods are investigational, and currently there is no agreement as to an optimal detection protocol. Given the diversity of the processing and examination of sentinel lymph node biopsies among laboratories, you should be familiar with the protocol details specific to your own institution. At the same time, there are generic guidelines that are widely applicable across institutions and assorted tumor types.

The sentinel lymph node biopsy specimen should be carefully examined to determine the number of lymph nodes. The size of each should be recorded. Each lymph node should be processed separately. Each node is serially sectioned along the longitudinal or transverse plane into 3- to 4-mm slices. Small lymph nodes that cannot be easily sectioned should be submitted in toto. Examine the cut surface of each slice for the presence of grossly visible tumor nodules.

Your gross assessment of the lymph node dictates the degree of sectioning by the histopathology laboratory. If tumor is visualized grossly, routine H&E staining of a single level is sufficient to document the presence of tumor and its possible extension beyond the lymph node capsule. If tumor is not grossly visible, the lymph node slices should be sectioned at multiple levels. There is currently no standard to guide the extent of tissue sectioning. At a minimum, one section from each of three levels of the tissue block should be obtained for routine H&E staining. Regardless of whether immunohistochemistry is part of a specific protocol, the histopathology laboratory should place intervening unstained sections on sialinated slides in an effort to minimize loss of potentially diagnostic material and provide a source of unstained sections should the need for immunohistochemistry arise.

Handling Radioactive Specimens Obtained by Sentinel Lymphadenectomy

The process of clinical lymphatic mapping and the identification of sentinel lymph nodes relies on nodal uptake of radioactive tracers. Fortunately for pathology personnel, the amount of radiation associated with sentinel lymphadenectomies is low. Even with frequent handling of these specimens, radiation exposure usually does not approach statutory exposure limits. Given the exceedingly low radiation exposure, most authorities now agree that quarantining these specimens does not enhance the safety of pathology personnel and only serves to delay the final diagnosis. Accordingly, sentinel lymph node biopsies should be processed immediately on receipt from the operating room using customary universal precautions. Nonetheless, if you have a question about a particular specimen, you should call your institution's radiation safety officer.

Sentinel Lymph Node Biopsy for Evaluating Metastatic Disease

1. Record the number of lymph nodes and their dimensions.
2. Serial section each lymph node along its longitudinal or transverse plane into 3- to 4-mm slices.
3. If a metastatic implant is grossly visible, have the histopathology laboratory cut and stain one representative section to document the presence of tumor.
4. If a metastatic implant is not grossly visible, have the histopathology laboratory cut multiple sections from at least three levels. At least one section from each level should be stained with H&E. Additional unstained sections should be stored on treated slides for future immunohistochemical studies as needed.

Important Issues to Address in Your Surgical Pathology Report

- What procedure was performed?
- How many lymph nodes from each anatomic level harbor metastatic tumor, and how many lymph nodes from each level were microscopically examined?
- What is the size of the largest metastatic implant?

- Does the metastasis extend beyond the nodal capsule into the surrounding perinodal fat? (This is particularly important to note for metastatic squamous cell carcinomas of the head and neck and metastatic carcinomas of the breast.)
- For sentinel lymph node biopsies, was the metastasis detected by routine histopathology, immunohistochemistry, molecular-genetic analysis, or some combination of these techniques?

III The Head and Neck

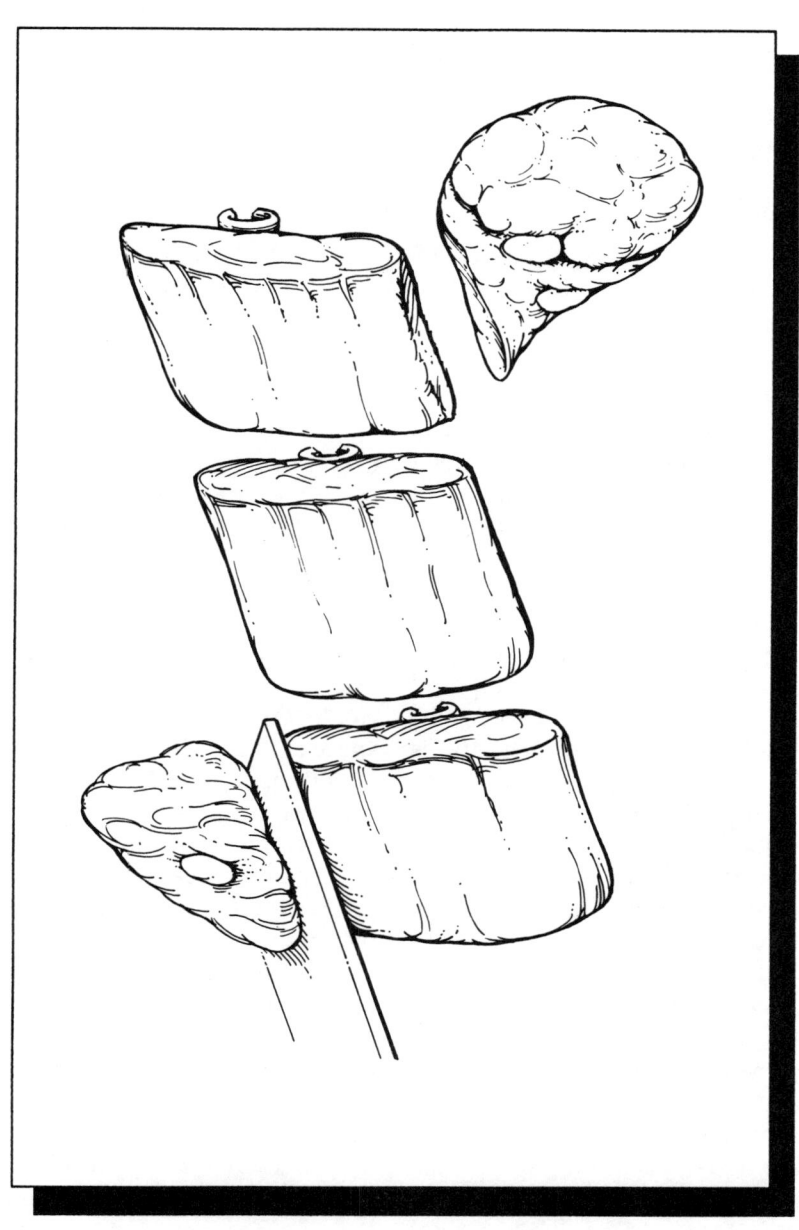

6 Larynx

The Anatomy

The patterns of spread of carcinomas of the larynx depend on their site of origin and on well-defined anatomic barriers. A detailed understanding of laryngeal anatomy is therefore an essential part of the dissection of any laryngeal specimen. Take time to look over the figures and refresh your memory of laryngeal anatomy.

The most important thing to remember about laryngal anatomy is that the larynx is composed of three anatomic regions: the supraglottis, the glottis, and the subglottis. The supraglottis is the portion of the larynx superior to the ventricles. It is composed of the epiglottis, the arytenoids, the aryepiglottic folds, and the false cords. The glottis is composed of the true vocal cords and their anterior and posterior attachments, the anterior and posterior commissures. The subglottis begins 1 cm below the free edge of the vocal cords and extends inferiorly to the trachea. These three anatomic regions should be kept in mind throughout your description and dissection of the larynx.

The important mucosal landmarks to identify in the larynx are illustrated and include the mucosa of the epiglottis, the aryepiglottic folds, the false vocal cords, the ventricles, the true vocal cords, and the subglottis. Some specimens may also include the base of the tongue with its overlying mucosa. These mucosal surfaces cover the cartilaginous framework of the larynx. This framework includes the cartilage of the epiglottis, the thyroid cartilage, and the cricoid cartilage. The epiglottis is attached to the thyroid cartilage by the thyroepiglottic ligament. The shield-shaped thyroid cartilage forms the anterior and lateral walls of the larynx. The cricoid cartilage is shaped like a signet ring, and it forms the posterior wall of the larynx. Situated in the back of the larynx are the two arytenoid cartilages. These are pyramidal in shape and rest along the upper border of the cricoid cartilage. Although the hyoid bone is not technically part of the larynx, it is often included in laryngectomy specimens.

Three additional anatomic landmarks need to be defined because cancers that invade these landmarks frequently escape from the larynx. The *pre-epiglottic space* is the triangular space anterior to the base of the epiglottis. The pre-epiglottic space is filled with fatty connective tissue, and it is bounded posteriorly by the epiglottis, inferiorly by the thyroepiglottic ligament, anteriorly by the thyrohyoid membrane, and superiorly by the hyoepiglottic ligament. The *paraglottic space* is a less well-defined area composed of loose connective tissue, which lies between the thyroid cartilage and two membranes that form the structural base for the vocal folds, the conus elasticus and quadrangular membrane. The *anterior commissure* is the anterior dense ligamentous attachment of the true vocal cords to the thyroid cartilage. The thyroid cartilage lacks an internal perichondrium; therefore, carcinomas may invade the thyroid cartilage at the level of the anterior commissure. Carcinomas may also escape the larynx inferiorly via the cricothyroid membrane.

Finally, although the pyriform sinuses are technically part of the hypopharynx, one should be aware of them because they are frequently resected with the larynx. The pyriform sinuses are small pouches that extend inferiorly from the intersection of the aryepiglottic folds, glossoepiglottic folds, and pharyngeal wall. Depending on the size and location of the tumor, laryngeal specimens may also include other portions of the hypopharynx (including the posterior pharyngeal wall and the pharyngo-esophageal junction) and the thyroid gland.

Total Laryngectomy

The easiest way to orient a total laryngectomy specimen is to identify the epiglottis. The epiglottis is present anteriorly at the most superior aspect of the larynx, and the flap of the epiglottis closes posteriorly. If the epiglottis is not present, then the thyroid cartilage can be used to orient the specimen. The superior horns of the thyroid cartilage are located superiorly and project posteriorly, while the V-shaped apex of the thyroid cartilage points anteriorly.

After the specimen has been oriented, ink the soft tissue and mucosal margins. The mucosal margins essentially form two rings. The inferior ring is formed by the trachea, and the superior ring is formed by the circular opening of the larynx into the pharynx. After the margins have been inked, cut through the posterior wall of the larynx in the midline using a pair of scissors. This posterior midline approach will fully expose the mucosal surfaces of the larynx without disrupting the anatomic structures located along its anterior and internal walls. The larynx can then be cracked open posteriorly by expanding the posterior opening with your thumbs. The easiest and safest way to do this is to push hard on the superior horns of the thyroid cartilage. The posterior aspect of the larynx can then be kept open using a small wooden stick. The opened larynx should be photographed to document the location and size of the tumor. Depending on the preferences of your laboratory, the larynx can be processed fresh or after fixation.

Continue your dissection by sampling the mucosal margins. Sampling the inferior mucosal margin is a relatively simple step. If this margin is not closely approached by tumor, it can be taken as a single shave section of the tracheal stump. If the tumor is close to the inferior margin, take perpendicular sections. Sampling the superior mucosal margin, on the other hand, is much more labor intensive. This mucosal margin spans a number of important laryngeal structures, and great care must be taken to sample the margin thoroughly and to designate each sampled margin as precisely as possible. As illustrated, the superior mucosal margin is formed (1) anteriorly by the mucosa of the base of the tongue, (2) laterally by the pyriform sinuses or lateral walls of the posterior hypopharynx, and (3) posteriorly by the posterior cricoid mucosa. Perpendicular sections of each of these three mucosal margins should be taken. Next, take the soft tissue margins. These can be taken as perpendicular sections from the anterior surface of the specimen and from any other areas where the soft tissues appear infiltrated by tumor.

Once all the margins are taken, turn your attention to the tumor. Keeping the three anatomic regions of the larynx (the supraglottis, glottis, and subglottis) in mind, carefully document the side, size, and exact location of any tumors. Also note whether the tumor is endophytic or exophytic. Submit sections of each identified tumor for histology to show its maximal depth of invasion as well as its relationship to grossly uninvolved mucosa. Next, carefully examine, document, and sample for histology the mucosa of the pyriform sinuses, the epiglottis, the aryepiglottic folds, the false cords, the ventricles, the true vocal cords, the anterior commissure, and the subglottis. In general, longitudinal sections are most informative. As illustrated, a single longitudinal section can be taken to include the false cord, the ventricle, and the true cord. Carefully examine the thyroid cartilage and the cricoid cartilage. These structures should be selectively sampled to document the presence or absence of tumor invasion. These sections may have to be submitted for decalcification. If a tracheostomy site is present it should be noted, and several sections of it should be submitted for histologic examination. Finally, remember the three additional anatomic landmarks discussed earlier. The pre-epiglottic space can be sampled by taking a midline section from the base of the epiglottis superiorly and anteriorly toward the hyoid bone. As illustrated, the paraglottic space is usually included in the histologic section of the true and false cords. Finally, a section of the anterior commissure should be submitted in cancers that involve the vocal cords.

If any organs were removed along with the larynx, their presence should be documented. Be especially diligent in your search for the thyroid gland. Often, only a portion of the gland is removed with the larynx, and it may be embedded within the anterior soft tissues and

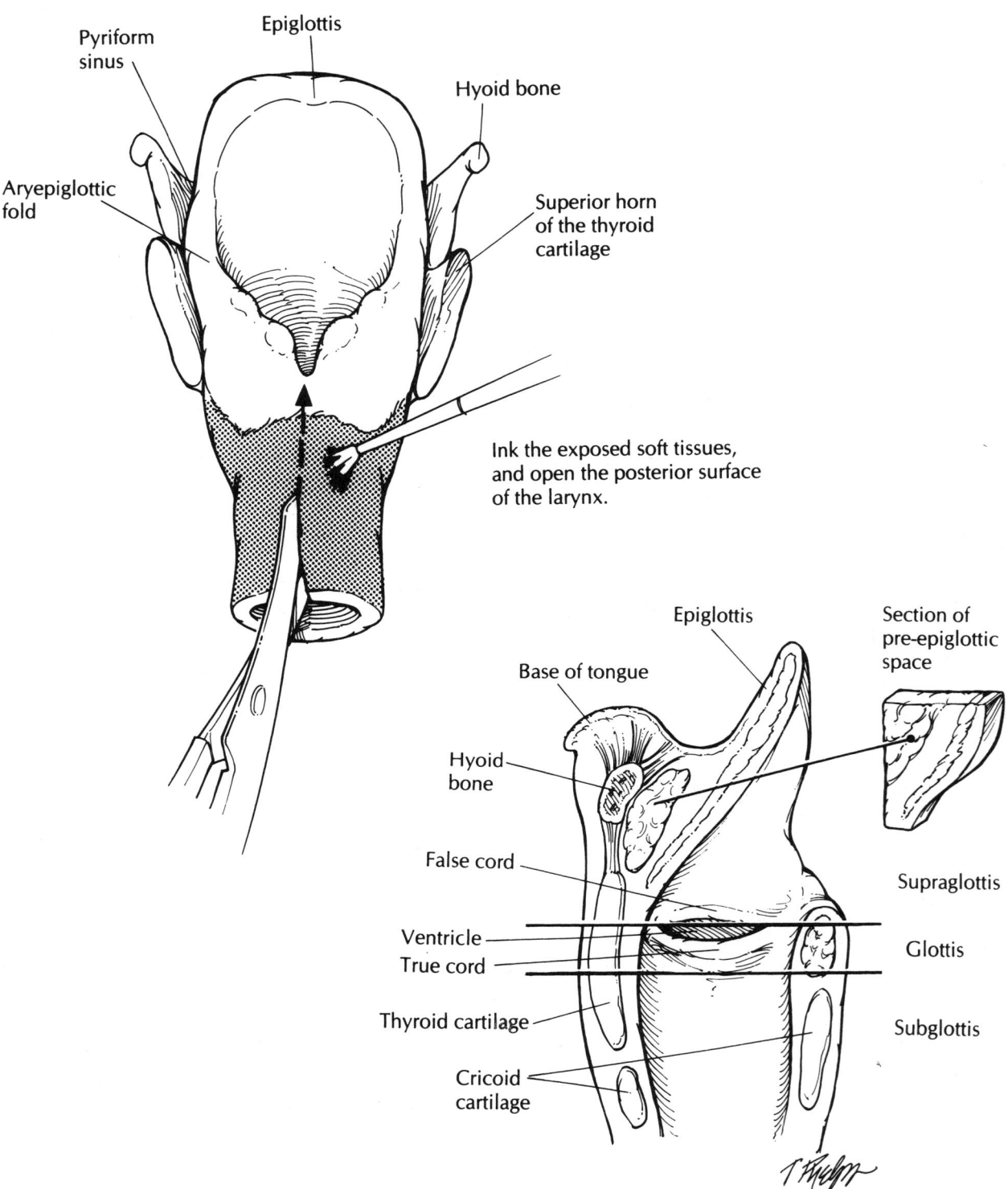

Ink the exposed soft tissues, and open the posterior surface of the larynx.

Although this is a plane of section you will not see, we find this diagram helpful, because it demonstrates the anatomy and the location of the pre-epiglottic space.

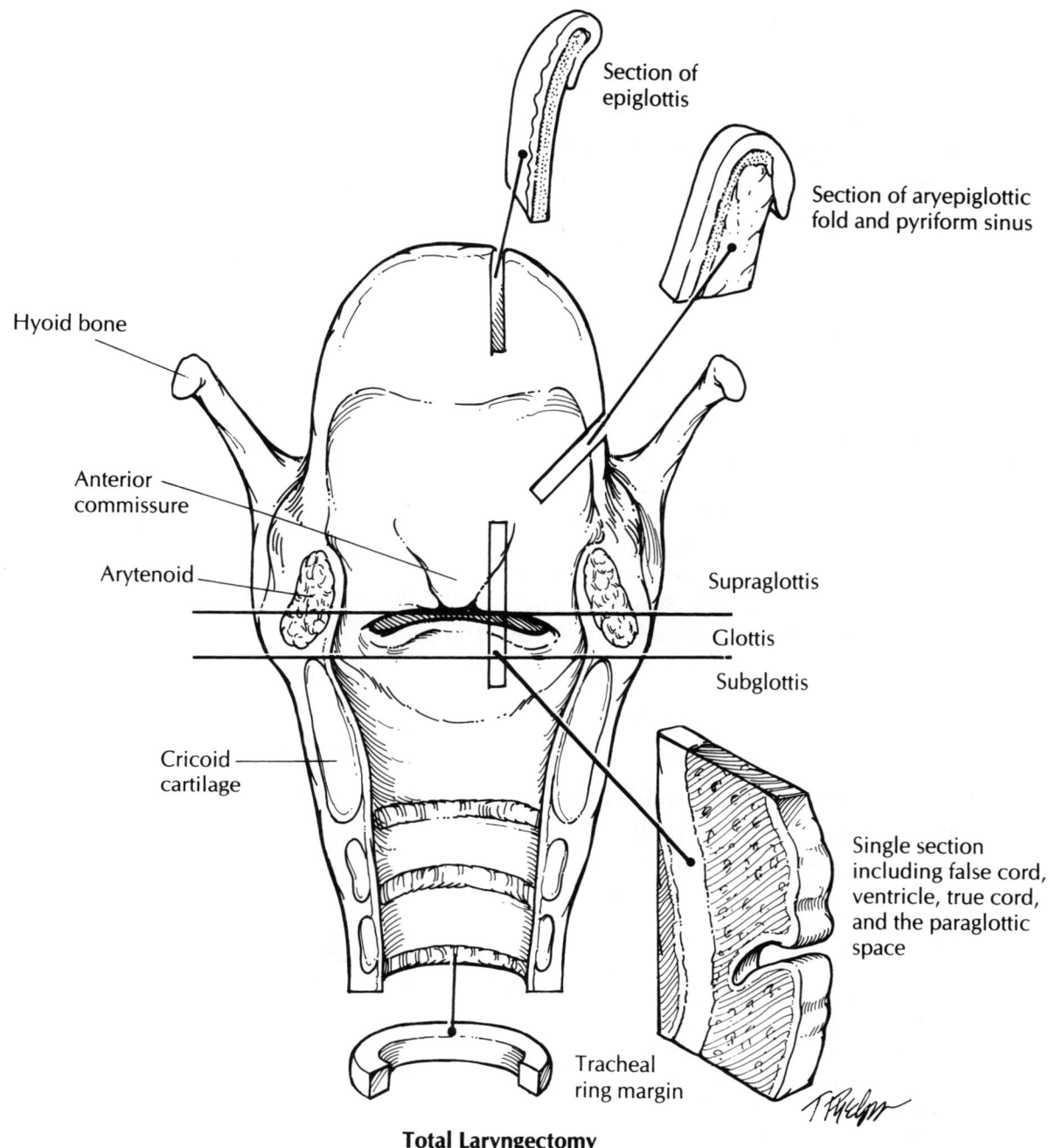

Total Laryngectomy

1. Orient the specimen. The epiglottis is present anteriorly at the most superior aspect of the larynx, and the flap of the epiglottis closes posteriorly.
2. Ink the margins, and then cut through the posterior wall of the larynx in the midline. Open the larynx by pushing hard on the superior horns of the thyroid cartilage.
3. Submit sections of the inferior (tracheal) and superior (base of tongue, pyriform sinus or lateral hypopharyngeal wall, and posterior cricoid) mucosal margins and anterior and posterior soft tissue margins.
4. Describe and submit sections of the tumor, keeping the three anatomic regions of the larynx in mind: the supraglottis, the glottis, and the subglottis.
5. Submit a section from both sides to include the false cords, the ventricles, and the true cords. Submit sections of the pyriform sinuses, the epiglottis, the aryepiglottic folds, the anterior commissure, the subglottis, the thyroid cartilage, the cricoid cartilage, and the hyoid bone. Submit sections of the pre-epiglottic space, the paraglottic space, and the anterior commissure.

strap muscles. If the thyroid gland is present, examine it as described in the thyroid section (see Chapter 36) and remember to look for parathyroid glands. If a radical neck dissection is attached, it can be removed and examined separately as described in the section on radical neck dissections (see Chapter 10).

Subtotal Laryngectomies

Portions of the larynx can also be resected. For example, a *hemilaryngectomy* is a voice-preserving procedure in which either the left or right thyroid cartilage, true vocal cord, false cord, and ventricle are removed in continuity. A *supraglottic laryngectomy* is a procedure performed for tumors of the supraglottic larynx in which the supraglottis is removed with a horizontal incision through the ventricles. The approach to these subtotal laryngectomy specimens should follow that for total laryngectomy. In addition, the new margins created by the procedure need to be sampled.

Important Issues to Address in Your Surgical Pathology Report on the Larynx*

General

- What procedure was performed, and what structures/organs are present?
- What is the exact location of the tumor? Specifically, what is the probable site of tumor origin (glottis, supraglottis, subglottis), and what compartments and structures (e.g., glottis, supraglottis, subglottis, hypopharynx, pre-epiglottic space, thyroid cartilage) does it involve by direct extension? Does the tumor cross the midline to involve both sides of the larynx?
- What are the tumor's size, grade, type, and growth pattern (exophytic or endophytic)? What is the depth of deepest tumor invasion?
- Is there perineural and/or vascular invasion?

- Are any soft tissue or mucosal margins involved?

Supraglottic Cancers

- If the hyoid bone is attached, is the tumor above or below the level of the hyoid?
- Does the tumor involve the false cord, the epiglottis, the aryepiglottic folds, and/or the arytenoids?
- Does the inferior edge of the tumor involve the anterior commissure and/or the roof of the ventricle?
- If the aryepiglottic fold is involved, how far down the pyriform sinus does the tumor extend?
- How far does the cancer extend superiorly toward the base of the tongue?
- Does the cancer involve the pre-epiglottic space?
- Does the tumor invade the cartilaginous framework?

Glottic Cancers

- Does the tumor involve one vocal cord or both, and what is the length of the cord involvement?
- Is the anterior commissure involved? If so, does the tumor extend anteriorly into the thyroid cartilage?
- How far inferiorly below the free edge of the true vocal cords does the tumor extend (in millimeters)?
- Does the tumor extend superiorly into the ventricle, false cord, or base of the epiglottis?
- Does the cancer involve the paraglottic space?

Subglottic Cancers

- What is the superior extent of the tumor? Does it involve the true vocal cord?
- What is the inferior extent of the tumor? How close is the tumor to the inferior margin?
- What is the maximal depth of invasion? Does the carcinoma penetrate the conus elasticus and extend into the paraglottic space?

---

*Modified from Kirchner JA, Carter D. The larynx. In: Sternberg SS, ed. *Diagnostic Surgical Pathology*, 2nd ed. New York: Raven Press; 1994:907–908.

7 Major Salivary Glands

The gross appearance of some salivary gland neoplasms is so characteristic that one can come close to establishing the diagnosis on the gross findings alone. Yet, all too often, salivary glands are simply inked, bread-loafed, and thrown into tissue cassettes. Take time to describe the appearance of any lesions encountered.

Examine the external surface of the specimen after it has been weighed and measured. Without help from the surgeon, it is usually not possible to distinguish the superficial from the deep lobe of the parotid. The surgeon sometimes uses a suture or tag to designate one or both lobes in total parotidectomy specimens. Carefully look for and tag with safety pins any large nerves that may have been resected with the gland. It is important to sample these nerves for histology, but they will not be identifiable after the specimen has been inked. After it has been oriented and inked, palpate the specimen and identify the tumor. Next, section the gland at 2- to 3-mm intervals. Measure the size of the tumor and describe its gross appearance. Is it well demarcated and encapsulated or poorly demarcated and infiltrative? Is the tumor solid or cystic? Are areas of cartilaginous differentiation appreciable grossly? How close is the tumor to the margins? Carefully examine the salivary gland parenchyma, keeping in mind that salivary gland tumors may be multinodular (e.g., recurrent pleomorphic adenomas) or multicentric (e.g., Warthin's tumor).

Salivary gland neoplasms should be thoroughly if not entirely sampled for microscopic examination. Sampling that is too limited runs the risk of: (1) missing focal areas of malignant transformation in a pre-existing adenoma; and (2) providing an incomplete representation of the overall microscopic appearance of these morphologically diverse neoplasms. Do not just scoop out the center of the tumor; instead, carefully submit sections showing the relationship of the tumor to the inked soft tissue margin, the tumor to the adjacent uninvolved gland, and, as noted, the tumor to any grossly identifiable nerves. Once the tumor has been described and submitted for histology, the rest of the gland can be examined and described. The parotid gland is unique among the major salivary glands in that it harbors a number of intraparenchymal lymph nodes. Thus, your search for lymph nodes should include the parotid parenchyma itself in addition to the periparotid soft tissues. These lymph nodes should be entirely submitted for histologic evaluation. Are any calculi present, and are the ducts of the salivary gland dilated? Submit representative sections of grossly uninvolved salivary gland.

Important Issues to Address in Your Surgical Pathology Report on Salivary Glands

- What procedure was performed, and what structures/organs are present? For parotid resections, which lobes have been removed?
- Is a neoplasm present?
- What are the type, size, and degree of differentiation of the tumor?
- Does the tumor infiltrate small or large nerves?
- Does the tumor involve any of the margins?
- If lymph nodes are present, how many are present, and how many are involved by tumor?
- Does the non-neoplastic portion of the salivary gland show any pathology?

8 Complex Specimens

Treat nature in terms of the cylinder, the sphere, and the cone, all in perspective.
Cézanne

While we have attempted to illustrate the dissection of the majority of the standard head and neck specimens received in the surgical pathology laboratory, you will occasionally be faced with a complex specimen that we have not illustrated. Without a game plan, these specimens can be overwhelming.

Our approach is a simple one based on four steps. First, identify the various components of the specimen (epithelium, bone, soft tissue, etc.). Second, think of each component as a geometric shape. Third, approach each component separately. Fourth, look for the relationships between any lesions and each component. This approach is illustrated below with the dissection of a portion of the tongue and mandible (partial glossectomy with partial mandibulectomy) resected for cancer.

Step 1. Identify the Various Components of the Specimen

In this case, the components include the soft tissue and muscle of the tongue, the epithelium of the oral cavity, and the bone of the mandible. This step helps ensure that important components of the specimen are not left out of the dissection, gross description, and tissue sampled for histology.

Step 2. Think of Each Component as a Geometric Shape

For example, as illustrated for the partial glossectomy with partial mandibulectomy specimen, the muscle of the tongue can be thought of as a cube, the bone of the mandible as a cylinder, and the epithelium as a flat two-dimensional square sheet.

Step 3. Approach Each Component Separately

The goal here is to take sections that will demonstrate each margin. The margins are easily remembered using the geometric shapes visualized for each component. For example, the muscle is thought of as a cube. You should therefore take perpendicular margins from each face of the cube. As illustrated, these include the anterior, posterior, medial, lateral, and inferior surfaces. The sixth surface, the superior surface, is covered by the epithelium, so this is not a margin. Similarly, the epithelium is thought of as a square sheet. Take perpendicular margins from the posterior, anterior, medial, and lateral edges of this square. Finally, the bone is thought of as a cylinder. Shave sections of the two ends of the cylinder—the anterior and posterior bone margins—should be submitted. Thus, in the case illustrated, the margins taken include anterior, posterior, medial, lateral, and inferior soft tissue margins; anterior, posterior, medial, and lateral epithelial margins; and anterior and posterior bone margins. Obviously, corresponding epithelial and soft tissue margins can be—and, indeed, usually are—included in the same section.

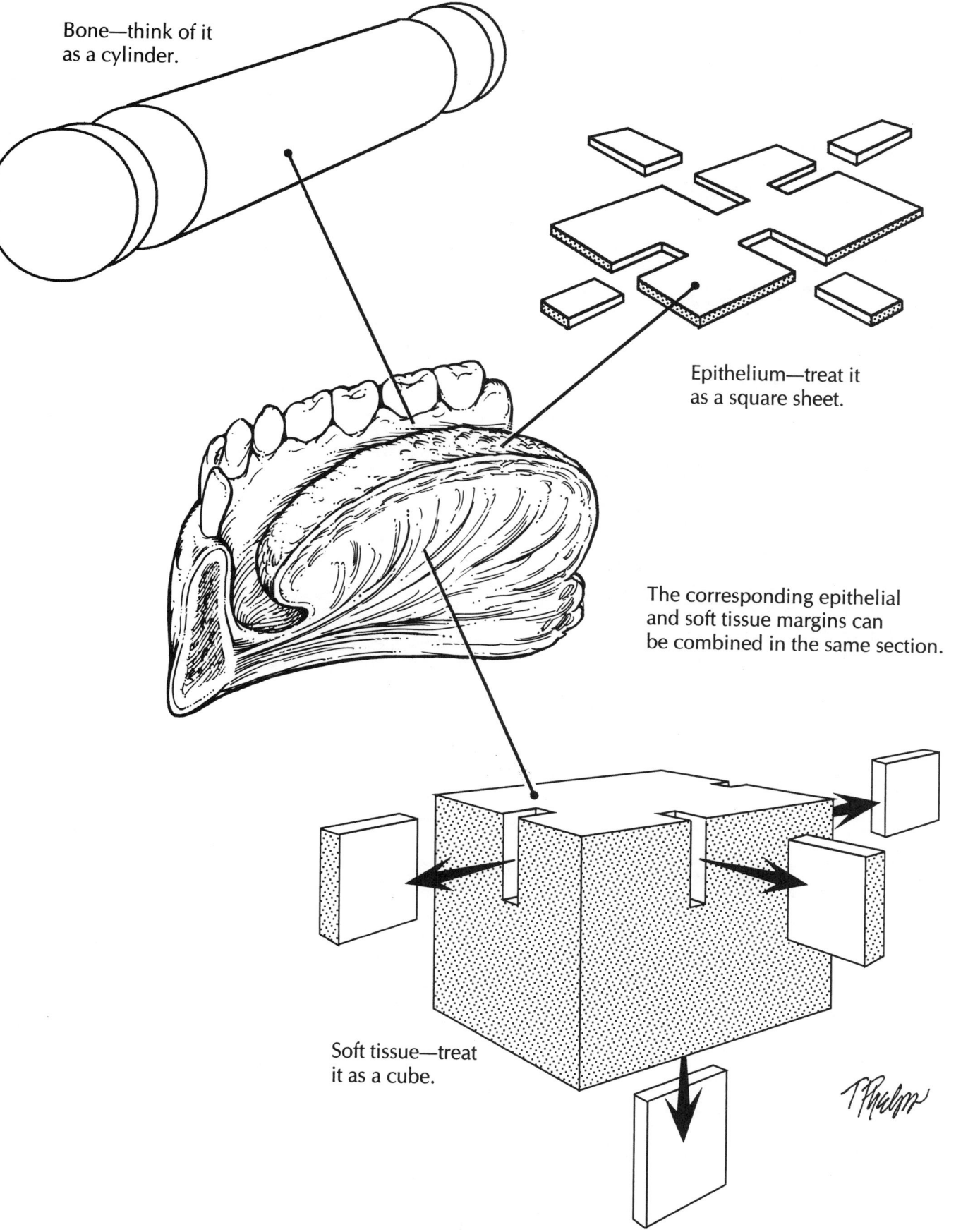

Step 4. Document the Relationship Between Any Lesions and Each Component of the Specimen

All lesions, as well as sections demonstrating the relationship of each lesion to each of the various components of the specimen, should be sampled. For example, in the specimen illustrated, sections should be taken showing the relationship of the tumor to the bone, of the tumor to the surface of the epithelium, and of the tumor to the muscle.

While we find this geometric approach to specimens helpful, you may wish to develop your own system for complex specimens. Whatever approach you choose, remember that your ultimate goal is to provide the clinician with the information needed for the appropriate management of the patient.

9 Maxilla

James J. Sciubba, D.M.D., Ph.D.

Resections of tumors involving the passages of the nose and paranasal sinuses present the ultimate challenge in surgical pathology dissection. These passages are walled by bony structures that defy efforts to section, expose, and sample. Moreover, the three-dimensional anatomy of these regions is inherently complex and difficult to reconstruct once the specimen has been removed from the patient. Nowhere are these difficulties more significantly encountered than during resection of the maxilla.

The maxillary sinus is somewhat pyramidal in shape and is surrounded on all sides by craniofacial bone. The daunting anatomic complexity of this region can be simplified by envisioning yourself in a room with a floor, a ceiling, and four walls. At your feet is the hard palate. Pass through this floor, and you enter the oral cavity. Above your head is a ceiling that forms the floor of the orbit. Pass through this ceiling, and you enter the orbital cavity. Turn medially, and you face a wall that is shared with the nasal cavity (i.e., the lateral nasal wall). Pass through this wall, and you enter the nasal chamber. The remaining walls are not shared with other chambers. Instead, the anterior and lateral walls form the bony surfaces of the face, which are bounded by the soft tissues and skin of the cheek. The posterior wall forms a boundary with the musculature and bony processes of the pterygoid complex. This conceptualization should help you discern the specific location of a tumor in the maxillary sinus and understand the paths of tumor spread into adjacent chambers and anatomic structures.

With this image in mind, orient the maxillectomy specimen. Remember that only a portion of the maxilla is generally removed during a cancer resection (i.e., partial maxillectomy). Consequently, only some of the surfaces are present, leaving the sinus exposed to visual inspection. The extent of the resection depends on the location and spread of the tumor. Specimen orientation is greatly facilitated by the recognition of a few key landmarks. Teeth, when present, identify the floor of the maxillary sinus (alveolar process) and help you discern the anterior and lateral aspects of the maxilla. The nasal choana are seen as smooth longitudinal folds or pouches of mucosa-lined tissues. These form the lateral wall of the nasal sinus and identify the medial aspect of the maxilla. Some specimens include the eye. In these cases, identification of the superior and anterior aspects of the specimen is obvious. If present, skin from the cheek marks the lateral and/or anterior aspect of the specimen. If you have done your best to identify these landmarks but still have trouble with orientation, do not hesitate to contact the surgeon.

Once you have confidently oriented the specimen, measure it in three dimensions. Identify and describe the anatomic boundaries of the specimen and note the presence of important anatomic structures (e.g., eye, skin, nasal choana, teeth). Ink the external margins of the soft tissue enveloping the maxilla, being careful not to let ink seep into the sinus. Without sectioning the specimen, look into the exposed maxillary sinus and try to identify the tumor. In addition to documenting the size of the tumor, determine its location within the maxillary sinus. Specifically, identify which walls are grossly involved by tumor. Determining the site of tumor origin helps guide further sectioning of the specimen to determine the path of tumor spread. For instance, a tumor arising from the floor of the sinus generally extends inferiorly and laterally into the palate and the alveolar process of the maxilla (infiltrating between and around molar teeth). More medially placed tumors are prone to extend into the nasal cavity. Tumors along the lateral wall may infiltrate the skin and soft tissues of the cheek. Tumors involving the roof of the sinus tend to extend into the orbital cavity, ethmoid air cells, ethmoid sinus, or cribriform plate. For tumors involving more than one chamber, try to determine the epicenter of the tumor. For example, if a tumor involves the floor of the maxillary sinus, try to distinguish between a maxillary sinus carcinoma that extends inferiorly into the palate and an oral cavity carcinoma that extends superiorly into the maxillary sinus.

Depending on your laboratory's preferences, the specimen can be dissected in the fresh state or be sectioned after fixation in formalin. After tissue has been obtained for special studies as needed, we recommend fixation before further processing. Tissue fixation facilitates the difficult process of stripping mucosal margins from underlying bone. Tissue fixation also minimizes tissue fragmentation and distortion should sawing be required to section through bone. Finally, adequate fixation is essential before the sample can be processed in demineralizing solutions should specimen decalcification be required.

Begin your dissection by sampling all of the margins including the soft tissues, bone, mucosa, and skin. The number and type of margin sections depend on the nature and extent of the resection. For example, if the medial wall of the sinus is removed, you need to sample the mucosa all along the nasal cavity margin. If the resection includes the orbit, you need to submit a shave section of the optic nerve. Before taking these sections, it is helpful first to tabulate all of the various chambers and tissue components present in the specimen so that no margin is overlooked. Sampling some of these margins can be challenging. For example, the presence of teeth and underlying bone are formidable barriers to well-oriented perpendicular sections that radiate from the edge of the specimen toward the center of the tumor. Instead of the standard perpendicular sections, the mucosal edges of the maxillary resection (particularly along the alveolar process of the maxilla) may have to be taken as thin parallel sections that are gently peeled off the underlying bone. Again, these sections are easier to obtain if the mucosa is well fixed. The soft tissue margins, in contrast, can be submitted as perpendicular sections. Be sure to include in your gross description details of the precise location and type of each margin. A photograph that indicates the location of each margin section is highly recommended.

After all of the margins have been sampled, bisect the specimen along a plane that passes through the epicenter of the tumor and best demonstrates the tumor's relationship to adjacent compartments. Before making this first cut, it may be useful to consult the preoperative imaging studies to determine the location of the tumor and its path of spread. This section may require the use of a band saw, particularly when the sections must pass through the dense bone of the alveolar process and palatal alveolus. A detailed description of the use of bone saws with an emphasis on safety issues is provided in Chapter 22. Teeth are particularly dense tissues, and they are difficult to section even with powerful bone saws. Unless there are indications to sample a tooth, sections through the alveolar process of the mandible should avoid the teeth. Direct the blade of the saw between the teeth. Make additional sections to further assess the extent of the tumor and its relationship to surrounding structures. When intact teeth are included within the portion of the specimen to be histologically evaluated, it may be prudent to remove the crowns of these teeth. This practice shortens the decalcification time and lessens decalcification-induced artifacts. Removal of crowns can be facilitated by use of a bone saw or dental drill with a stream or spray of coolant water.

Now that the tumor has been more fully exposed, describe its appearance and growth characteristics. Is the tumor exophytic, endophytic, erosive, and/or infiltrative? Measure and record its dimensions including its deepest level of invasion. Determine the anatomic structures and compartments the tumor involves. Is the tumor confined to the maxillary sinus? If there is invasion into bone, has the tumor extended beyond the bone and into an adjacent chamber?

When sampling the tumor, submit sections to demonstrate the relationship of the tumor to the surrounding mucosa and the underlying bone. In addition, submit sections to determine tumor spread into adjacent anatomic structures and compartments. For example, the nasal mucosa should be amply sampled for tumors involving the medial maxillary wall. If an eye is included in a resection of the superior wall of the maxilla,

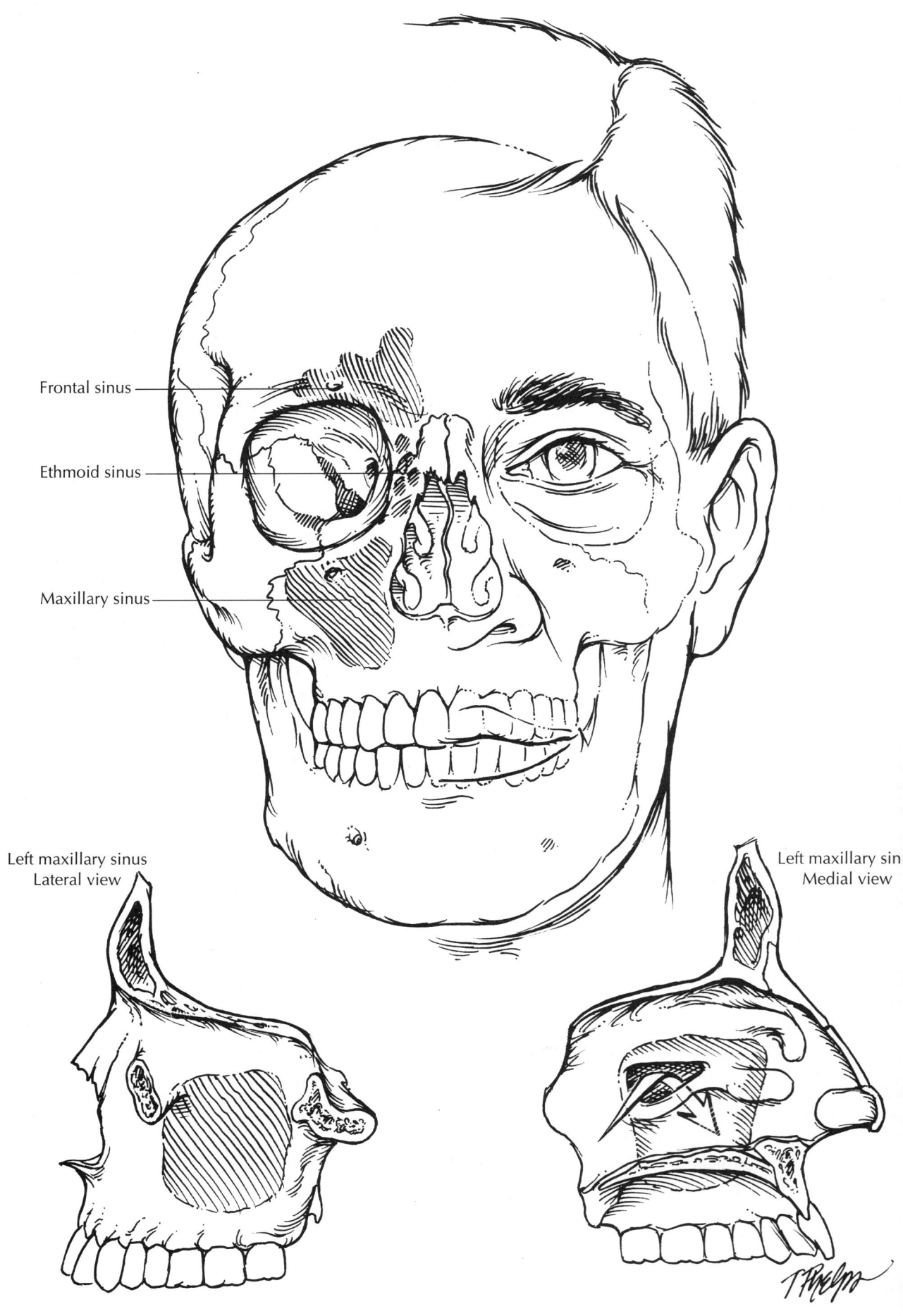

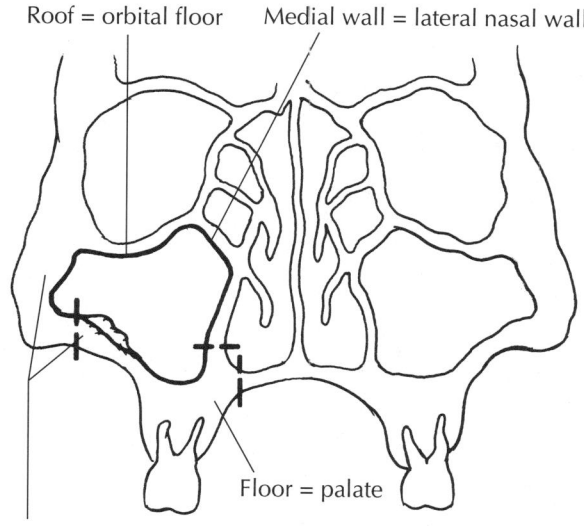

Walls of maxillary sinus
Roof = orbital floor
Medial wall = lateral nasal wall
Floor = palate
Lateral and anterial walls = facial tissues

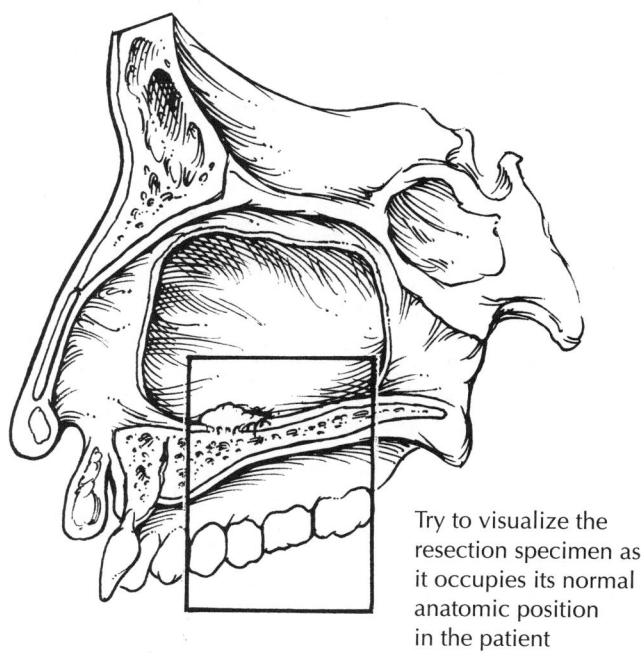

Try to visualize the resection specimen as it occupies its normal anatomic position in the patient

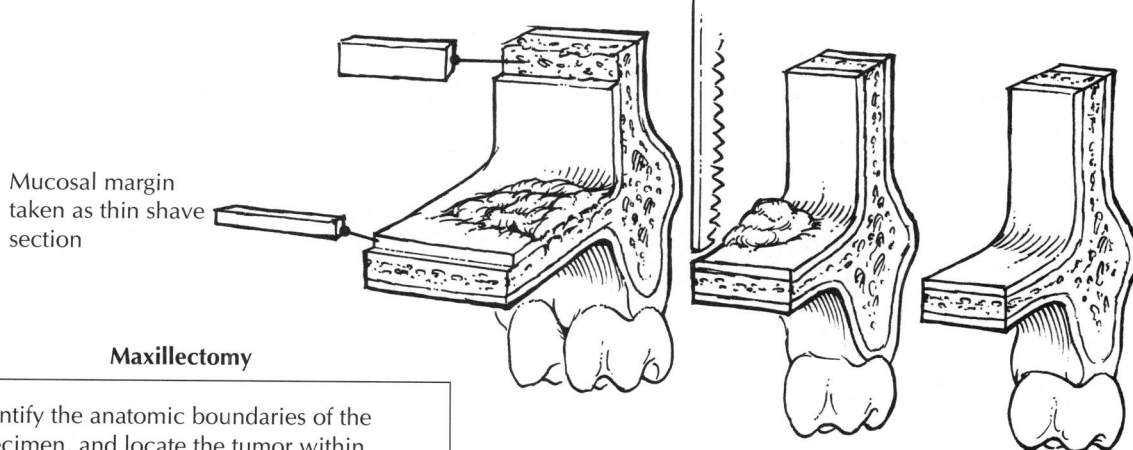

Mucosal margin taken as thin shave section

Maxillectomy

1. Identify the anatomic boundaries of the specimen, and locate the tumor within the maxillary sinus.

2. Ink the mucosal and soft tissue margins.

3. Sample all of the margins including the soft tissue, bone, mucosa, and skin. It may be most practical to submit the mucosal margins as thin shave (parallel) sections that are peeled off the underlying bone.

4. Section the specimen along a plane that best demonstrates the tumor's relationship to adjacent structures and compartments. These sections may require the use of a bone saw. Make additional sections to determine the tumor's size and extent of spread.

5. Submit sections of the tumor that demonstrate its relationship to adjacent anatomic structures and compartments.

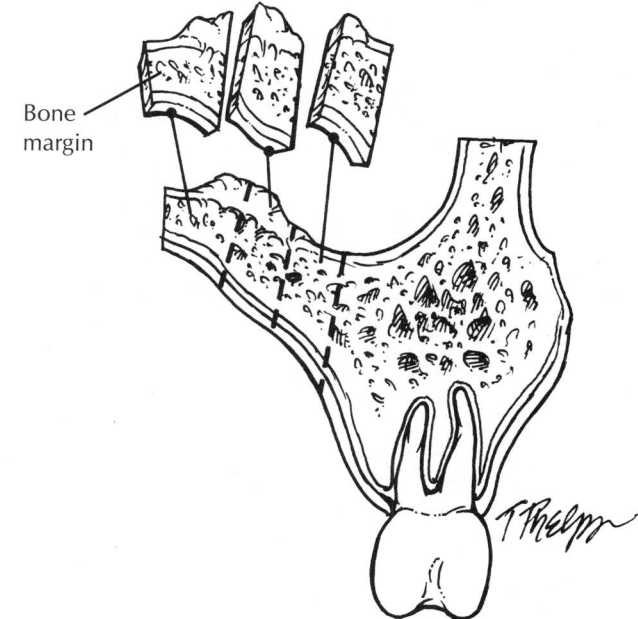

Bone margin

submit sections of the orbital contents. For the eye itself, one section (in addition to the optic nerve margin) is generally sufficient to document its presence and to demonstrate its relationship to the tumor. If there are reasons to perform a more thorough evaluation of the eye, follow the guidelines for enucleation specimens provided in Chapter 35.

Regional lymph nodes are usually removed separately by the surgeon and submitted as separate specimens. They should be anatomically oriented, and each level should be carefully dissected (see Chapter 10). Each lymph node should be submitted for histologic evaluation.

Important Issues to Address in Your Surgical Pathology Report on Maxillary Sinus Resections

- What procedure was performed, and what structures/organs are present?
- Is a neoplasm present?
- What is the probable site of tumor origin (maxillary sinus, maxillary bone, palate, nasal cavity)? For tumors of the maxillary sinus, from what surface does the tumor arise (inferior, superior, medial, lateral, anterior, posterior)?
- What is the size of the tumor (in centimeters), and what is the greatest depth of tumor invasion?
- What are the histologic type and grade of the tumor? Is an *in situ* component present?
- Does the tumor extend into bone? If so, does the tumor extend beyond the bony confines of the maxillary sinus to involve adjacent compartments and structures (e.g., nasal cavity, oral cavity, orbital cavity, skin, pterygoid complex)?
- Does the tumor involve the margins (mucosal, skin, bone, soft tissues)?
- Does the tumor involve regional lymph nodes? Include the number of nodes examined and the number of nodes involved.

10 Radical Neck Dissection

Neck dissections for the en bloc removal of cervical lymph nodes come in a variety of shapes and sizes. The radical neck dissection is the standard procedure to which all other neck dissections are compared. It includes resection of the sternocleidomastoid muscle, the internal jugular vein, the spinal accessory nerve, and the lymph nodes from levels I to V. The goal of the surgical pathologist in evaluating these specimens is simply to identify the number of lymph nodes involved by tumor at each level.

Start by orienting the specimen. The dissection is shaped like a Z. The pink-tan, lobulated submandibular gland is usually easy to identify, and it occupies level I, the most anterosuperior aspect of the specimen. The internal jugular vein, as its name implies, is present on the internal (medial) surface of the sternocleidomastoid muscle. Using these two anatomic landmarks, one can both orient the specimen and determine which side it was taken from. After orienting the specimen, measure its overall dimensions. Next, open the jugular vein along its length, and look for tumor involvement or thrombosis. Sample any abnormality in the vein.

The specimen can now be divided into its five levels and each level separately dissected for lymph nodes. First, dissect off level I, which includes the submandibular salivary gland and the triangle of soft tissues anterior to the sternocleidomastoid muscle. Next, remove level V, the triangle of fatty connective tissue posterior to the muscle. Finally, levels II, III, and IV can be separated off by dividing the sternocleidomastoid muscle into equal thirds. Level II, the upper jugular group, is composed of the lymph nodes around the upper third of the sternocleidomastoid muscle. Level III, the middle jugular group, is composed of the lymph nodes around the middle third of the sternocleidomastoid muscle, and level IV, the lower jugular group, is composed of lymph nodes around the lower third. Now search for the lymph nodes. The best place to look for lymph nodes in each level is in the fatty connective tissue. Lymph nodes usually will not be found within the sternocleidomastoid muscle itself. Section each lymph node at 2- to 3-mm intervals along its long axis. If the lymph node is grossly uninvolved by tumor, submit the entire lymph node for histologic examination. If the lymph node is grossly involved by tumor, measure the size of the implant and submit two sections of the metastasis. Be sure that these two representative sections include the lymph node capsule along with a rim of the perinodal fat so you will be able to determine the presence or absence of extranodal tumor spread. In addition, the salivary gland in level I should be measured, described, and serially sectioned. If any masses are found in the salivary gland, the gland should be dissected as described in Chapter 7. If no abnormalities are grossly apparent, simply submit a representative section for histology. Finally, representative sections of any tumor involving the sternocleidomastoid muscle or extranodal soft tissue should be submitted for histology. If a group of matted lymph nodes is present, it will be impossible to dissect out each individual lymph node. In these cases, submit two sections through each level involved to document the extensive nature of the tumor.

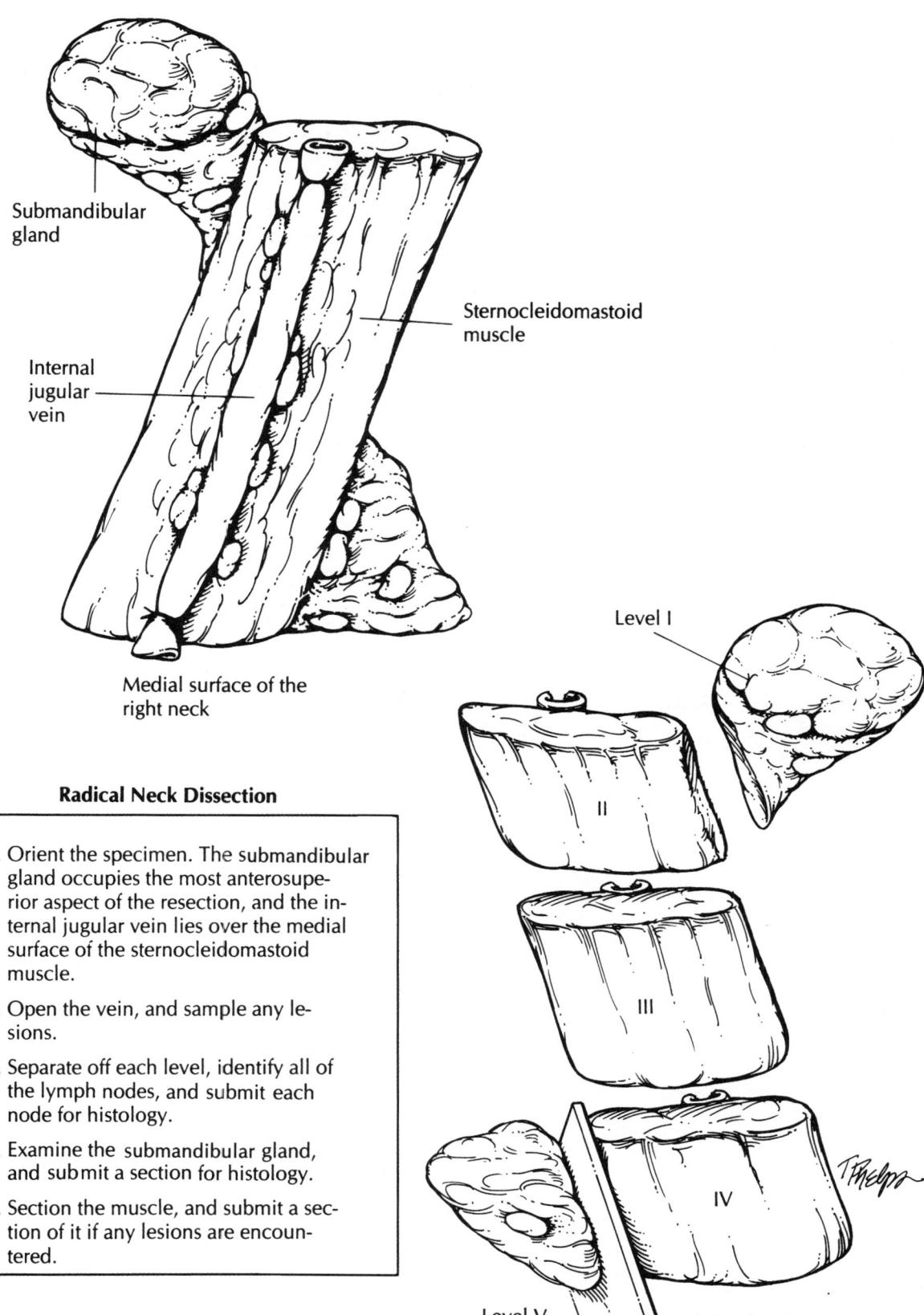

Radical Neck Dissection

1. Orient the specimen. The submandibular gland occupies the most anterosuperior aspect of the resection, and the internal jugular vein lies over the medial surface of the sternocleidomastoid muscle.
2. Open the vein, and sample any lesions.
3. Separate off each level, identify all of the lymph nodes, and submit each node for histology.
4. Examine the submandibular gland, and submit a section for histology.
5. Section the muscle, and submit a section of it if any lesions are encountered.

A number of variations of the neck dissection exist. These are well described by Robbins and co-workers.[2] In a *modified neck dissection*, for example, lymph nodes from levels I through V are removed, but one or more of the three major structures (internal jugular vein, spinal accessory nerve, sternocleidomastoid muscle) is not included in the dissection. *Selective neck dissections* differ from radical and modified neck dissections in that lymph nodes from only some of the five levels are removed. Each of these can be dissected using the same approach outlined above. First, orient the specimen. Without important land marks (e.g., submandibular gland, internal jugular vein), you will usually have to rely on the surgeon to designate each level. Second, identify the lymph nodes at each level. Third, submit each node for histology.

Important Issues to Address in Your Surgical Pathology Report on Radical Neck Dissections

- What procedure was performed, and what structures/organs are present?
- What is the total number of lymph nodes present at each level, and how many of these are involved by tumor?
- What is the size of the largest metastasis?
- Does the carcinoma extend beyond the lymph node and into extranodal soft tissue?
- Is the internal jugular vein thrombosed and/or infiltrated by tumor?
- Do the salivary glands, muscle, and soft tissues contain tumor or any other pathology?

IV   The Digestive System

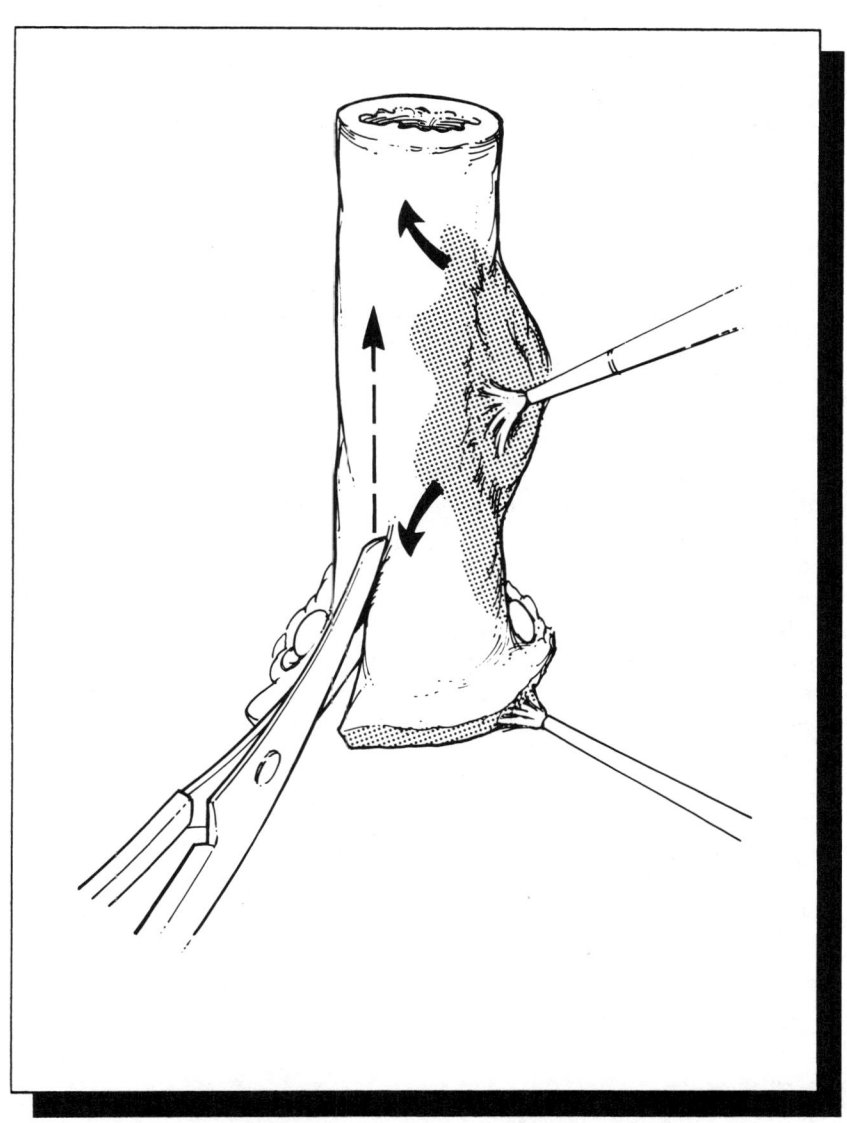

11 Esophagus

Elizabeth Montgomery, M.D.

Esophagectomies

Esophagectomies are almost always performed to resect neoplastic processes. The nature and extent of the neoplastic process, however, may be quite variable. Lesions may range from microscopic alterations in patients with a long history of Barrett's esophagus to large fungating carcinomas in patients presenting with obstruction and dysphagia.

Esophagectomy specimens (either segmental esophagectomy or esophagogastrectomy) are anatomically simple structures consisting essentially of a straight muscular tube. Orientation is seldom difficult, since a cuff of stomach is usually resected in continuity with the distal portion of esophagus. After measuring the dimensions of the specimen, ink its outer surface and the mucosal margins. The esophagus, you will recall, does not have a serosa. Rather, the surface of the soft tissues investing the esophagus represents a true soft tissue margin.

Next, open the esophagus to expose the mucosal surface. As illustrated, this step involves cutting through the wall of the esophagus from one end of the specimen to the other. A common mistake is to cut directly across the tumor. This can be a costly error, since it distorts the appearance of the tumor and disrupts the tumor's relationship with underlying structures. Fortunately, this can easily be avoided by first localizing the tumor and then cutting through the esophageal wall on the opposite side. The key, of course, is to pay close attention to the location of the tumor before heedlessly wielding the scissors. Begin by palpating the unopened esophagus. Areas of induration often divulge the location and extent of an infiltrating tumor. Next, cut the esophagus in a stepwise fashion: Inspect the lumen with a probing finger, and then advance the scissors one cautious cut at a time.

Once the specimen is opened, observe the appearance and thickness of the esophageal wall. If strictures are present, measure the luminal circumference of the esophagus at the point of narrowing and at the point of maximal dilatation proximal to the stricture. Carefully inspect the mucosa. If a tumor is not seen, try to identify the site of a previous biopsy. Biopsy site changes can be subtle. Look for focal areas of mucosal hemorrhage, ulceration, scarring, and puckering. Identify the gastroesophageal junction (GEJ), the point at which the tubular esophagus joins the saccular stomach. It is usually located 1 to 2 cm from the proximal edges of the gastric folds. Keep in mind that the GEJ does not always correlate with the squamocolumnar mucosal junction. Rather, the squamocolumnar junction normally may occur anywhere within the distal 2 to 3 cm of esophagus. The gastric mucosa is velvety red, and it contrasts sharply with the smooth gray appearance of the squamous epithelium lining the esophagus. Proximal extension of the squamocolumnar junction beyond the distal 2 to 3 cm of the esophagus is abnormal and suggestive of Barrett's esophagus.

If a tumor is apparent, note its dimensions (give three dimensions) and its location with respect to the squamocolumnar and gastroesophageal junctions. Note the configuration of the tumor (exophytic/fungating, endophytic/ulcerating, diffuse infiltrative).

If the tumor is at the gastroesophageal junction, it is classified as esophageal if the epicenter is in the esophagus, as gastric if the epicenter is in

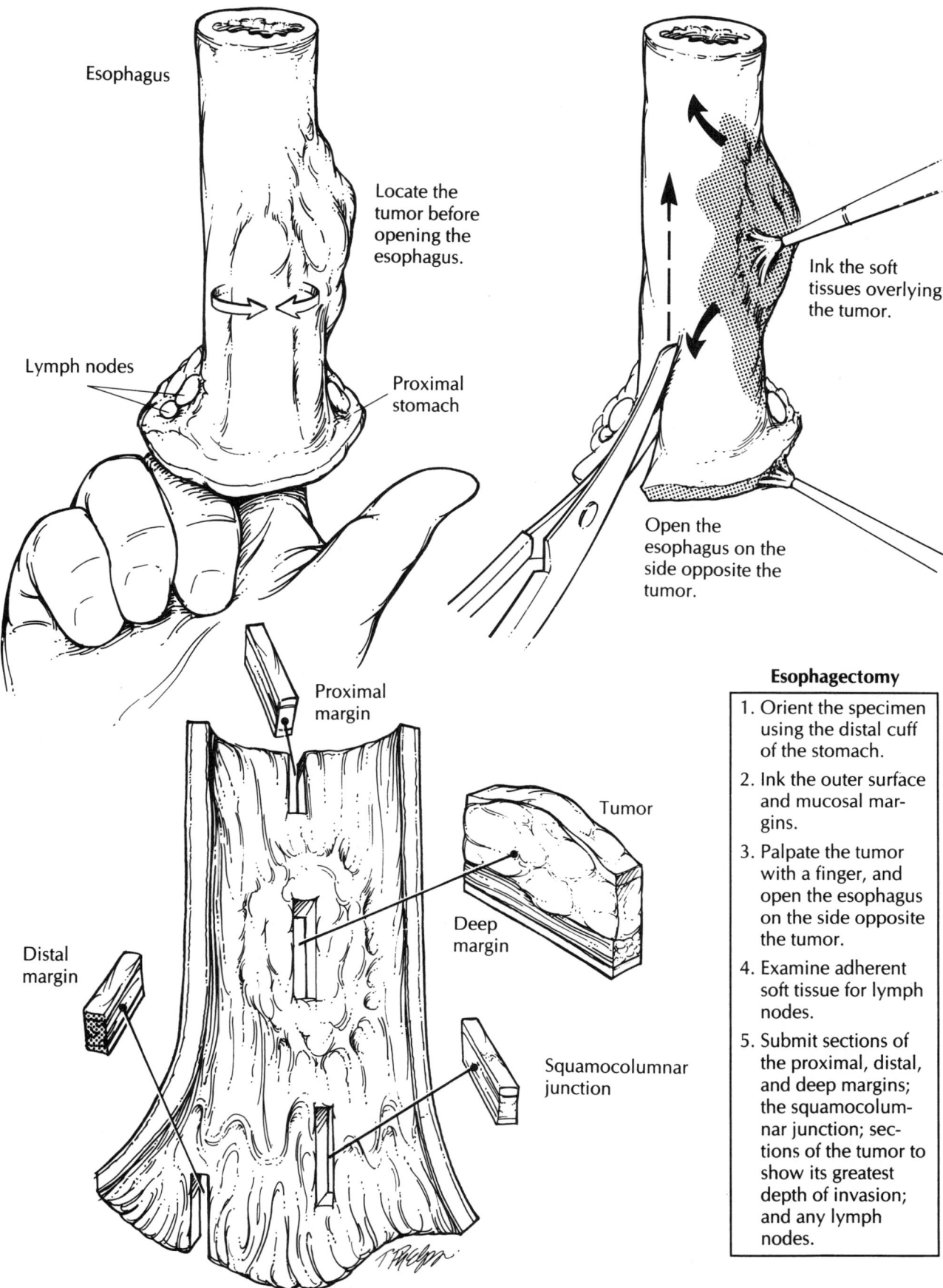

the stomach, and as a gastroesophageal junction primary tumor if the epicenter is at the junction of the tubular esophagus and the saccular stomach. This distinction is of clinical significance, as staging criteria differ according to the site: The AJCC staging system recognizes N0 and NI for esophageal cancers, whereas N0, N1, N2 and N3 designations are used for staging gastric cancers.

The following should be noted: (1) the proportion of tumor located in the esophagus versus that in the stomach; (2) the greatest dimensions of each individual component; (3) the anatomic site of the center of the tumor. (If more than 50% of the tumor involves the esophagus, the tumor is staged as esophageal, whereas if more than 50% involves the stomach, the tumor is staged as gastric.); and 4) the distance of the tumor's edges from the margins of resection. The distance of the tumor to the resection margin should always be measured in the fresh specimen; fixation causes the mucosa to retract, giving the appearance that the mucosal margins are closer to the tumor than they actually are. Photograph the opened specimen to document the gross findings. Before placing the specimen in formalin, ask yourself if fresh tissue should be submitted for special studies. Pin the specimen flat onto a wax tablet, and submerge it in formalin until well fixed.

Once the specimen is fixed, section through the full thickness of the tumor and the underlying wall to determine the level and depth of tumor extension. Submit at least two full-thickness sections of the esophagus at the level where it appears most deeply penetrated by the tumor. Be sure that these sections include the inked soft tissue surface (radial margin) so that this margin can be assessed. Also take sections of tumor to demonstrate its relationship to the adjacent mucosa, and liberally sample areas of Barrett's mucosa. In those cases where a tumor is not grossly apparent, three specific areas should be entirely submitted for histologic evaluation: (1) the squamocolumnar junction; (2) areas of abnormal mucosa such as the red velvety changes seen in Barrett's mucosa; and (3) previous biopsy sites. Sample the proximal and distal resection margins using perpendicular sections if the tumor is close or shave sections if the tumor is far removed.

Carefully dissect the soft tissues investing the esophagus for lymph nodes. Most of these lymph nodes will be found in the region of the gastroesophageal junction. Submit each lymph node found for histologic evaluation.

Important Issues to Address in Your Surgical Pathology Report on Esophagectomies

- What procedure was performed, and what structures/organs are present?
- In which portion of the esophagus does the tumor arise (cervical, upper thoracic, midthoracic, lower thoracic)?
- What are the histologic type and grade of the tumor?
- What are the size, location, and depth of maximum invasion of the tumor? Is it *in situ*? If invasive, into which level does it invade (lamina propria or submucosa, muscularis propria, adventitia, or adjacent structures)?
- Is there invasion into the stomach? Is there lymphatic/vascular space invasion?
- Does the tumor involve any resection margins? Specifically, what is the status of the proximal (esophageal), distal (stomach), and deep (radial) margins.
- What is the condition of the non-neoplastic/preoplastic esophagus? For example, are there changes of Barrett's esophagus, dysplasia, inflammation, or infection?
- Is there evidence of metastatic disease? Record the number of lymph nodes examined and the number of lymph node metastases.

12 Stomach

Elizabeth Montgomery, M.D.

Total and Partial Gastrectomies

Stomach specimens come in a variety of shapes and sizes depending on the pathologic process for which the stomach is removed. For example, a small portion of stomach may be removed for peptic ulcer disease, while the entire stomach and even adjacent organs can be resected when an infiltrating cancer is present. Regardless of the specimen's size and shape, a wise approach is to regard every stomach resection as though it potentially harbors a malignant neoplasm. Do not be betrayed by the innocent-looking ulcer. Instead, take care to evaluate the resection margins, adequately sample the lesion, and diligently search for lymph nodes. With this approach, the dissection should always be adequate, even in that rare instance when a carcinoma is incidentally discovered in a benign-appearing ulcer.

The dissection of a stomach specimen begins with a basic understanding of the stomach's anatomy. This understanding is important for two reasons: First, the anatomic regions of the stomach are functionally and histologically distinct; thus, each region of the stomach should be individually assessed. Second, anatomic landmarks can be used to orient most stomach specimens. The four divisions of the stomach are the cardia, fundus, body, and antrum. The cardia is the rim of the stomach that surrounds the gastroesophageal junction (GEJ). The fundus is the dome-shaped region of the stomach that sweeps superior to the GEJ. The body accounts for the major portion of the stomach. It narrows distally as it merges with the antrum. The antrum is the distal third of the stomach and includes the pyloric sphincter. The anatomic boundaries separating these regions are not distinct, at least not in the unopened specimen. Once the mucosal surface is exposed, however, the demarcation between the body and antrum can be easier to appreciate. For example, the body shows prominent rugal folds, whereas the mucosa of the antrum is comparatively flat. This flattened antral surface forms a V. The nadir of the V rests on the lesser curvature and points toward the proximal portion of the stomach. Other landmarks that are useful in orienting the specimen include the greater curvature, the broad and convex inferior aspect of the stomach; the lesser curvature, the concave superior aspect of the stomach; and the pyloric ring, a thick muscular collar at the outlet of the stomach. In more limited stomach resections, these landmarks may not be present and correct orientation relies upon the surgeon's designation.

Begin your examination by clearly marking the stomach resection margins. Keep in mind that these margins may be difficult to reconstruct once the specimen has been opened. One simple method is to ink the margins and then place four safety pins—two on either side of the greater curvature at both the proximal and distal margins. By cutting the specimen between these safety pins, you can easily reconstruct the opened specimen simply by juxtaposing the two pins.

To facilitate handling of the stomach, remove the bulky omenta (when present) suspended from the greater and lesser curvatures of the stomach. Do not discard this fat. Instead, set it aside for later dissection. Next, open the stomach along its entire length, cutting between the safety pins at each stomach orifice. To avoid cutting across the lesion, insert a probing finger into the lumen, and explore the inner surface of the

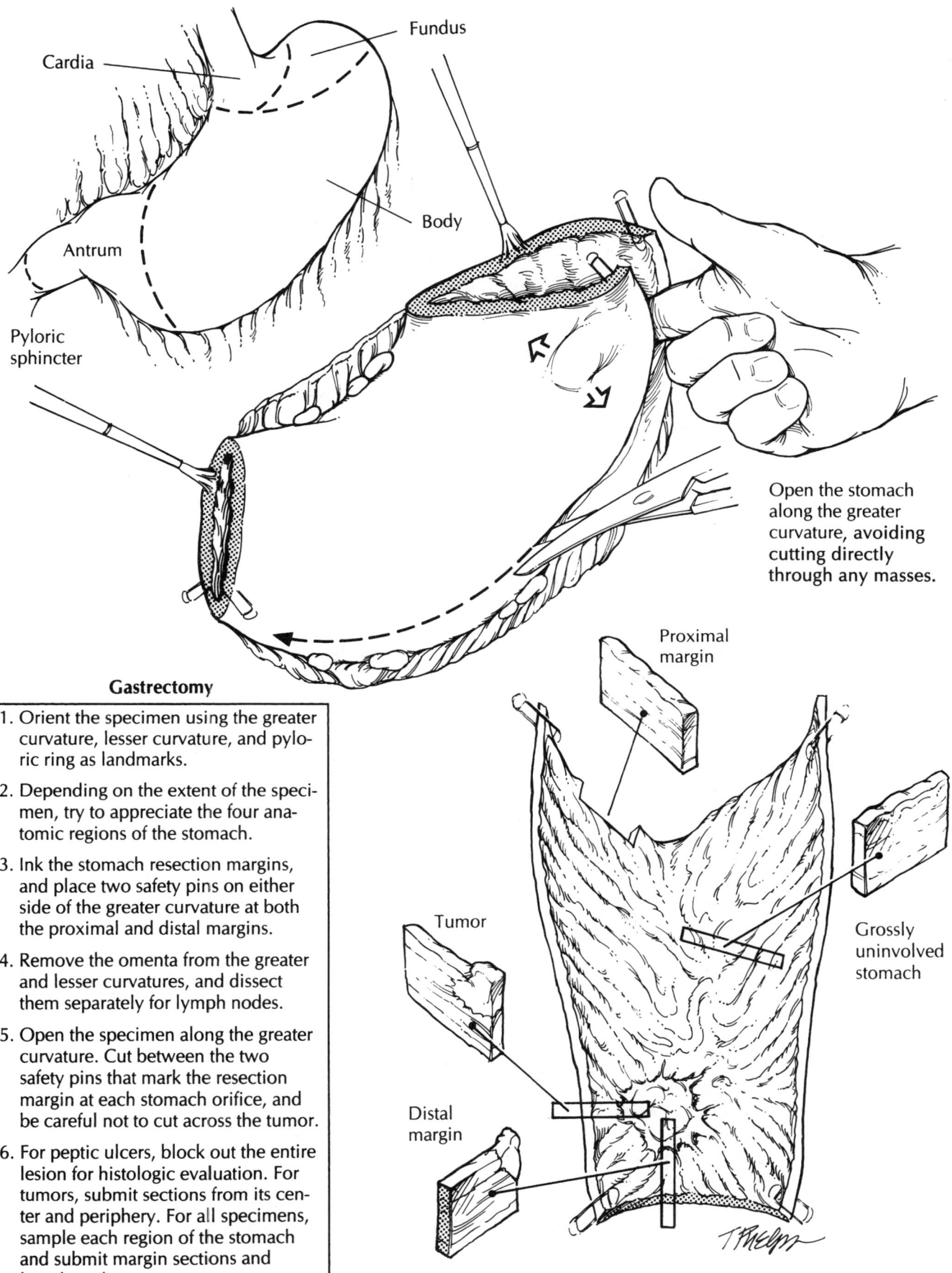

Gastrectomy

1. Orient the specimen using the greater curvature, lesser curvature, and pyloric ring as landmarks.
2. Depending on the extent of the specimen, try to appreciate the four anatomic regions of the stomach.
3. Ink the stomach resection margins, and place two safety pins on either side of the greater curvature at both the proximal and distal margins.
4. Remove the omenta from the greater and lesser curvatures, and dissect them separately for lymph nodes.
5. Open the specimen along the greater curvature. Cut between the two safety pins that mark the resection margin at each stomach orifice, and be careful not to cut across the tumor.
6. For peptic ulcers, block out the entire lesion for histologic evaluation. For tumors, submit sections from its center and periphery. For all specimens, sample each region of the stomach and submit margin sections and lymph nodes.

stomach ahead of the advancing scissors. Be flexible in your approach. Whenever possible, cut along the greater curvature, but always be ready to tailor the dissection to avoid cutting through a tumor. When the line of excision along the greater curvature is obstructed by a tumor, the lesser curvature may serve as an alternative route for opening the stomach.

Once the stomach is opened, evaluate each of the three layers of the stomach—the mucosa, wall, and serosa. Do the gastric folds appear thickened or effaced? Assess the number, size, location, and appearance of any lesions. For ulcerative lesions, carefully note those features that are helpful in distinguishing benign ulcers (e.g., sharply defined margins, smooth and flat borders, straight walls, clean base) from gastric carcinomas (e.g., irregular margins, thickened and heaped-up borders, shaggy base). Important measurements include not only the dimensions of the lesion but also the distance from the lesion to the resection margins. This distance, known as the *gross clearance*, should be measured while the specimen is fresh, because the mucosa tends to retract during fixation.

The precise location of the tumor should be documented. For tumors involving the gastroesophageal junction, every effort should be made to assign a precise site of origin. The gastroesophageal junction is the junction of the tubular esophagus and saccular stomach regardless of the type of epithelium lining the esophagus. Assess the proportion of tumor in the esophagus versus the stomach and find the anatomic location of the tumor's epicenter. If more than 50% of the tumor involves the esophagus the tumor is classified as esophageal, whereas it is classified as gastric if more than 50% involves the stomach.

Next, examine and describe the wall and the serosa of the stomach. Are any mural nodules noted? Is the wall diffusely thickened or focally indurated? Are any serosal lesions noted? Is the serosa retracted? Collect fresh tissue samples for special studies as needed, then pin the specimen flat on a wax tablet, and submerge it in formalin until well fixed.

"Better safe than sorry" is a wise policy when sampling the stomach. Consider again the prudence of viewing each lesion with the suspicion that it represents a malignant neoplasm. Thoroughly sample all lesions, evaluate every margin, and diligently search for lymph nodes. For lesions that are clinically believed to be peptic ulcers, submit the entire ulcer in a sequential fashion so that an underlying malignancy is not missed. When a tumor is apparent, section through it to determine whether it extends into or through the stomach wall. Be sure to describe its gross configuration (exophytic/polypoid, infiltrative, diffusely infiltrative, expansile/noninfiltrative, ulcerating, or annular). Submit sections from the center of the tumor to determine its maximum depth of invasion. Also submit sections from the tumor's periphery to demonstrate the transition between the tumor and the adjacent gastric mucosa. When the stomach appears diffusely thickened by an infiltrative process (e.g., linitis plastica) submit sections from all four regions of the stomach. Margins should generally be sampled using perpendicular sections when the tumor is close, and shave sections when the tumor is far removed. Submit all lymph nodes. Keep the greater and lesser omental node groups separate. A good place to find lymph nodes is at the point where the omenta attach to the stomach.

The grossly uninvolved stomach should also be sampled for histologic evaluation. Depending on the extent of the resection, these sections should represent all four regions of the stomach, the squamocolumnar junction, and if present the contiguous esophagus. For extended resections that include adjacent colon, spleen, liver, and/or pancreas, sections should be taken to determine the presence of direct tumor extension, tumor metastases, and the adequacy of surgical excision (i.e., the status of the margins).

Photography plays an important role in the evaluation of stomach specimens. Sections taken for histology can be mapped with considerable detail on Polaroid or digital photographs of the specimen. This is a useful method for correlating the histologic features with the anatomic region of the stomach.

Important Issues to Address in Your Surgical Pathology Report on Gastrectomies

- What procedure was performed, and what structures/organs are present?
- What are the location (cardia, fundus, body, or antrum), size, type, and histologic grade of the neoplasm?

- Is there invasion into the esophagus or stomach? Is there blood/lymphatic vessel invasion? Is there perineural invasion?
- What is the extent of the neoplasm? Specify into which level of the wall of the stomach the tumor invades (e.g., mucosa, submucosa, muscularis propria, subserosal soft tissues, or serosa). Does the tumor extend beyond the serosa to involve adjacent structures?
- Does the tumor involve the soft tissue and/or mucosal margins? What is the distance of the mucosal margin from the edge of the tumor?
- What is the condition of the non-neoplastic stomach (e.g., changes of *Helicobacter pylori* gastritis or presence of intestinal metaplasia, dysplasia, atrophy, adenomas, or ulceration)?
- Is there evidence of metastatic disease? Record the number of lymph nodes examined and the number of lymph node metastases.

13 Non-Neoplastic Intestinal Disease

Robb E. Wilentz, M.D.

Small Biopsies

Proper tissue orientation is a critical part of the histologic evaluation of biopsies of the gastrointestinal tract. Tissue orientation is a two-step process that involves the coordinated actions of the endoscopist and the histotechnologist. The endoscopist should mount the biopsy mucosal-side up on an appropriate solid surface (e.g., filter paper) and place it in fixative. This first step should be done immediately, in the endoscopy suite, so that the specimen does not dry out en route to the surgical pathology laboratory. The histotechnologist can then embed and cut the biopsy specimen perpendicular to the mounting surface. If the specimen is free-floating, great care must be taken to identify the mucosal surface for proper embedding. Multiple sections should be cut from each tissue block for histologic evaluation. Step sections are preferred to serial sections so that intervening unstained sections are available for special stains as needed.

Resections of Small and Large Intestine for Inflammatory Bowel Disease

Given the structural simplicity of the intestinal tract and the ease with which the bowel can be opened, there is a strong tendency to rush into these dissections without thinking ahead. The approach to the non-neoplastic bowel specimen requires an effective strategy that gives careful consideration to an organized gross description, specimen photography and fixation, and details of dissection and tissue sampling.

The Organized Gross Description

A good gross description not only describes all the relevant gross findings but presents these findings in an organized fashion. This can be a difficult task in bowel resections, where the specimen may consist of more than one structure (e.g., ileum, appendix, cecum, and colon). Organize your gross description. First, describe the specimen after it has been examined and at least partially dissected. This will make it possible to collect all of the gross findings and integrate them into an organized statement. Second, always describe each component of the resection as an individual unit. For example, describe the mucosa, wall, and serosa of the ileum and then move on to the appendix, cecum, and finally the colon. Third, focus on the mucosa. Begin by describing the distribution of mucosal alterations (e.g., diffuse, discontinuous) and then describe the specific characteristics of these changes (e.g., ulcerated, granular). Of course, no gross description is complete without a description of the wall, serosa, and mesentery; but for inflammatory bowel disease, a less detailed description of these layers will generally suffice.

Specimen Dissection

Given the structural simplicity of the bowel, opening these specimens is generally straightforward. When possible, the small intestine should be opened adjacent to the mesentery. In contrast, the large intestine should be opened on the antimesenteric border along the anterior (free) teniae coli. Remove the mesentery before fixing the bowel. Treat the mesenteric soft tissues as though

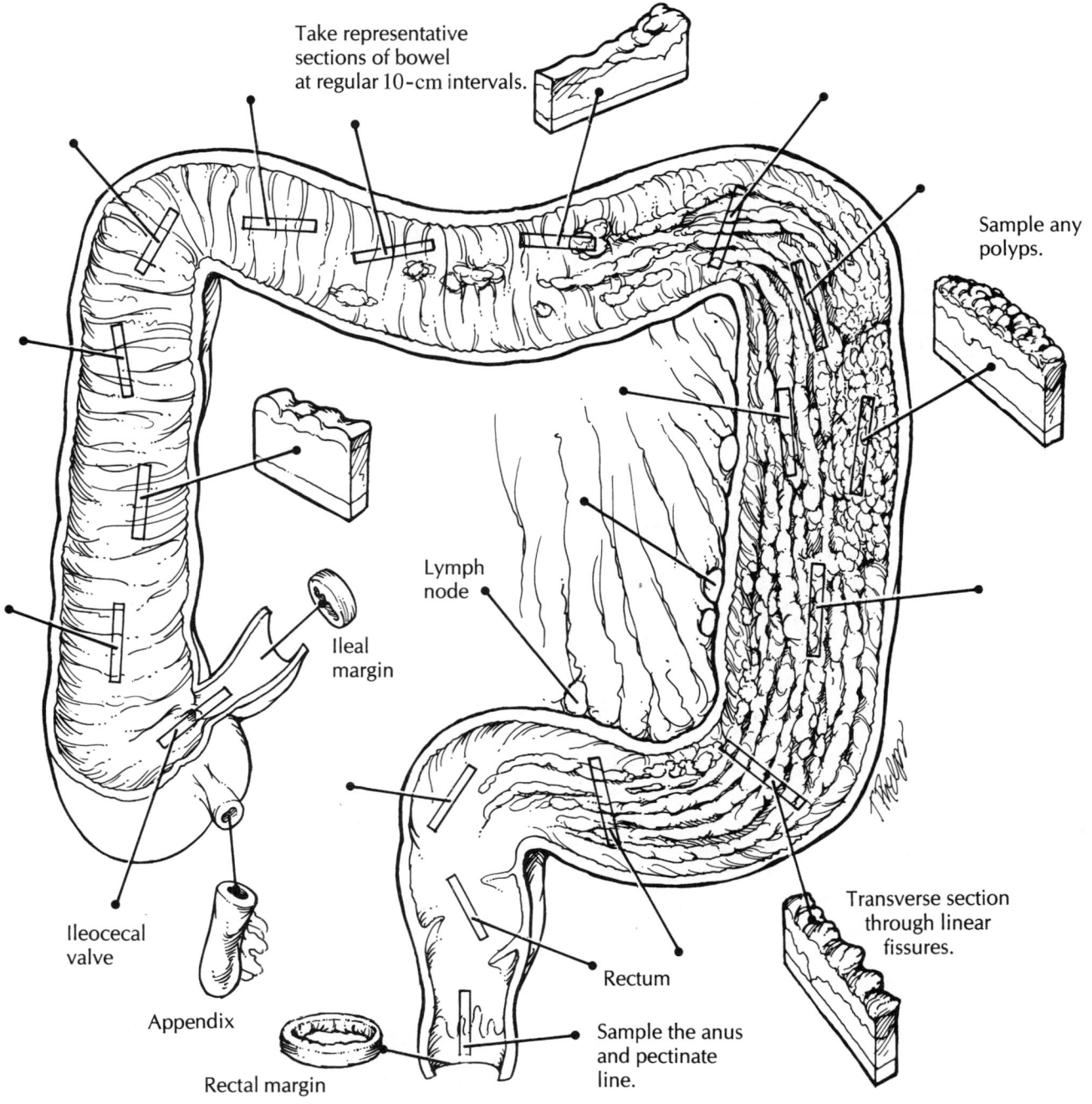

Resections for Inflammatory Bowel Disease

1. Orient the specimen. The large intestine can be distinguished from the small intestine by its larger diameter and by the presence of longitudinal muscle bands (teniae coli), sacculations, and the appendices epiploicae.
2. Identify and measure all components of the specimen (do not forget to look for the appendix).
3. Remove the mesentery. Open the small bowel along its mesenteric border, and open the large bowel along the anterior teniae coli. Rinse the bowel, pin it flat on a cork or wax tablet, and submerge it in formalin until well fixed.
4. Describe the specimen in a systematic fashion. Include a description of the mucosa, wall, and serosa of each component of the specimen.
5. Sample all areas of the bowel by submitting sections at regular 10-cm intervals. Also include sections of the appendix, ileocecal valve, margins, mesenteric vessels, any focal lesions, and representative lymph nodes from all regions of the bowel.

a carcinoma will be discovered in the bowel resection, keeping in mind that carcinomas may arise in the setting of long-standing inflammatory bowel disease. For total colectomies, remove the mesentery as six separate portions, and designate these as proximal ascending, distal ascending, proximal transverse, distal transverse, proximal descending, and distal descending. Although only representative lymph nodes need to be submitted, the six portions should be clearly labeled and saved for easy retrieval if more extensive lymph node sampling is later required.

Specimen Fixation

In general, the bowel should be fixed before it is photographed, described, and sectioned. Subtle mucosal alterations (e.g., erosions, ulcerations, areas of hemorrhage) that may not be apparent in the fresh specimen are often well defined once the specimen is fixed. In most cases, the specimen can be opened and pinned on a solid surface as a flat sheet and then submerged in formalin. Some specimens may be so distorted that they cannot be easily opened and pinned flat without the risk of cutting across structures (e.g., fistulae, diverticula) and disrupting important relationships. These distorted specimens may be best handled by infusing formalin into the lumen of the bowel and then clamping both ends of the specimen. Whether the bowel is submerged or infused, fecal material should first be rinsed from the mucosal surface (a more formidable challenge in the unopened specimen) using a gentle stream of an isotonic solution.

Specimen Photography

Photographs of the specimen should be liberally taken to document further the gross findings, especially the distribution and nature of the mucosal alterations. Photograph the specimen after it has been opened and fixed. Photographs of the unopened bowel are generally useless. Fixation tends to both accentuate the mucosal alterations and reduce the amount of reflected light. Always position the specimen anatomically on the photography table. Total colectomies, for example, should be positioned so that the ascending colon is to the anatomic right, the descending colon is to the left, and the transverse colon is to the top and center. Finally, include close-up photographs to illustrate the details of the mucosal pathology.

Tissue Sampling

To evaluate the distribution of inflammatory changes in the specimen, all areas of the bowel should be sampled for histologic evaluation. One method that consistently ensures adequate sampling is to submit representative sections at 10-cm intervals, beginning at the distal end of the specimen and proceeding proximally in a step-wise fashion. This not only will ensure that the mucosa is well sampled but will also provide information on the distribution of the disease process. Of course, sections of any focal lesions such as ulcers or polyps should be submitted in addition to these interval sections. Sections should also be taken of the appendix and the ileocecal valve when these structures are present. When no tumor is grossly apparent, the resection margins may be taken as shave sections. In addition to sampling the mesentery for lymph nodes, submit sections of mesenteric blood vessels and of any focal lesions such as fistula tracts or areas of fat necrosis. Indicate the site from which all sections were taken on the Polaroid or digital photographs. Take longitudinal sections (i.e., parallel to the teniae coli). Exceptions are permitted when, for example, a linear ulcer is best demonstrated by a transverse section through the bowel.

Once these principles regarding gross description, fixation, dissection, and sampling are mastered, the inflammatory bowel specimen can be handled with relative ease. The initial step is to identify the structures that are present in the resected specimen. The large intestine is readily distinguished from the small intestine by its larger diameter and the presence of longitudinal muscle bands (the teniae coli), sacculations (the haustra), and the appendices epiploicae. In addition, the small intestine shows mucosal folds that stretch across the entire circumference of the bowel, whereas the mucosal folds of the large intestine are discontinuous. Several features may be helpful in appreciating the various regions of the large intestine. The cecum is usually quite apparent, and it can be used to identify the origin of the ascending colon. The transverse colon can be recognized by its large mesenteric pedicle attachment, while the sigmoid colon has a relatively short mesenteric pedicle. When a portion of rectum is included in the specimen, it can be distinguished from the sigmoid colon by the absence of a peritoneal surface lining.

The initial description should be limited to a list of the structures present and the dimensions of each. Further handling of the bowel is facilitated by removing the mesenteric fat. As described previously, these soft tissues should be removed according to their anatomic location, and each portion should be clearly labeled so it can be easily identified and retrieved. Most prosectors have an easier time finding mesenteric lymph nodes while these tissues are still in the fresh state. Remember, most of the lymph nodes are found at the junction of the bowel and mesenteric fat. Open the bowel along its entire length, cutting the small bowel along its mesenteric attachment and the large bowel along the anterior teniae. Gently rinse any fecal material from the mucosal surface using a stream of isotonic solution. Pin the opened bowel flat on a solid surface, and submerge it in formalin.

Once the specimen is fixed, complete the examination of the mucosa, noting in the gross description the distribution and characteristics of the mucosal alterations. Place the bowel in its correct anatomic position, and photograph it. Take a Polaroid or digital photograph of the entire specimen, so that the sites from which histologic sections were taken can be indicated on the image, and take close-up views of focal lesions.

Remember to section all regions of the bowel by using a method of stepwise sectioning at regular (i.e., 10-cm) intervals. Specific bowel sections should include the proximal and distal resection margins, the ileocecal valve, the appendix, and any focal lesions. If a neoplasm is not found, sampling of representative lymph nodes from each level will suffice. Sampling of the mesentery should also include a section of the mesenteric blood vessels and sections of any focal lesions.

Important Issues to Address in Your Surgical Pathology Report on Non-Neoplastic Intestinal Disease

- What procedure was performed, and what structures/organs are present?
- What disease processes are present, and what is their location?
- For inflammatory processes, are any diverticula, strictures, fistulae, or perforations present?
- Does the mucosa show any preneoplastic or neoplastic changes? (See Chapter 14.)
- Do the lymph nodes show any evidence of an inflammatory process or metastatic disease? Record the number of lymph nodes examined and the presence or absence of lymph node metastases.
- What is the status of the mesenteric vessels?

14 Neoplastic Intestinal Disease

Elizabeth Montgomery, M.D.

Polypectomies

Polyps of the gastrointestinal tract are usually removed endoscopically by a single incision at the base of the polyp stalk. Although these specimens lack the size and complexity of more extended bowel resections, they are delicate structures that require meticulous processing. First, obtain relevant clinical information such as the patient's history, the endoscopic findings, and the anatomic site from which the polyp was removed. Next, turn your attention to the specimen itself. The polypectomy specimen poses three important questions to the surgical pathologist: (1) Are adenomatous changes present? (2) Is infiltrating carcinoma present, and if it is does it infiltrate into the stalk? (3) Do any of the neoplastic changes extend to the resection margin at the base of the stalk? Clearly, the polypectomy specimen must be carefully oriented and processed so that these issues can be addressed.

The key to orienting the polyp is to find its stalk. This may require careful inspection, since a short stalk is often overshadowed by the much larger head of the polyp. After finding the stalk, mark its base (i.e., the resection margin) with either ink or colored tattoo powder. Measure the height and diameter of the polyp. Next, place the specimen in formalin for fixation. Given the soft and spongy consistency of the fresh polyp, sectioning the polyp is greatly facilitated if it is well fixed.

Once fixed, the specimen should be sectioned in a way to show the relationship of the stalk to the head of the polyp. As illustrated, this relationship is usually best demonstrated by trisecting the polyp into two lateral caps and one median section that includes the stalk and the center of the head. The median section should demonstrate the largest cross-sectional area of the head of the polyp, its interface with the stalk, and the surgical margin. The importance of trisecting the polyp is readily apparent if one pauses to consider the impact of this method on the histologic sections. Serial sections into the median section of a trisected polyp will approach the point of interest, the center of the polyp. To avoid missing a small focus of carcinoma, submit the entire specimen for histologic evaluation.

Important Issues to Address in Your Surgical Pathology Report on Polyps

- What procedure was performed, and what structures/organs are present?
- What is the histologic type of the polyp (e.g., adenomatous, hyperplastic, hamartomatous, inflammatory)?
- For adenomatous polyps, is the polyp architecturally tubular, villous, or tubulovillous?
- If a carcinoma is present, what is the depth of invasion of the tumor? (Specify the presence or absence of invasion of the stalk and of the submucosa at the base of the stalk or base of a sessile polyp.) Specify whether there are any poorly differentiated areas.
- Is there evidence of vascular invasion?
- What is the status of the resection margin at the base? Measure (in millimeters) the distance from the deepest part of the invasive carcinoma component to the nearest polyp margin. Does the adenomatous epithelium or the infiltrating carcinoma extend to this margin?

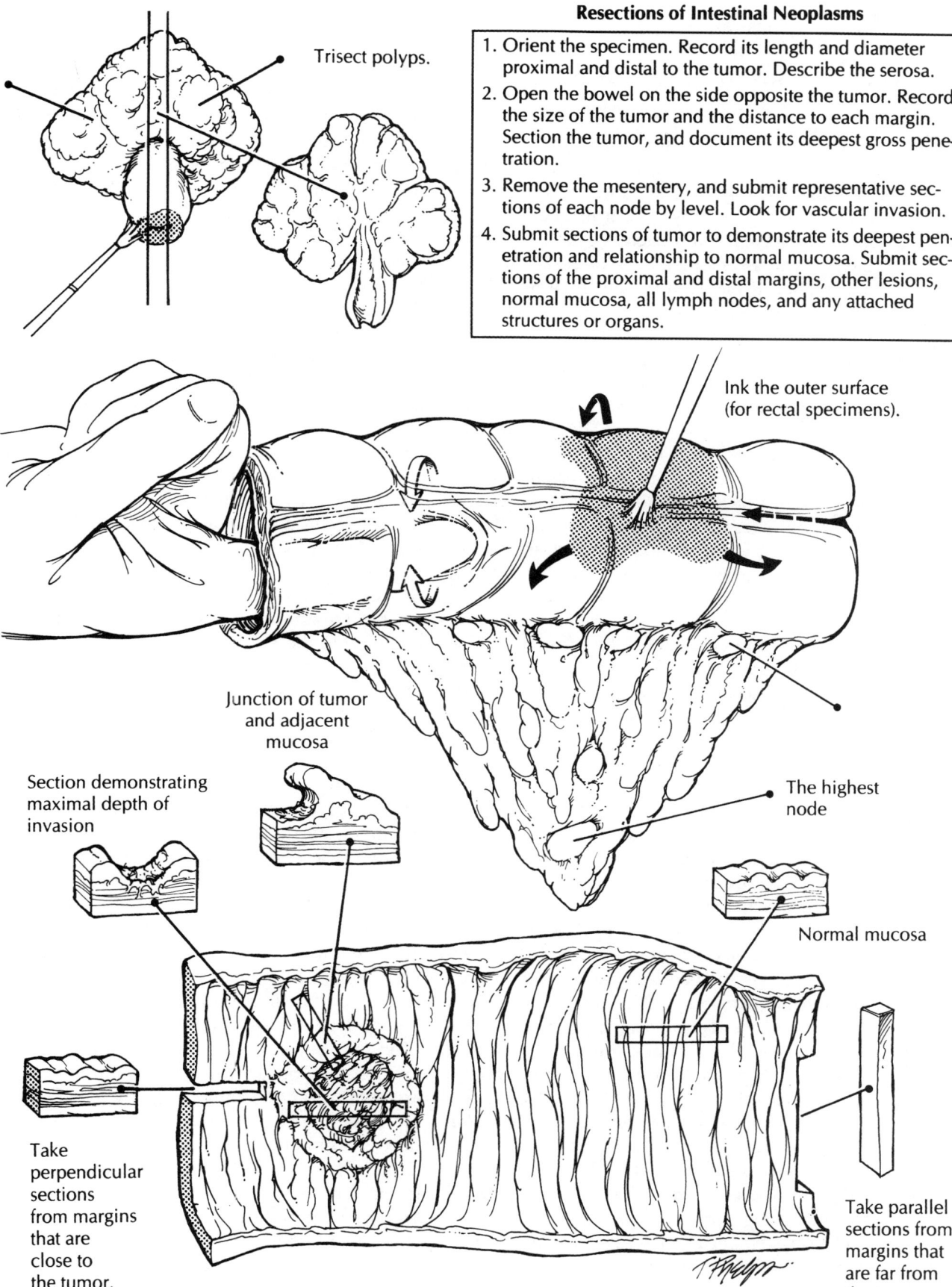

Resections of Intestinal Neoplasms

The pathologic evaluation of resected intestinal neoplasms plays an integral part in determining the patient's prognosis and in selecting the appropriate adjuvant therapy. As is true for other specimens, a systematic approach to your dissection is the best way to ensure that all of the appropriate information is included in your final report.

Start with the patient's history. This should include both the patient's clinical history (Crohn's disease, ulcerative colitis, polyps, family history) and the relevant endoscopic findings. Next, identify the segment of bowel that was resected, and orient the specimen. As described in Chapter 13, the large intestine is readily distinguished from the small intestine by its larger diameter and the presence of longitudinal muscle bands (the teniae coli), sacculations (the haustra), and the appendices epiploicae. In addition, the small intestine shows mucosal folds that stretch across the entire circumference of the bowel, whereas the large intestinal mucosal folds are discontinuous. The rectum can be distinguished from the colon by the absence of a peritoneal surface covering the rectum. Record the length and the diameter of the bowel. The diameter should be recorded both proximal and distal to any lesions. Look for and document the presence and appearance of any other structures, such as the appendix. Next, describe the serosa. Are any diverticula, gross perforations, or serosal nodules present?

As noted above, the rectum lacks a serosal lining. Therefore, the outer surface of the rectum represents a true soft tissue margin, and these soft tissues should be inked. Otherwise, only the proximal and distal margins need to be inked. When opening the bowel, make every effort not to cut through the tumor. First, localize the tumor by palpating the specimen and probing the lumen of the bowel with your finger, then open the bowel on the side opposite the tumor. If a tumor cannot be appreciated grossly, simply open the small intestine adjacent to the mesenvery, the colon along the anterior (free) teniae, and the rectum along the midline anteriorly. Once the specimen has been opened, gently rinse off the intestinal contents using a stream of isotonic saline.

Next, systematically describe the opened specimen. Start with the tumor. Document its location relative to the margins and to any landmarks, such as the ileocecal valve or the pectinate line. Describe the size of the tumor in its longitudinal and transverse dimensions, as well at its gross configuration (endophytic, pedunculated, sessile, diffusely infiltrative, or annular). It is especially critical to document tumor size for anal carcinomas, since it is tumor size rather than depth of invasion that serves as the key feature for assessing "T" when staging the tumor. Multiple cancers should be looked for, described, and labeled separately. After the tumor has been described, make multiple parallel 2- to 3-mm sections through the tumor, and note its deepest gross penetration. It is also important to note if bowel perforation (a hole in the bowel wall) is associated with the tumor. Also note the distance from the tumor to the soft tissue or *radial margin*. This is the distance from the outermost part of the tumor to the lateral margin of resection along a radius drawn from the center of the lumen of the bowel through the deepest penetration of the tumor. The soft tissue margin is only important for rectal cancers and for colon cancers located on the mesenteric aspect of the bowel.

After the tumor has been described, turn your attention to the remainder of the bowel. Be systematic in your description. For example, begin with the mucosa, wall, and serosa of the proximal portion of the specimen and then proceed distally. When describing the mucosa, note diverticula, changes of inflammatory bowel disease, polyps, and ischemic changes. A systematic approach to your gross dictation will ensure that all important findings are included.

We like to examine the soft tissues for lymph nodes in the fresh state because the nodes are easier to palpate and because they retain their pink color, which contrasts to the yellow fat. The next step, therefore, is to dissect the mesentery. Look for and sample any lymph nodes adjacent to the point of ligation of the vascular pedicle, and designate these as the highest lymph nodes. Next, cut the mesentery close to the bowel, maintaining anatomic orientation. Do not remove any areas in which the tumor directly extends into the mesenteric fat. Sample these as a part of the deep margin after the specimen has been fixed. Then divide the detached mesenteric fat into groups: those proximal to the tumor, those at the level of the tumor, and those distal to the tumor. If any great vessels are present, identify and separately designate the nodes adjacent to them. Thinly section the mesenteric fat at each level, and examine and palpate each section for lymph nodes. Submit for histology each identified node. When looking for the nodes, remember that they are frequently present at the junction of the bowel wall and the mesentery. When submitting the lymph nodes for histologic processing, remember to designate the level from which they were taken. Also examine the veins and arteries in the mesentery for thrombi. If any are present, submit a representative section of the involved vessel for histologic examination. After the mesentery has been examined, separately bundle each level for fixation and storage. Should you ever have to return to the mesentery, the orientation will be preserved. The specimen can now be pinned to a wax tablet and fixed overnight.

After the specimen is well fixed, it can be sampled. Start with the tumor. Submit at least two sections: one from the edge of the tumor to show the junction of tumor and normal bowel, and one from the point of deepest tumor penetration into the wall of the bowel. If the tumor does not grossly appear to involve the bowel wall, then submit the entire base of the lesion to demonstrate the presence or absence of invasion. Submit the proximal and distal margins. If the tumor is close to a margin, these sections should be perpendicular (longitudinal), and if the tumor is far from a margin, these sections can be parallel (transverse). Next, sample any other lesions. When sampling polyps, remember to include both the head and stalk in your sections. Submit representative sections of normal bowel mucosa and wall, and submit representative sections of all remaining structures/organs, such as the appendix and terminal ileum. Remember that longitudinal sections are better than transverse sections when sampling the colon wall.

Important Issues to Address in Your Surgical Pathology Report on Resections for Intestinal Neoplasms

- What procedure was performed, and what structures/organs are present?
- What is the location of the tumor?
- What are the dimensions of the tumor?
- What is the gross configuration of the tumor (endophytic, pedunculated, sessile, diffusely infiltrating, annular)?
- What are the histologic type and grade of the neoplasm?
- What is the maximum depth of invasion of the tumor? Is it *in situ* (high-grade dysplasia), or does it extend into the lamina propria, submucosa, muscularis propria, or through the muscularis propria into subserosa? Does the tumor extend into other organs, or does it extend into the visceral peritoneum?
- Is there bowel wall perforation?
- Is any vascular invasion identified?
- What is the status of the margins (proximal, distal, and radial)?
- How many lymph node metastases were identified, and how many lymph nodes were sampled at each level?
- Are there mesenteric deposits? For staging purposes, tumor nodules in the pericolorectal fat without histologic evidence of residual lymph node are classified as regional node metastases if they have the form and smooth contour of a lymph node. Nodules with irregular contours are believed to reflect microscopic venous invasion using AJCC criteria.
- Are any other lesions noted (e.g., adenomas, intestinal inflammatory disease, dysplasia)?

15 Appendix

Elizabeth Montgomery, M.D.

Simple Appendectomies

The appendix is a common specimen in the surgical pathology laboratory. The dissection of these specimens is not complex, since most appendectomies are performed for simple acute appendicitis. Even so, the appendix is all too often not examined appropriately. Cursory examination of the appendix is a pitfall to be avoided. Instead, develop the habit of thoroughly examining every appendix. Regard every appendiceal specimen as an opportunity to uncover unsuspected pathologic processes.

The major objectives in dissecting the simple appendectomy specimen are to document the presence or absence of inflammation and to search for incidental neoplasms. These objectives are met by examining each component of the appendix—the serosa, wall, mucosa, and lumen—in a sequential manner. Begin by inspecting the outer surface of the appendix and the attached mesoappendix. Inflammatory processes often convert the glistening, smooth, tan serosa into a surface that is dull, shaggy, and discolored. Carefully look for perforations. Small transmural perforations that are not easily seen can sometimes be demonstrated by gently infusing formalin into the lumen of the appendix using a syringe. Document the dimensions of the specimen, and then section the appendix so that the wall, the mucosa, and the lumen can be evaluated. As illustrated, bread-loaf the body of the appendix using thin transverse sections, and bivalve the distal 2-cm tip of the appendix using a longitudinal section. Inspect the wall for masses, strictures, edema, and other inflammatory changes. Finally, evaluate the mucosa and the luminal contents for fecaliths, pus, and collections of mucus. If a neoplasm is present, submit a shave margin from the base of the appendix, and be sure to document the size of the tumor, the distance from the tumor to the surgical margin, and the layers of the appendix that are involved. When the lumen is obstructed, attempt to identify the nature of the obstruction, keeping in mind that most tumors of the appendix are discovered in specimens resected for other reasons.

Sections for histologic evaluation should include a transverse section through the base and body and a longitudinal section of the tip. Include a portion of the attached mesoappendix. For a normal-appearing appendix removed by incidental appendectomy, one section each from the base, body, and tip placed into a single tissue cassette will suffice. For an inflamed appendix, additional sections may be required to demonstrate points of perforation or luminal obstruction. If a mass or mucocele is present, the entire appendix should be submitted in a sequential fashion. The most proximal section from the base of the appendix represents the margin of resection.

Important Issues to Address in Your Surgical Pathology Report on Appendectomies

- What procedure was performed, and what structures/organs are present?
- What are the nature and extent of any inflammatory processes present (e.g., acute appendicitis, abscess formation, gangrene)? Be sure to mention the presence or absence of perforations and peritonitis.
- What are the type, grade, size, location, and extent of any incidental neoplasms identified? Is the tumor present at the resection margin?

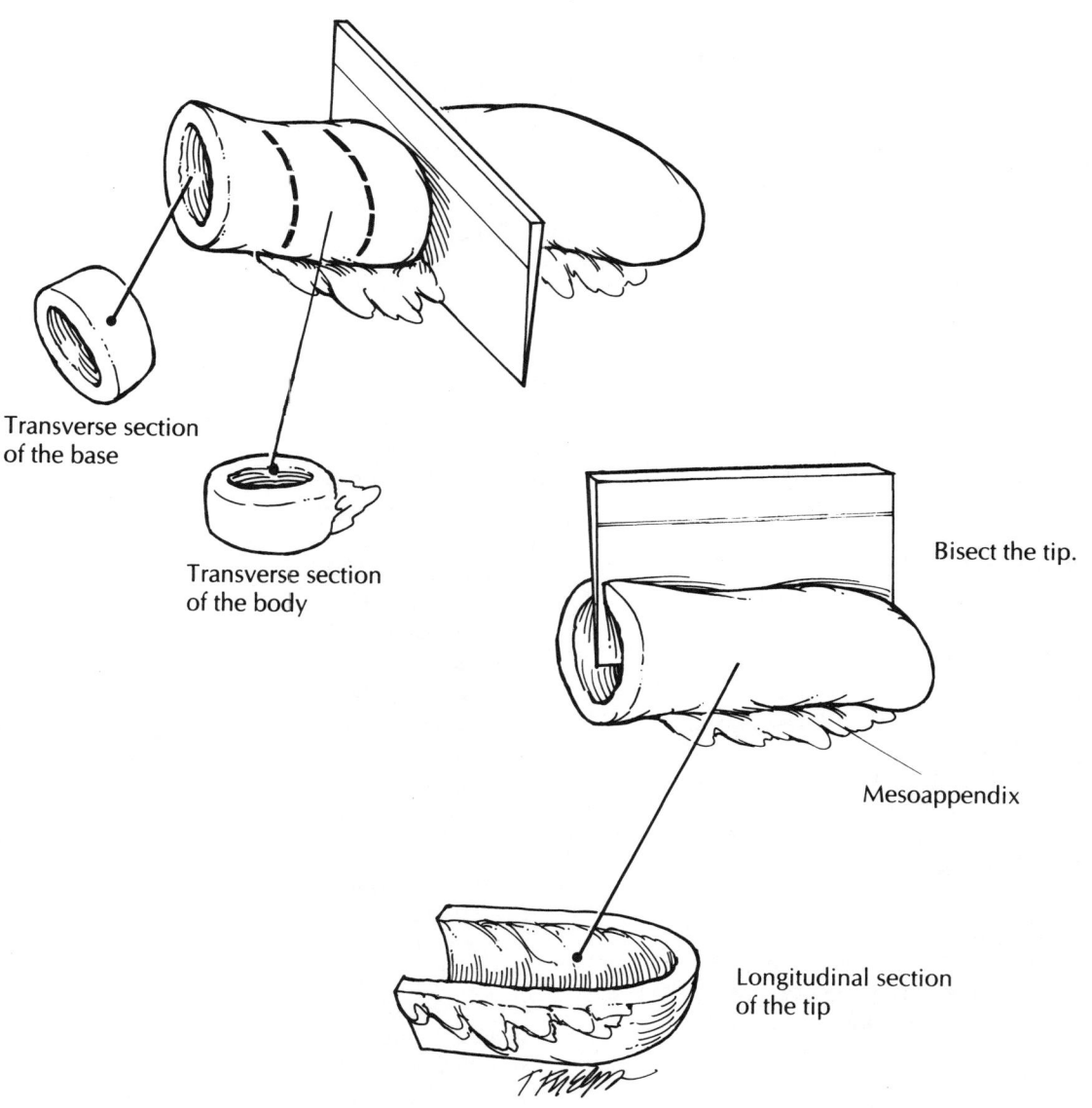

Appendectomy

1. Orient and measure the appendix. Carefully look for perforations.
2. Serially section the body of the appendix using transverse sections. Bivalve the tip using a longitudinal section.
3. Describe and measure any tumors.
4. Submit sections of the base, body, and tip of the appendix for histologic evaluation. The entire appendix should be submitted for all tumors and mucoceles.

16 Liver

Michael S. Torbenson, M.D.

Biopsies

Biopsies of the liver come in two forms: the delicate needle-core biopsy and the larger wedge biopsy. In either case, the specimen should be measured and submitted in its entirety for routine histology. Thin-core biopsies are particularly susceptible to desiccation. Therefore, unless special studies are indicated, biopsies should be placed in fixative in the operating room. The core biopsy can be embedded whole, while the wedge biopsy may be thick enough to warrant sectioning before submitting to the histology laboratory. When sectioning the wedge biopsy, identify the smooth capsule, and then cut the liver at 0.2-cm intervals perpendicular to this surface. Multiple slides should be prepared from each tissue block for histologic evaluation. Step sections are preferred to serial sections so that the intervening sections are available for special stains. If a storage disease is suspected, then a small portion of the biopsy should be placed in glutaraldehyde for electron microscopy.

Partial Hepatectomy

Focal lesions in the liver can be removed by partial liver resections. The extent of these resections varies from small wedges to the removal of an entire lobe. Regardless of its size, the partial liver resection is not structurally complex. Typically, it consists of a focal lesion surrounded by a variable rim of non-neoplastic liver parenchyma. Several faces of the specimen are covered by a peritoneal lining, but at least one surface shows exposed hepatic parenchyma. This exposed surface is the surgical resection margin. This margin has to be correctly identified and oriented. Identification of the resection margin is seldom problematic. Unlike the smooth contour of the peritoneal-lined liver capsule, the resection plane exposes liver parenchyma—which may be fragmented or bloody—and shows cautery effect. On the other hand, orientation of the margin can be very difficult, given the paucity of anatomic landmarks in these limited resections. If the surgeon needs to know the precise location at which a tumor involves or approaches the surgical margin, orientation will require the surgeon's assistance.

Once the margin is identified and the specimen oriented, weigh the specimen, and measure it in each dimension. Examine its contours and surfaces. A bulge in the surface of the liver and/or retraction of the serosa can help localize an intraparenchymal mass. Livers resected for traumatic ruptures should be carefully examined for lacerations of the capsule. Next, rinse the blood from the cut margin, blot it with paper towels, and then ink the dry resection margin. As illustrated, serially section the liver perpendicular to the resection margin. The initial section should pass through the center of the tumor to demonstrate the closest approach of the tumor to the resection margin. Continue sectioning the liver parallel to this first cut at thin (e.g., 0.5-cm) intervals. Examine all cut surfaces for additional nodules.

Record the number, size, location, color, consistency, and circumscription of all lesions. Note the presence or absence of necrosis, hemorrhage, and scarring. Measure the distance from all lesions to the surgical resection margin. If intrahepatic

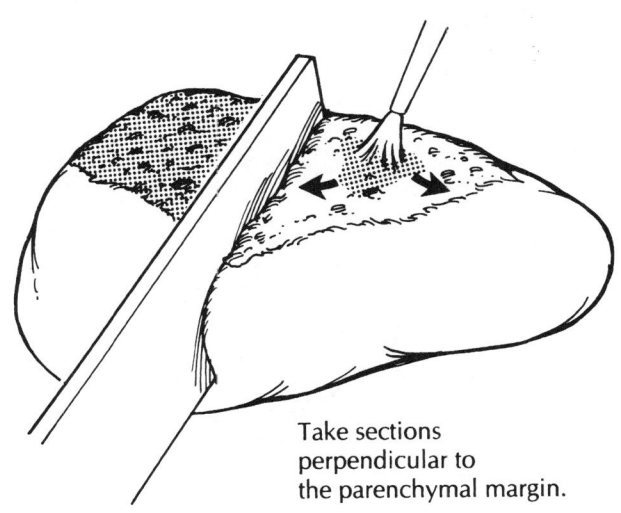

Take sections perpendicular to the parenchymal margin.

Partial Hepatectomy

1. Weigh and measure the specimen.
2. Identify and ink the liver resection margin.
3. Serially section the liver perpendicular to the resection margin at 0.5-cm intervals.
4. Document the distance from the resection margin to the edge of the tumor.
5. For metastatic lesions, submit sections from the periphery of the tumor and of the margin. Sample primary liver tumors more extensively, including perpendicular sections from the resection margin at points most closely approached by tumor. Representative sections of non-neoplastic liver should also be submitted, including a section as far away from the mass as feasible to evaluate background liver fibrosis.

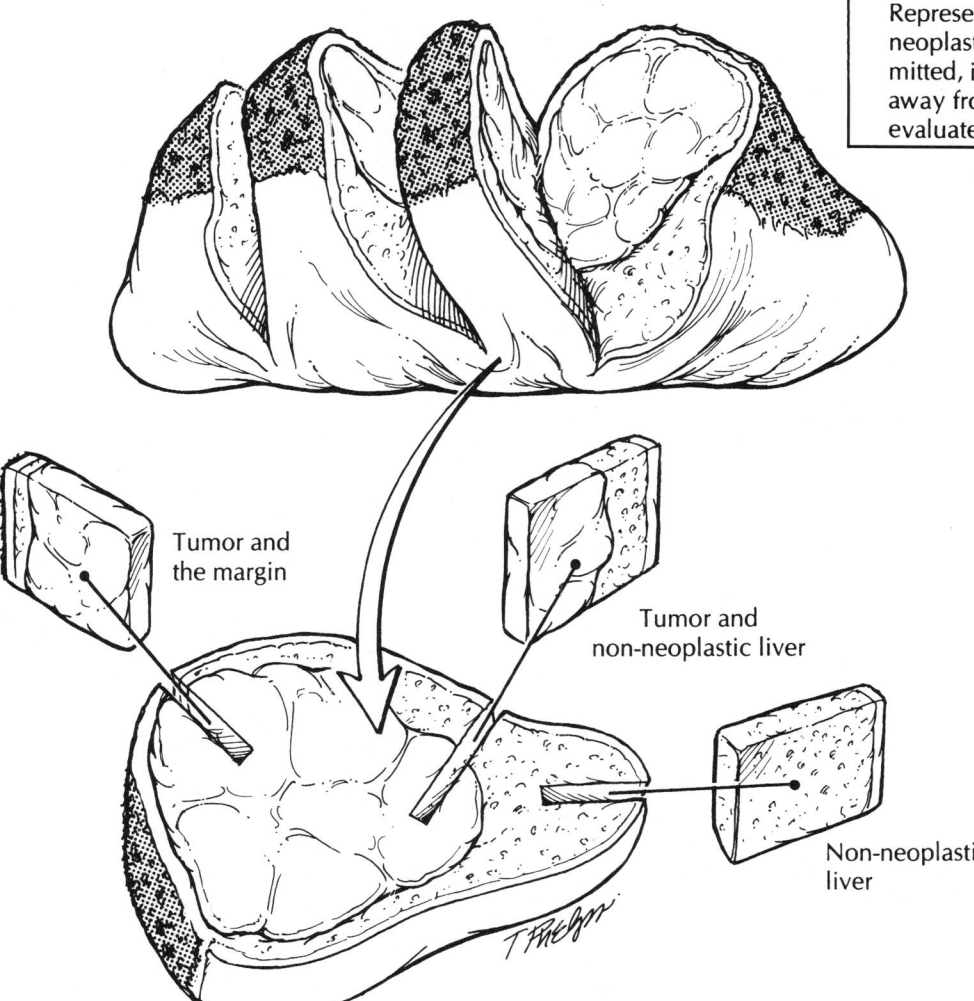

Tumor and the margin

Tumor and non-neoplastic liver

Non-neoplastic liver

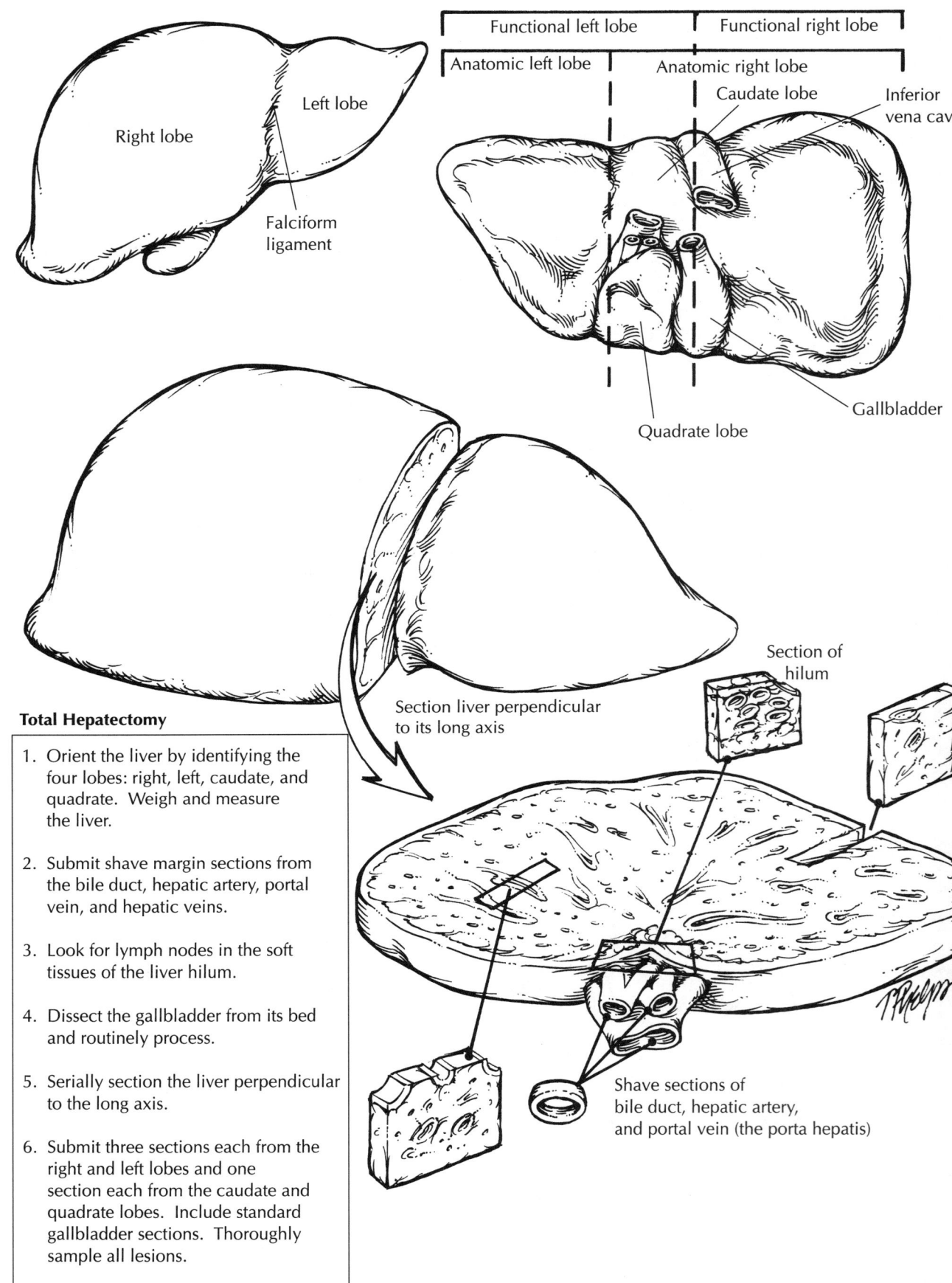

Total Hepatectomy

1. Orient the liver by identifying the four lobes: right, left, caudate, and quadrate. Weigh and measure the liver.

2. Submit shave margin sections from the bile duct, hepatic artery, portal vein, and hepatic veins.

3. Look for lymph nodes in the soft tissues of the liver hilum.

4. Dissect the gallbladder from its bed and routinely process.

5. Serially section the liver perpendicular to the long axis.

6. Submit three sections each from the right and left lobes and one section each from the caudate and quadrate lobes. Include standard gallbladder sections. Thoroughly sample all lesions.

blood vessels are apparent, examine them for tumor thrombi. Remember to describe the appearance of the non-neoplastic hepatic parenchyma. Is the lesion arising in a background of cirrhosis? Is there intraparenchymal hemorrhage associated with an overlying laceration of the capsule?

Sections of tumors should be taken to demonstrate the relationship of tumor to the surrounding liver parenchyma and of the tumor to the resection margin. Sections from the periphery of the tumor are generally much more informative than are those from the center of the tumor. The periphery of a tumor demonstrates the interface with adjacent tissues, and the periphery of a tumor is often less necrotic than the center. Sample the resection margin using perpendicular sections from the areas closest to the edge of the tumor. Depending on the extent of the resection, several representative sections of the non-neoplastic liver parenchyma should also be submitted for histologic evaluation. These sections of uninvolved liver parenchyma are generally more informative when taken far from the nodule. In particular, sections taken adjacent to a tumor can significantly overestimate the degree of fibrosis.

Important Issues to Address in Your Surgical Pathology Report on Partial Hepatectomies

- What procedure was performed, and what structures/organs are present?
- How many tumor nodules are present? What are their sizes? Are they confined to one lobe?
- What are the type and histologic grade of the neoplasm? Is the tumor of liver origin or a metastasis from another site?
- Is vascular invasion identified?
- Is the surgical margin involved by tumor? If not, what is the distance from the margin to the edge of the tumor?
- Does the tumor involve lymph nodes? Include the number of nodes examined and the number involved by tumor.
- What is the condition of the non-neoplastic liver? Is the non-neoplastic liver cirrhotic? Is there evidence of hepatitis?

Liver Explants

Entire liver resections are encountered in hospitals where liver transplantations are performed. The aim of these dissections is to document the cause of the patient's hepatic failure and, in the cases of liver tumors, to stage the tumor and assess the margins at the porta hepatis. Not infrequently, the cause of the hepatic failure is infectious. Be very careful in handling these specimens, and as always strictly observe universal precautions. It is not unreasonable to take the margins, thinly section the specimen (see figure), and submerge the entire specimen in formalin before further processing.

To sample all regions of the liver adequately and to evaluate the important structures of the porta hepatis, you will need to remember the basic anatomy of the liver. As illustrated, the liver is made up of four lobes. Viewed from above, the anatomic right and left lobes are separated by the falciform ligament. The two central lobes are best appreciated by examining the undersurface of the liver. The caudate lobe sits between the portal vein and the inferior vena cava. The quadrate lobe is between the gallbladder fossa and the ligamentum teres and is separated from the caudate lobe by the portal vein. Sometimes the liver is more simply divided into functional right and left lobes by a plane that passes from the gallbladder bed through the inferior vena cava. The major structures forming the porta hepatis are the bile duct, hepatic artery, and portal vein. These three structures maintain a consistent relationship one to another. The duct is most anterior and to the right, the artery is to the left, and the vein is most posterior.

Weigh and measure the liver, and record the appearance of its external surface. If the gallbladder is present, record its size as well. Begin the dissection at the liver hilum. Avoid the temptation to section the liver parenchyma before the hilar structures have been located, identified, and sampled. First, identify and submit a shave section (complete cross section) of the common hepatic duct, the hepatic artery, the portal vein, and hepatic veins. Typically, the hilar vessels and bile duct have been surgically clipped or sutured by the surgeon and can thus be easily located. The portal vein and hepatic veins are frequently transected quite close to the liver, with little extrahepatic tissue remaining. In these cases, the margins may have to be of the initial intrahepatic portion of these vessels. Remember to check for thromboemboli. In cases of chronic extrahepatic biliary tract disease, the extrahepatic bile duct may be difficult to recognize. If this is the case,

make a cut in the liver parallel to the porta hepatis, about 1 cm away from the porta hepatis. Now locate a large bile duct (by its green-yellow color) and insert a probe back toward the porta hepatis to reveal the extrahepatic bile duct. Look for lymph nodes in the hilar soft tissues, and sample each of these for histologic evaluation. Take a section perpendicular to the hilum that captures the soft tissue of the porta hepatis and the underlying liver. This section provides a look at many larger bile ducts and peribiliary glands. Next, dissect the gallbladder from its bed, and process it as you would a routine cholecystectomy (see Chapter 17).

Now that the porta hepatis has been carefully examined and sampled, section the liver parenchyma. Using a long, sharp knife, section the liver as illustrated. Record the color and consistency of the liver parenchyma. Is the liver nodular, fibrotic, or necrotic? Are any focal lesions present?

In addition to the sections taken of the porta hepatis, all lobes of the liver should be represented in a routine sampling of the explanted liver. Three sections each from the right and left lobes and one section each from the caudate and quadrate lobes are generally sufficient, but more sections may be required to sample all areas that have a distinct appearance. Additional sections should also be taken of any focal lesions.

Important Issues to Address in Your Surgical Pathology Report on Liver Explants

- What procedure was performed, and what structures/organs are present? How much does the liver weigh?
- What are the nature and extent of the disease that underlies the liver failure?
- Are there any thromboemboli in large vessels?
- Is the gallbladder present? Are calculi or any other pathologic processes identified?
- Is a neoplasm present? What are its type, grade, size, and location? Does the tumor involve the structures of the porta hepatis? Are the margins at the porta hepatis involved by tumor?
- How many lymph nodes were examined, and how many of them harbor a metastasis?

17 Gallbladder and Extrahepatic Biliary System

Susan Abraham, M.D.

The biliary system forms a conduit whereby bile produced by hepatocytes is transmitted to and concentrated in the gallbladder and finally excreted into the duodenum. Bile is first secreted into bile canaliculi, which form the smallest branches of the biliary system. Canaliculi drain into interlobular bile ducts, which join to form progressively larger intrahepatic ducts until the left and right hepatic ducts emerge from the liver in the region of the porta hepatis. Slightly distal to the porta hepatis, the left and right hepatic ducts join to form the common hepatic duct. The common hepatic duct is then joined on its right side by the cystic duct of the gallbladder to form the common bile duct. The distal common bile duct usually joins with the pancreatic duct within the head of the pancreas and empties into the duodenum at the ampulla of Vater. The exact anatomy and lengths of the various extrahepatic ducts vary among individuals. The common hepatic duct ranges from 1 to 5 cm in length, the cystic duct from 2 to 6 cm, and the common bile duct from 5 to 10 cm. The usual diameter is 4 to 5 mm for the cystic duct and 5 to 7 mm for the common bile duct.

Cholecystectomies

The gallbladder is one of the more frequently encountered specimens in the surgical pathology laboratory. It is usually removed for stones and/or an inflammatory condition, but it rarely does harbor a neoplasm.

The gallbladder is a saccular structure composed of a fundus, body, and neck. It progressively narrows to form the cystic duct. Even though this structural anatomy is straightforward, take a moment to orient the specimen and identify a few important features. First, note that the usual gallbladder has two very different external surfaces. One side of the gallbladder is smooth and glistening, whereas the other is rough. The distinction between these two surfaces is important. The smooth surface is lined by peritoneum. In contrast, the rough surface is where the adventitia of the gallbladder has been dissected from the undersurface of the liver, and it represents a surgical margin. (Rarely, a gallbladder is entirely buried within the liver parenchyma or is attached to the liver only by a mesentery.) Second, the lymphatics of the gallbladder drain into a lymph node located along the cystic duct. When present in the specimen, this cystic duct lymph node can be identified by palpating the soft tissues investing the cystic duct.

State whether the gallbladder is received fresh or in fixative. Measure the specimen, and describe the external surfaces. One important issue to address at the onset of the dissection is whether the specimen is received intact. Not uncommonly, a gallbladder is opened in the operating room and the stones removed. Receipt of a previously opened gallbladder should be documented in the gross description. If the specimen is still intact, open the gallbladder lengthwise through its serosa-lined surface. Using a small pair of scissors, begin at the fundus; next, extend the cut through the body and neck of the gallbladder and then through the cystic duct. The lumen of the cystic duct should be examined, even though the duct may be tortuous and difficult to open. The direction in which the gallbladder is opened is important. Do not begin at the opening of the cystic duct because a probe or scissors forced into this opening could dislodge stones.

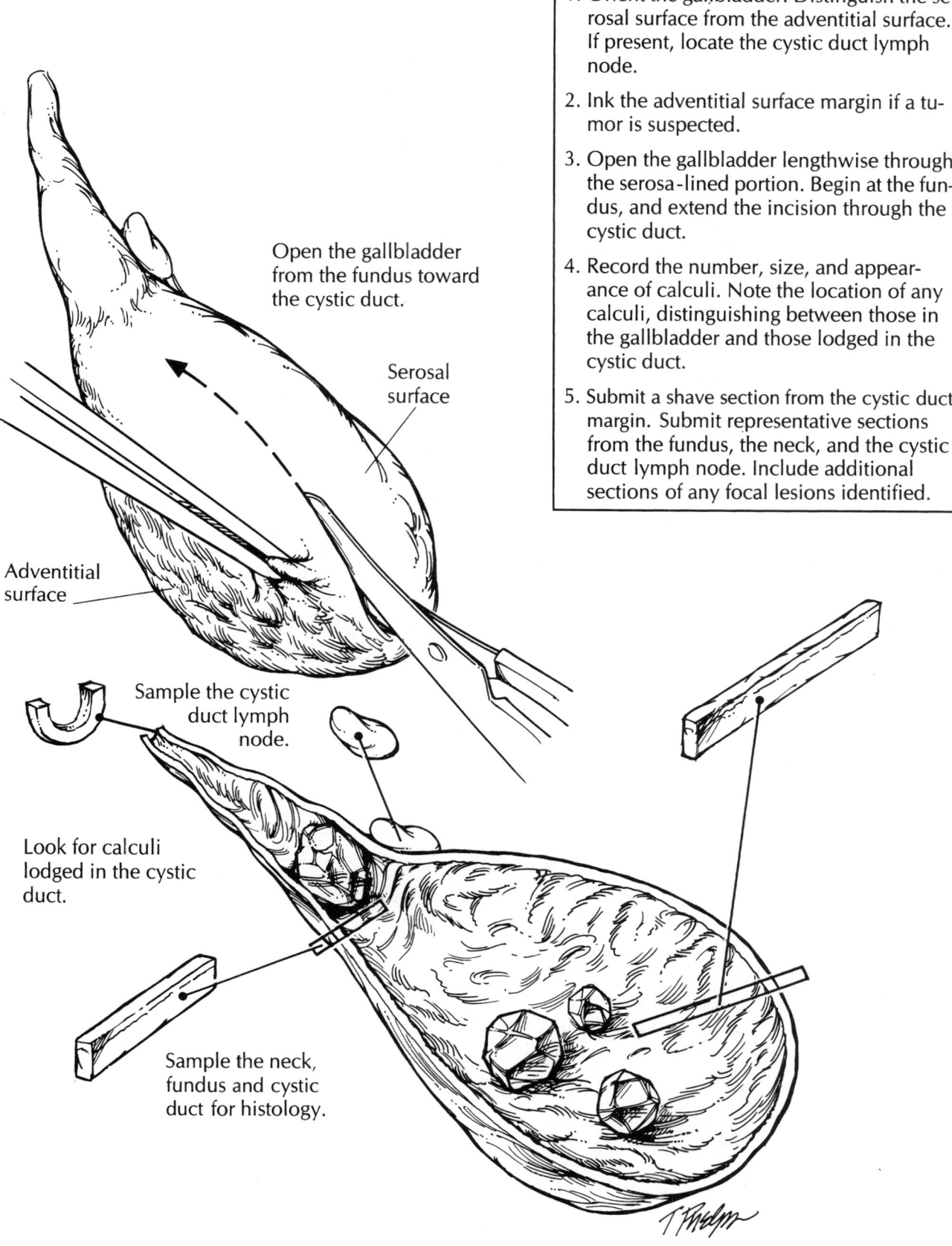

Cholecystectomy

1. Orient the gallbladder. Distinguish the serosal surface from the adventitial surface. If present, locate the cystic duct lymph node.

2. Ink the adventitial surface margin if a tumor is suspected.

3. Open the gallbladder lengthwise through the serosa-lined portion. Begin at the fundus, and extend the incision through the cystic duct.

4. Record the number, size, and appearance of calculi. Note the location of any calculi, distinguishing between those in the gallbladder and those lodged in the cystic duct.

5. Submit a shave section from the cystic duct margin. Submit representative sections from the fundus, the neck, and the cystic duct lymph node. Include additional sections of any focal lesions identified.

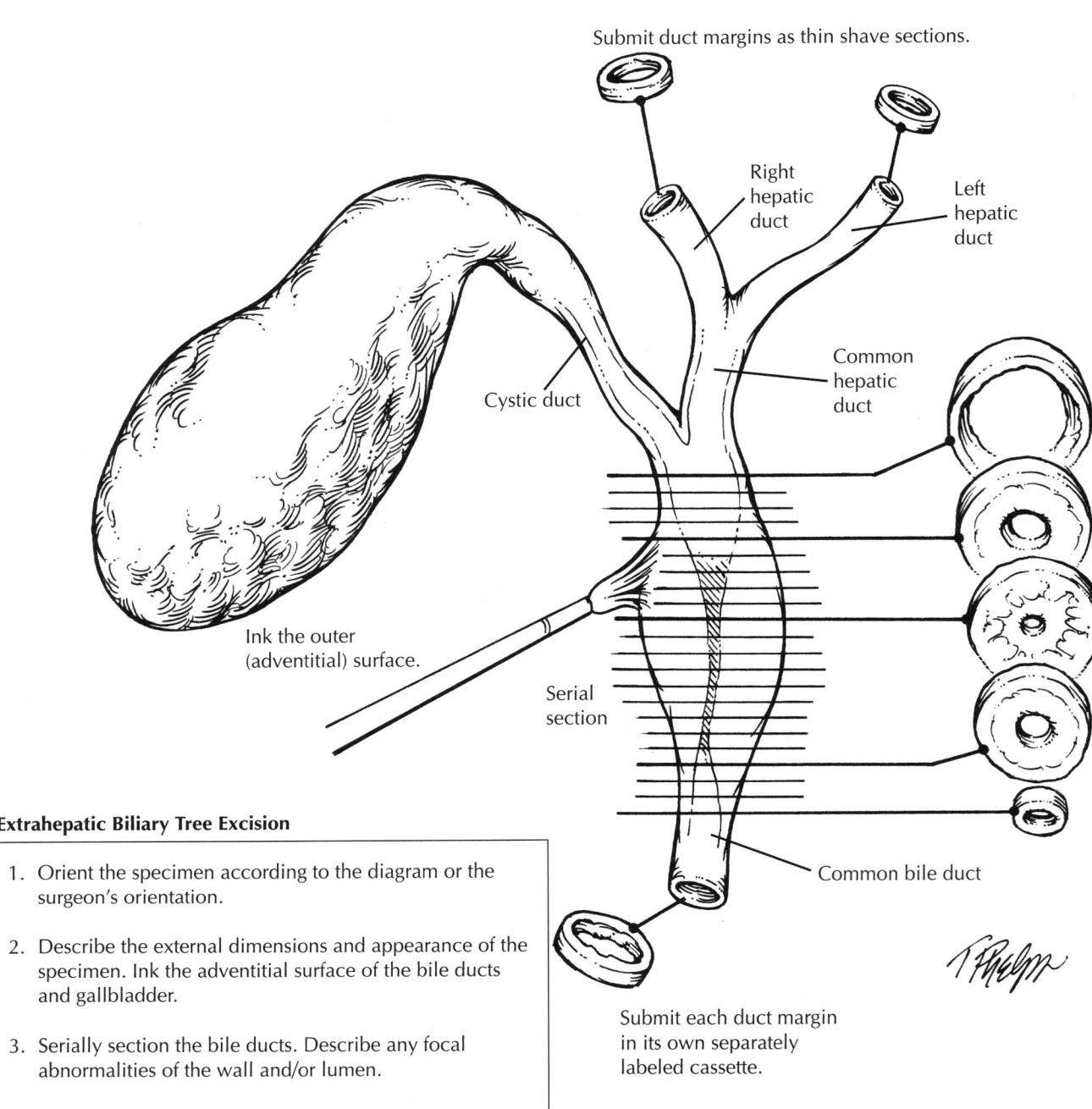

Extrahepatic Biliary Tree Excision

1. Orient the specimen according to the diagram or the surgeon's orientation.

2. Describe the external dimensions and appearance of the specimen. Ink the adventitial surface of the bile ducts and gallbladder.

3. Serially section the bile ducts. Describe any focal abnormalities of the wall and/or lumen.

4. Sample each duct margin (i.e., left hepatic duct, right hepatic duct, common bile duct) as a thin shave section.

5. Entirely submit the bile ducts for histologic examination. Carefully label each duct margin, and separately submit each margin in its own labeled tissue cassette.

6. If the gallbladder is included, submit routine sections including sections of the adventitial margin and the cystic duct lymph node.

After the specimen has been opened, note the contents of the gallbladder and the cystic duct. Is the usual thin, dark green bile present; or is it hemorrhagic, viscous, or sludgy? Is the lumen filled with pus (an infected gallbladder) or replaced by clear white mucoid material (mucocele)? Look for calculi, and determine whether they are present within the lumen of the gallbladder or within the cystic duct. Record the appearance of any calculi. Are they round or faceted? What is their color? Use a sharp blade to cut the calculi in half, and note the appearance of their cut surfaces. How many calculi are present? When numerous calculi are present, there is a tendency to record the size of the largest one. Instead, record the full range of sizes, keeping in mind that the smaller calculi are more apt to become lodged in the cystic duct than are the larger ones.

Next, measure the thickness of the gallbladder wall, and describe the appearance of the mucosa. The mucosa is normally bile-stained and has a fine, honeycombed appearance. A frequent mucosal abnormality is cholesterolosis, in which there are numerous yellow punctate deposits or interlacing linear yellow streaks on the mucosa ("strawberry gallbladder"). If a neoplasm is suggested by the presence of an exophytic or ulcerative lesion, the external adventitial surface should be inked, as it represents an important surgical margin. Describe the location of the neoplasm, its dimensions, and its configuration (e.g., exophytic, ulcerating, diffusely infiltrating with associated wall thickening). If liver parenchyma is attached to the adventitial surface of the gallbladder, does the tumor appear to invade the liver?

The gallbladder is best sampled after it has been allowed to fix. For routine specimens, submit one representative full-thickness section from the fundus, one through the body/neck of the gallbladder, and one cross section of the cystic duct margin. Additional sections are required when focal lesions are present. If a neoplastic process is suspected, obtain full-thickness sections of the tumor to demonstrate its maximum depth of invasion. Also submit sections from the periphery of the tumor to demonstrate its relationship to the surrounding uninvolved mucosa. To assess the status of the margins when a neoplasm is suspected, submit a shave section from the cystic duct margin and perpendicular sections from the inked adventitial surface. When present, the cystic duct lymph node should always be submitted for histologic evaluation.

Local or Segmental Biliary Resections

The extrahepatic bile ducts are most commonly encountered as part of a pancreaticoduodenectomy (including the distal common bile duct) and partial or total hepatectomy (including portions of the proximal extrahepatic biliary tree). Examination of the bile ducts in these specimens is described elsewhere in this book. Local or segmental resections of the extrahepatic bile ducts are less common but may be performed for carcinoma of the extrahepatic bile ducts, isolated strictures, or choledochal cysts.

The specimen should first be oriented, preferably as indicated by the surgeon or by noting its relationship to the gallbladder. Note if the specimen is received fixed or unfixed, whether it has been previously incised, and whether other tissues or organs accompany the bile duct. Measure the length and diameter of each portion of the biliary tree that is present. Describe the appearance of the external surface, including the presence of any mass lesions or adhesions. In general, the proximal and distal bile duct margins and the periductal soft tissue (forming the circumferential margin of the excision) should then be inked because of the high likelihood of carcinoma.

It is best not to attempt to open the ducts longitudinally, since small papillary lesions in the ducts could easily be dislodged and the mucosa disrupted by the scissors. Instead, make serial cross sections at 2- to 3-mm intervals with a scalpel, keeping the cross sections oriented with regard to the segment of the biliary tree and the proximal and distal margins. The resulting cross sections can then be examined for the presence of any obstructing lesions in the lumen, the presence of a mass, or the presence of a stricture. If a stricture is present, describe its location and measure its length, the sizes of the bile duct lumen at, above, and below the stricture, and the thickness of the bile duct wall in the region of the stricture and elsewhere. Carcinoma of the bile ducts can infiltrate diffusely into the bile duct wall and thereby mimic a benign stricture, or it can have a papillary or nodular configuration. If a calculus,

papillary lesion, or mass is seen, describe its location, whether it obstructs the lumen, and whether there is obvious penetration of the bile duct wall and involvement of any adjacent structures. In general, the specimen should then be submitted in its entirety in serial cross sections, keeping the proximal and distal shave margins separate. (Surgically resectable carcinomas of the bile ducts are unlikely to be too large to submit in toto, and segmental bile duct resections without a grossly obvious tumor would have to be completely embedded anyway.)

Choledochal cysts should also be inked along the external surface. Measure the dimensions of the cyst and describe its configuration (e.g., fusiform or saccular). Carefully incise the cyst with a scalpel and drain the contents into a container. Note the volume and type of the fluid present (bile, blood, fibrin, mucoid material, pus). After draining the cyst contents, open the cyst longitudinally with a small pair of scissors and examine the inner lining. Specifically, describe the appearance of the lining (often denuded, bile-stained, and shaggy) and the presence of any visible islands of residual mucosa. Are any masses or suspicious lesions present? The risk of carcinoma developing within choledochal cysts increases with age, and up to 15% of choledochal cysts in adults harbor a carcinoma. If a suspicious lesion is present, describe its dimensions, color, consistency, associated necrosis, and how deeply it penetrates the cyst wall.

Representative full-thickness sections of the cyst should be taken. They should include approximately one section per centimeter of cyst wall diameter as well as proximal and distal shave margins. If any suspicious lesions are present, additional sections are needed, including full-thickness sections of the lesion at its deepest extent and sections that demonstrate the interface between the lesion and the adjacent cyst wall.

Important Issues to Address in Your Surgical Pathology Report

- What procedure was performed, and what structures/organs are present?
- What are the contents of the gallbladder, bile duct, or choledochal cyst (e.g., bile, pus, blood, mucus)? When calculi are present, note their type (pigment, cholesterol, mixed), number, and the range of sizes. Are any calculi lodged in the cystic duct or present in a bile duct?
- What are the nature and severity of the inflammatory processes (e.g., acute or chronic cholecystitis, xanthogranulomatous cholecystitis, primary or secondary sclerosing cholangitis)? For a cholecystectomy, be sure to mention the presence or absence of perforations and peritonitis.
- Is a neoplasm present? What are its location, size, histologic type, histologic grade, and depth of invasion (mucosa, gallbladder muscularis or bile duct fibromuscular layer, perimuscular or periductal soft tissue)? Is there angiolymphatic invasion or perineural invasion? Does the tumor extend into adjacent organs? For gallbladder carcinomas, it is important to note whether there is invasion into the liver, and whether this invasion is more than 2 cm. Are the adventitial/hepatic bed margin and the cystic duct margin free of tumor? For bile duct carcinomas, are the periductal soft tissue margin and the proximal and distal bile duct margins free of tumor?
- Are there preneoplastic changes in the surrounding mucosa (intestinal metaplasia, dysplasia)?
- How many lymph nodes were examined, and how many of them harbored a metastasis?

18 Pancreas

The pancreas can intimidate even the most experienced pathologist. The complexity of the anatomy of the pancreas and the importance of a good dissection in establishing the correct diagnosis make the arrival of a resected pancreas in the surgical pathology laboratory a particularly stressful event. This stress can, however, be greatly reduced if you familiarize yourself with a few basic aspects of the anatomy of the pancreas, and if you take a simple, logical approach to your dissection.

Pancreaticoduodenectomies

The Whipple procedure (pancreaticoduodenectomy) has emerged as an effective and safe treatment for neoplasms of the head of the pancreas, duodenum, distal common bile duct, and ampulla of Vater. The orientation of these specimens can be greatly simplified if you remember that the specimen is composed of four basic components: (1) the duodenum, (2) the ampulla of Vater, (3) the bile duct, and (4) the pancreas.

Begin by orienting the duodenum: Two features of the duodenum can be used to identify its proximal and distal ends. First, the free proximal end is almost always shorter than the free distal segment of the resected duodenum. Second, a small part of the stomach is occasionally attached to the proximal end. Next, identify the bile duct. As illustrated, the common bile duct can be recognized by its greenish color and characteristic tubular appearance. Also, if the gallbladder is present, use the insertion of the cystic duct to identify the common bile duct. The remaining components of the pancreas can be identified using the duodenum and bile duct as guides. The pancreas itself sits at the base of the junction of the bile duct and duodenum. The head of the pancreas sits within the duodenal C loop. The pancreatic neck margin can be recognized as the cut oval pancreatic surface with a central duct. Although the uncinate process of the pancreas is more difficult to identify, it can be visualized if you keep the anatomy of the pancreas in mind. As illustrated, the pancreas sits like a slightly curled hand enveloping the superior mesenteric artery and the portal vein. The thumb of the curled hand corresponds to the uncinate process of the pancreas and the flat fingers to the neck, body, and tail. Although the superior mesenteric vessels are not present in the resected specimen, remember that they were dissected from the pancreas right at the groove between the thumb and index finger.

After the major external landmarks have been identified, measure the dimensions of each, and ink the surface of the pancreas and the proximal and distal duodenal margins. Begin the dissection by opening the duodenum along the side opposite the pancreas. Look for and document any duodenal masses, ulcers, or areas of puckering of the duodenal mucosa. Before cutting the specimen any further, submit sections of the margins. These should include: (1) a shave section of the bile duct margin; (2) a shave section of the pancreatic neck margin; (3) a perpendicular section of the uncinate margin taken to include the vascular groove; (4) a perpendicular section from the proximal duodenal margin; and (5) a shave section from the distal duodenal margin. Next, using a pair of scissors, open the common bile duct. Because the extrapancreatic (proximal) portion of the duct is usually dilated, you may find it easier to start the incision at the proximal end. Extend the incision longitudinally down through the ampulla of Vater, and note any strictures or exophytic masses in the bile duct and in the ampulla of Vater. Similarly, if the gallbladder is present, open it from its dome through the cystic duct to the point where it opens into the common bile duct. Note any calculi, strictures, or masses, and take a representative section of the gallbladder for histology (see Chapter 17).

After the duodenum and bile duct have been opened, you can now section the pancreas. This can be accomplished in a variety of ways, but we like to bread-loaf it into 2-mm slices perpendicular to the long axis of the duodenum. Use a long sharp knife to cut through the pancreas, leaving each slice attached to the specimen at the duodenum.

Now that the various components of the specimen have been exposed, there are five questions to answer: First, is a neoplasm present? Most of the cancers will be obvious, but if you have trouble finding the tumor, look carefully at the bile duct and pancreatic parenchyma. Often, the bile duct is strictured at the level of the tumor, and tumors involving the pancreas usually disrupt the gland's normal lobular architecture. Second, if a tumor is present, where is it located, and what is its probable site of origin (pancreas, bile duct, ampulla of Vater, or duodenum)? Third, what is the size of the tumor (measured in centimeters)? Fourth, what is the gross appearance of the neoplasm (solid or cystic)? Finally, how many lymph nodes are present, and are the lymph nodes grossly abnormal? The answers to each of these five questions will help identify and stage the neoplasm, and each answer should be carefully documented in the gross description. At this point, you may wish to fix the specimen overnight in formalin.

After the specimen has been well fixed, carefully paint the mucosa of the common bile duct with orange ink or tattoo powder. This simple step will help in the interpretation of microscopic slides, because without the paint in the bile duct, it can be almost impossible to distinguish the bile duct from the pancreatic duct microscopically. Next, submit sections for histology. The sections will flow naturally if you remember the four basic components of the specimen (the pancreas, duodenum, bile duct, and ampulla). Submit sections of the pancreatic parenchyma, the bile duct, the duodenum, the ampulla, and representative sections of all masses. Submit one section of pancreatic parenchyma for each 1 cm of maximum pancreatic length. As illustrated, a section that we find particularly helpful is a section parallel to the long axis of the bile duct that includes the duodenum, ampulla, bile duct, and pancreas all in one. If a mass is present, be sure to include sections that demonstrate the relationship of the mass to each of the four components of the specimen and sections that demonstrate the relationship of the neoplasm to the anterior and posterior soft tissue margins. Next, submit a representative section of each lymph node. Although the lymphatic drainage of the pancreas is complex, we have not found detailed accounts of the exact location of each lymph node submitted to be helpful. Instead, we prefer to spend time making sure that we find all of the nodes. A good place to look for nodes is in the peripancreatic fat at the junction of the pancreas and duodenum. They may also be found in the mesentery and around the bile duct.

Distal Pancreatectomies

Distal pancreatectomies are much easier to handle than are pancreaticoduodenectomies. The anatomy is simple, and there are fewer margins to sample. First, find the proximal and distal ends of the pancreas. The spleen helps identify the distal aspect of the gland, and the cut surface of the pancreas is the proximal end. Next, weigh and measure the specimen, and submit a shave section of the proximal pancreatic margin. Ink the surface of the gland, and then bread-loaf it into 2-mm slices using a long sharp knife. These slices should be made perpendicular to the long axis of the gland. Examine the pancreatic parenchyma carefully, paying particular attention to the pancreatic duct. Is the duct dilated or stenotic? Are there any masses or calculi in it? What is the consistency of any fluid in the duct? Note the size, location, and gross appearance of any masses. Submit representative sections of any tumors and of the pancreatic parenchyma. Examine the peripancreatic soft tissues for lymph nodes, note their gross appearance, and submit a representative section of each. If the spleen is present, weigh it, measure it, section it, and submit representative sections, as described in the discussion of the spleen (see Chapter 42).

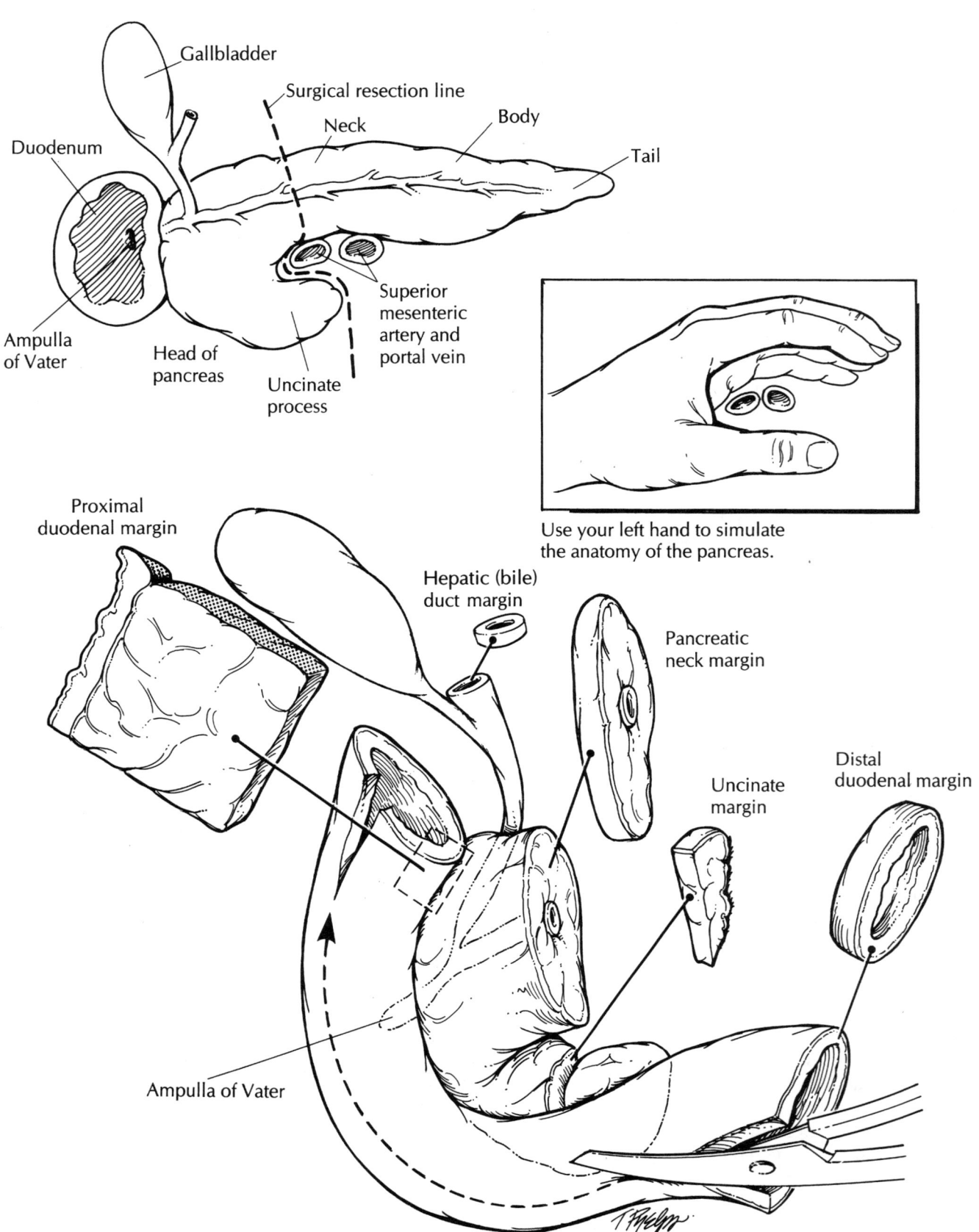

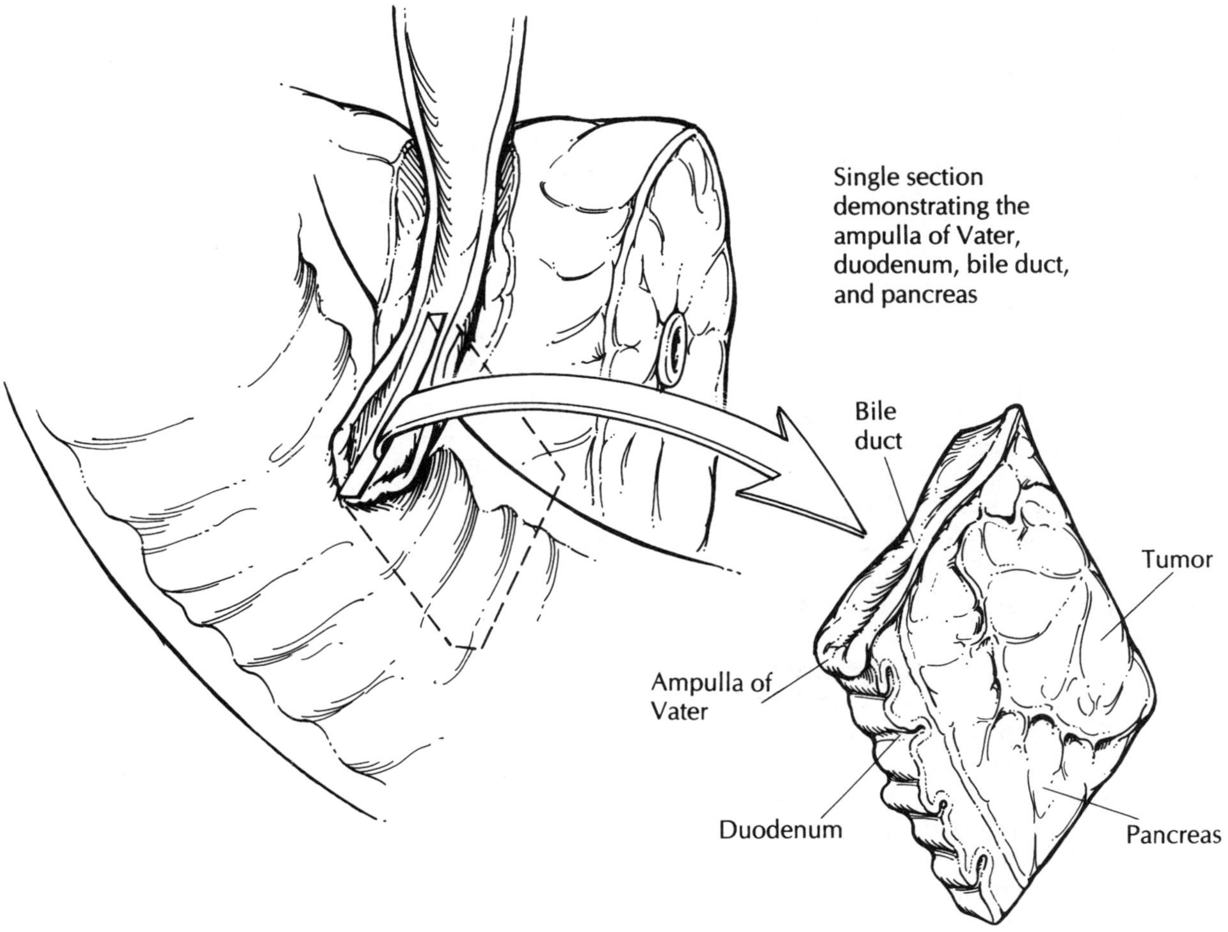

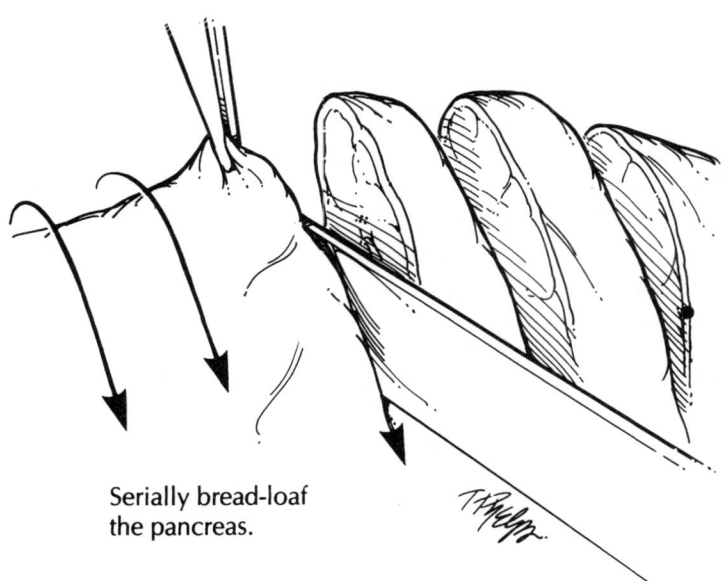

Single section demonstrating the ampulla of Vater, duodenum, bile duct, and pancreas

Bile duct
Tumor
Ampulla of Vater
Duodenum
Pancreas

Serially bread-loaf the pancreas.

Pancreaticoduodenectomy

1. Remember the four basic components of the specimen: the duodenum, the ampulla of Vater, the bile duct, and the pancreas.
2. Orient the specimen. The distal portion of the duodenum is usually longer than the proximal portion.
3. Shave the distal duodenal, bile duct, and pancreatic neck margins. Take perpendicular sections of the proximal duodenal and uncinate margins.
4. Open the duodenum on the side opposite the pancreas. Open the bile duct, and paint it with orange tattoo powder or orange ink.
5. Section the pancreas at 2-mm intervals.
6. Submit the five margin sections and sections of the tumor, the pancreatic parenchyma, the bile duct, the duodenum, the ampulla of Vater, and each lymph node.

Like the pancreaticoduodenectomy specimen, your final report should document the presence or absence of a neoplasm; the type, grade, and size of the tumor; the status of the margins; any lymph node metastases; and the presence or absence of vascular, perineural, and soft tissue invasion.

Cystic Tumors

Cystic masses in the pancreas should be handled as described above. In addition, remember to do the following: (1) Describe the character of the cyst contents. Is the fluid clear or cloudy? Is it serous, mucinous, necrotic or bloody? A good description of the cyst contents can be invaluable in determining the tumor type. (2) Document whether the cyst is unilocular or multilocular. How large are the cysts, and are there any mural nodules? (3) If the cyst is lined by mucinous epithelium, then the entire cyst should be submitted for histologic diagnosis. Keep in mind that otherwise benign-appearing mucinous cystic neoplasms can harbor small invasive cancers. (4) Finally and importantly, document the relationship of the cyst to the pancreatic ducts. This can be important because intraductal papillary mucinous neoplasms, by definition, involve the duct system, whereas mucinous cystic neoplasms usually do not.

Ampullectomy

The ampulla of Vater is formed by the confluence of the pancreatic and distal common bile ducts as they pass through the wall of the duodenum and open into the duodenal lumen. Small neoplasms of the ampulla of Vater are occasionally resected in a procedure known as an ampullectomy. In these instances the specimen usually consists of a small disk of duodenal tissue about the size of a quarter. The underside of the disk is composed of transected sections of the pancreatic and bile ducts, the disk itself is traversed by the ducts, and the upper surface is lined by duodenal mucosa, in the center of which is the papilla of Vater.

Identify the bile and pancreatic ducts and submit a shave section of each duct margin. Next, ink the edges of the disk (the duodenal margins) and the aspects of the deep margin not sampled when the duct margins were taken. Then simply bread-loaf the specimen in 2-mm slices along the axis that best demonstrates the relationship between the tumor and the duodenal margin it most closely approaches. Document the gross appearance (e.g., papillary, endophytic), size, and location of any masses; then submit the entire specimen for histologic evaluation.

Important Issues to Address in Your Surgical Pathology Report on Pancreatic Resections

- What procedure was performed, and what structures/organs are present?
- Is a neoplasm present?
- What is the probable site of origin of the tumor (bile duct, pancreas, ampulla of Vater, or duodenum)?
- What is the size of the tumor (in centimeters)?
- What are the histologic type and grade of the neoplasm? Is an *in situ* component identified?
- Does the tumor extend into the peripancreatic soft tissues? If so, does it extend anteriorly or posteriorly?
- Does the tumor infiltrate blood vessels, lymphatics, or nerves? Does the tumor extend into the pancreas, duodenum, ampulla of Vater, common bile duct, or spleen?
- Does the tumor involve any of the margins (pancreatic neck, uncinate, bile duct, soft tissue, and proximal and distal duodenal)?
- Does the tumor involve regional lymph nodes? Include the number of nodes examined and the number of nodes involved.
- Do the non-neoplastic portions of the pancreas and duodenum show any pathology?

V The Cardiovascular/Respiratory System

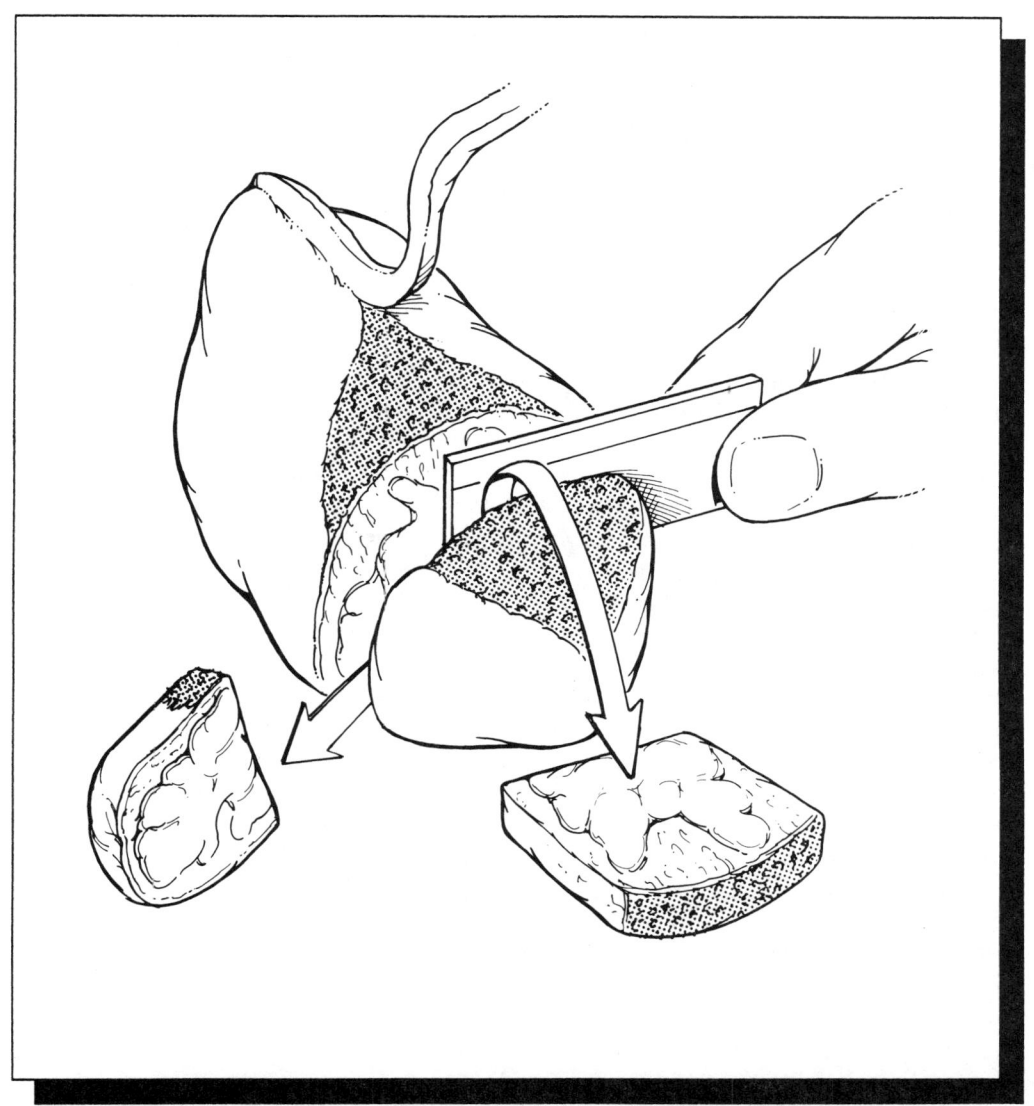

19 Heart, Heart Valves, and Vessels

E. Rene Rodriguez, M.D.

The Explanted Heart

The examination of hearts explanted from heart transplant recipients provides a unique opportunity to study cardiac pathology. Moreover, in some instances it influences posttransplant therapy and prognosis.

The specimen should be emptied of clotted blood and weighed before examination. Document the general shape (globular or normal) and consistency (firm or floppy) of the heart, and identify the major structures (ventricles, atria, pulmonary artery, root of the aorta). In most instances the atria are partially or completely missing, and this should be recorded. The pulmonary artery and valve as well as the aortic root and valve may be intact or partially torn during the resection of the heart. Document the anatomy. Do the great vessels emerge from the heart in their normal anatomic location? If you suspect a congenital heart disease, you should work carefully with the clinician and review appropriate preoperative imaging, as the clinical history guides your dissection. Further examination of the heart is simplified if you approach the three layers of the heart (epicardium, myocardium, endocardium), the valves, and the coronary vessels systematically.

Start with the epicardium. Examination of the external surface of the heart should document the presence or absence of petechiae, adhesions (fibrous or fibrinous), scar (focal or extensive), calcification, and grafts (vascular or synthetic material). If grafts are present, document their location and the status of the anastomoses. Grossly examine the valves as best you can before sectioning the heart. Document any thrombi or vegetations. In most instances transverse sectioning of the heart at 1-cm intervals from the apex to just below the atrioventricular apparatuses allows the diagnosis of hypertrophy and/or dilatation, and it demonstrates the greatest surface area of the sectioned myocardium. Examine the myocardium carefully. The size and location of recent or remote infarcts, focal punctate lesions, hemorrhages, fibrosis, or frank necrosis should be noted. Examination of the myocardium should be guided by the patient's clinical history, as some pathologic conditions affect specific areas of the heart. For example, sarcoidosis tends to begin in the basal portion of the heart close to the atrioventricular apparatus; on the other hand, right ventricular dysplasia affects the right ventricular free wall during early stages and spreads to the left ventricle late in the disease. Next, turn your attention to the endocardium and valves. Are the endocardial surfaces smooth, or are focal lesions noted? Examine the atrioventricular and semilunar valves, as described later under Heart Valves. Lastly, the coronary arteries can be examined. Do this systematically. Start at the orifice of the left main coronary artery and serially section the vessel proceeding down the left anterior descending and left circumflex arteries as far as possible. Similarly, section the right coronary artery from its orifice to its distal branches. Document the course of these vessels. Are they in their normal anatomic location? As described in detail under Arteries and Veins, examine the lumen of each vessel for thrombi; examine the intima for evidence of intimal proliferation, hemorrhage, or atheromatous plaques; and document the location and percentage narrowing caused by any lesions. For example, your report could include "there is 90% stenosis of the left anterior descending coronary arteries just proximal to the take-off

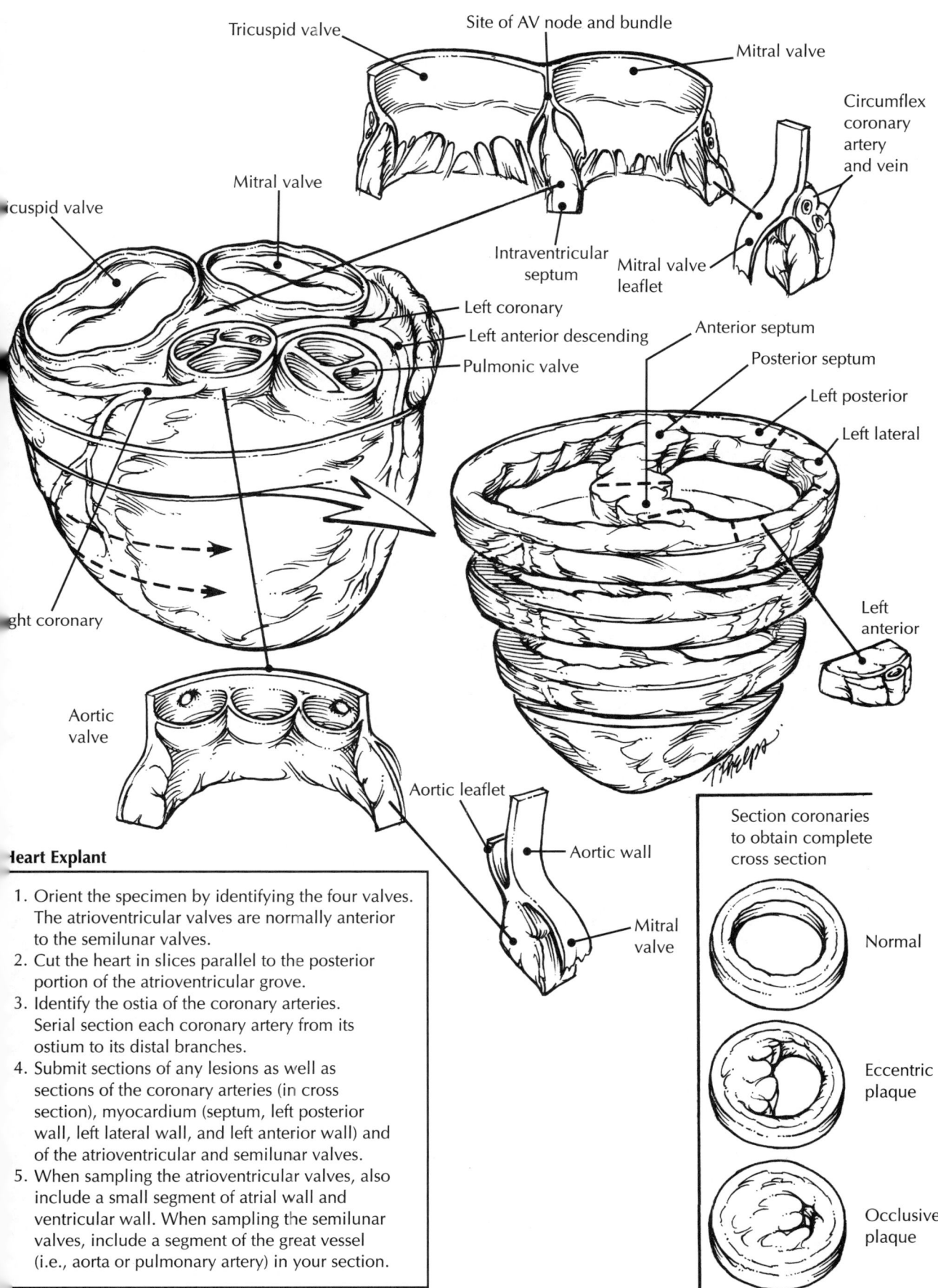

Heart Explant

1. Orient the specimen by identifying the four valves. The atrioventricular valves are normally anterior to the semilunar valves.
2. Cut the heart in slices parallel to the posterior portion of the atrioventricular grove.
3. Identify the ostia of the coronary arteries. Serial section each coronary artery from its ostium to its distal branches.
4. Submit sections of any lesions as well as sections of the coronary arteries (in cross section), myocardium (septum, left posterior wall, left lateral wall, and left anterior wall) and of the atrioventricular and semilunar valves.
5. When sampling the atrioventricular valves, also include a small segment of atrial wall and ventricular wall. When sampling the semilunar valves, include a segment of the great vessel (i.e., aorta or pulmonary artery) in your section.

of the first diagonal branch." It is not uncommon to receive specimens with one or more metal stents within the coronaries. If stents are present, describe their presence and location. Section the vessel close to the stent and inspect its lumen. Sectioning through the stents is not feasible in common pathology practice.

The heart can now be sampled. Samples of myocardium for electron microscopy should always be procured. Also in modern pathology practice, pieces of each ventricle should be frozen in optimal controlled temperature (OCT) compound and also snap-frozen for any molecular diagnostic test that may be needed later. Sections submitted in formalin for histopathologic examination should include a minimum of four sections of the ventricles (interventricular septum, anterior wall, lateral wall, and posterior wall); a section of any valve lesions; a section of the mitral and aortic valves; and representative sections of each of the coronary arteries. The section of the anterior wall can often be taken to include the left anterior descending coronary artery. Sample any additional area showing gross pathologic changes. Examination of the atrioventricular conduction system is often possible, whereas in most instances examination of the sinoatrial node is not. It is easy to sample the conduction system if needed (see The Conducting System). Remember that atherosclerosis and some valve lesions can be quite calcified, and therefore decalcification should be performed as necessary.

The Conduction System

Histologic examination of the conduction system is difficult and time-consuming, and it is usually fruitless unless the patient has a clinical history of a complete heart block. Nonetheless, in some instances examination of the conduction system can provide critical insight into the underlying nature of the patient's pathology.

In general, the sinoatrial node is not present in the explanted heart. Examination of the atrioventricular (AV) node was well described by Hutchins:[3] From the right side of the heart, identify the ostium of the coronary sinus, the septal leaflet of the tricuspid valve, the membranous interventricular septum, and a line approximately 2 cm below the insertion of the septal leaflet of the tricuspid valve. Remove the block of tissue contained within these landmarks by cutting into the septum from the right side. This block of tissue can then be serially sectioned for histologic examination.

Endomyocardial Biopsy

Endomyocardial biopsy is still the gold standard for monitoring the allograft. Biopsies are also frequently performed to determine the etiology of heart failure in nontransplanted patients. The tissue is usually procured with a bioptome through either the jugular or the femoral vein. There is evidence that with three pieces only 95% of inflammatory infiltrates are detected. However, if four pieces are examined, up to 98% of infiltrates are detected. The working formulation for heart allograft monitoring therefore recommends examination of at least four pieces of tissue.[4] Documenting the number of biopsy specimens received is therefore important. The specimens are handled differently depending on the timing or the reason for the biopsy.

Following a few simple rules ensures optimal preservation of the tissue for diagnostic analysis. Minor modifications to these rules for specific tests or research protocols can be made without disrupting the work flow in the heart biopsy suite. Some helpful hints include the following.

1. Plan ahead. Take into account that the working formulation recommends "four to six undivided pieces of tissue," "one piece frozen," and "no tissue routinely fixed for electron microscopy." Commonly, the fixative of choice is 10% phosphate-buffered formalin. Alternatively, fixation can be done in glutaraldehyde for microscopy or in other fixatives that preserve antigens for immunohistochemistry studies.

2. The tissue should not be handled with forceps or divided with a scalpel. The tip of an intravenous catheter or syringe needle is usually a good instrument for picking up the biopsy. Squeezing the tissue can produce artifacts that upon microscopic examination render it uninterpretable.

3. The tissue should be fixed immediately in the desired fixative that has been allowed to reach room temperature. Cold fixative enhances contraction band artifacts. The tissue should not be allowed to sit for long periods of time on filter paper, gauze, or any other surface impregnated with saline. Saline is a poor solution

for preserving the morphology of myocardium, as it readily creates artifacts.

4. During the first six weeks after transplantation, at least one piece of tissue should be frozen. The working formulation recommends that the tissue be frozen in OCT compound (Miles Inc., Diagnostics Division, Elkhart, IN, USA).[4] We prefer to freeze the tissue using isopentane, which should be chilled to −20°C in a small 1.8-ml cryogenic vial. The biopsy tissue is then immersed in this prechilled isopentane cryovial, the cap is tightened, and the container is immersed in liquid nitrogen. At this point the tissue can be processed for immunofluorescence or stored at −80°C for future study.

5. In the nontransplanted patient, one or more pieces of tissue can be snap-frozen for special studies (e.g., immunohistochemistry, *in situ* nucleic acid hybridization, polymerase chain reaction).

For transplant biopsies the working formulation[4] recommends: "a minimum of three step levels through the paraffin block with at least three sections of each level." Similar handling is adequate for nontransplant specimens. Slides should be stained routinely with hematoxylin and eosin; additional unstained slides should be obtained for other stains to avoid having to "face" the paraffin block again and thus minimize tissue loss due to technical handling.

For heart transplant biopsies the working formulation does not require routine submission of tissue from cardiac allograft biopsies for electron microscopy. However, for diagnostic "cardiomyopathy work-up" biopsies, it is important to procure at least one specimen and fix it in glutaraldehyde. If the biopsy is received in formalin and there are more than four biopsy pieces, one may be transferred to glutaraldehyde and submitted for electron microscopy. In cases of suspected adriamycin toxicity, consideration should be given to submitting all of the tissue for electron microscopy.

Cardiac Tumors

Resections of cardiac tumors are not common surgical pathology specimens. Despite their infrequency, these specimens are easily tackled using the standard approach to tumor dissection.

Describe the number and sizes of the tissue pieces received and the presence of epicardium, endocardium, or muscle. Document the size of any masses. The color and texture of the mass are also important to note, as they may indicate the predominant presence of fibrous tissue, myxoid stroma, adipose tissue, or muscle. Intracavitary masses can be pedunculated or sessile and should be described accordingly. The resection margin(s) should be inked and sampled, and the status of these margins should be documented in your final report, as it is useful information for the surgeon. As with any tumor, adequate sampling requires representative sections of areas that may show distinct gross features, such as fibrosis, necrosis, hemorrhage, or a recognizable normal structure (e.g., valve, trabeculae). If the mass is large, one cassette for every centimeter of maximal diameter of the tumor should be adequate. A piece of the tumor may be frozen and stored for special studies, and submission of fresh tissue may be indicated if cytogenetic or flow cytometric analysis is to be performed. Sampling the tumor for these analyses should avoid areas of frank necrosis. If the tumor is heavily calcified, it should be handled similar to a bone specimen for the slicing, sampling, and decalcifying procedures.

Pericardium

The pericardium includes the parietal and visceral pericardium. The parietal pericardium consists of the tough fibrocollagenous tissue sac covering the heart. Its inner surface is lined by mesothelial cells. Usually there are very few blood vessels coursing through it. The visceral pericardium is a more delicate, thinner fibrous layer covering the heart and epicardial fat. In general, the pericardial specimens submitted to surgical pathology are samples of the parietal pericardium, which can become very thick as a result of inflammatory and/or neoplastic infiltration.

In addition to the overall dimension of the piece of tissue received, it is important to record the average thickness of the pericardial sample. Document the presence or absence of adipose tissue, areas of hemorrhage, nodules, and the status of the surface (e.g., smooth, shiny, ragged, fibrinous, granular). Note whether there are fibrin deposits, fibrous collagenous bands, cystic spaces, or papillary projections. Rarely, frank abscesses are demonstrated on gross examination.

Adequate sampling may vary according to the size of the specimen and the clinical information. Careful gross examination aids in determining what should be sampled for histology. A thickened pericardial sample (i.e., pericardial thickness of more than 3 mm) should be fixed and cut perpendicular to the inner surface of the pericardial sac, which in most cases is easily identified. Serial slices may be submitted to maximize the surface area. If the pericardial sample is thin (less than 2 mm in thickness) one should make sure that the sections are embedded "on edge" to perform an adequate histologic examination.

Heart Valves

For years, almost all valvular heart disease has been ascribed to chronic rheumatic heart disease. As a result, excised heart valves are among the most neglected specimens in the surgical pathology laboratory. Failure to pay appropriate attention to resected valves can be a disservice to the patient. Careful examination of heart valves not only will help in the clinical management of these patients but may also help in the development of improved prosthetic heart valves.

As is true for any specimen, clinical information is essential for the appropriate classification of heart valve disease. The results of echocardiography and cardiac catheterization, as well as the surgeon's operative findings, should all be obtained before you begin your examination. Although there is some overlap, the examination of native, mechanical, and bioprosthetic heart valves each presents unique challenges.

Native Heart Valves

Although we tend to think of heart valves as consisting only of the valve leaflets, remember the other components of the valve. The atrioventricular valves (mitral and tricuspid) are composed of an annulus, leaflets, chordae tendineae, and papillary muscles. The semilunar valves (the aortic and pulmonic) are made up of three cusps, each with a sinus. These cusps meet at three commissures. Remembering these basic components of each valve is essential, because, although some native heart valves can be removed intact by the surgeon, the majority are fragmented during removal.

Before handling an excised valve, check to see if cultures are needed. In addition, a photograph of the inflow and outflow aspects of a valve can help document the cause of the disease. Similarly, a radiograph of the specimen may help establish the extent and distribution of calcifications. Begin by documenting whether the valve is in one piece or is fragmented. Note the dimensions of the valve as well as the dimensions of the valve orifice. Next, systematically examine each component of the valve. Start with the leaflets. Count and record the number of leaflets. Note the edges of the leaflets, and look for any evidence of rolling or commissural fusion. Next, examine the leaflets themselves. Document the presence or absence of myxoid changes, fibrosis, calcifications, thrombi, and vegetations. If the leaflets are fibrotic, are they diffusely or focally involved? If calcifications or thrombi are present, document their location, size, and apparent impact on valve function. If vegetations are noted, are they friable or firm? Next, for atrioventricular valves, examine the chordae tendineae and papillary muscles. Are the chordae normal, or are they shortened, thickened, stretched, fused, or ruptured? Are the papillary muscles normal, or is there evidence of recent or remote myocardial infarction? If a portion of the annulus is present, examine it as well. Once you have completed your gross description, submit a section for histology. The section should include the valve leaflet, the free edge of the valve, and if present the chordae and papillary muscle. It may be necessary to decalcify this section.

Mechanical Heart Valves

Numerous different types of mechanical heart valves have been developed over the years. The majority of these valves have three main components (1) a cloth ring, which is used by the surgeon to sew the valve in place; (2) an occluder or poppet (ball or disk); and (3) components that limit the movement of the poppet or allow the occluder to tilt. Despite the similarities, the various types of mechanical heart valves have several important differences, and different valves are prone to different complications. Therefore, before beginning your examination of a mechanical heart valve, we recommend that you identify the type of valve by referring to a valve identification guide such as "Cardiac Valve Identification

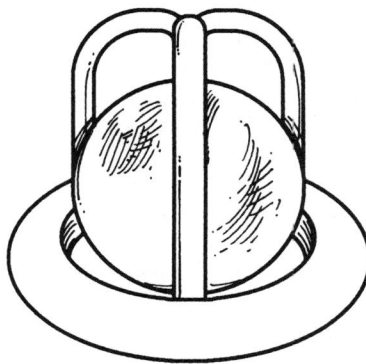

Starr-Edwards
(Ball-in-cage mechanical)

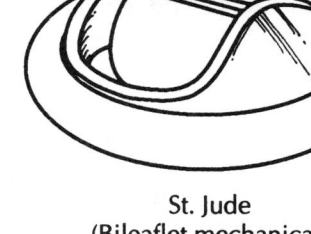

St. Jude
(Bileaflet mechanical)

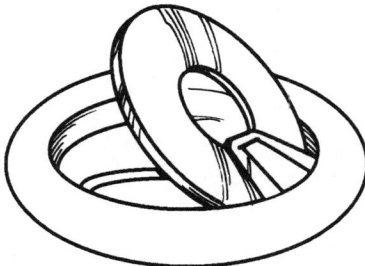

Bjork-Shiley
(Monoleaflet mechanical)

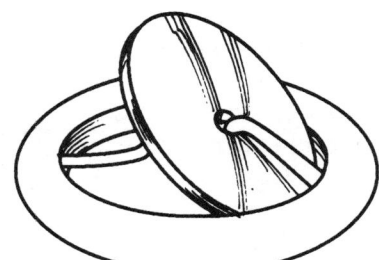

Medtronic-Hall
(Monoleaflet mechanical)

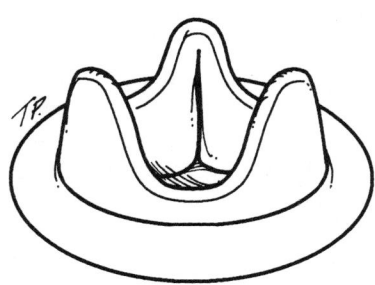

Carpentier-Edwards and
Hancock porcine
(Tissue valves)

Common Prosthetic Cardiac Valves

1. Identify the type of valve.
2. Look for, document the presence of, and sample for histology any thrombi, vegetations, or fibrous tissue proliferations.
3. Document the movement of the valve.
4. Examine and document the condition of each component of the valve: (1) the valve ring, (2) the occluder or poppet, and (3) components that limit the movement of the poppet or allow the occluder to tilt.
5. *Save the valve.* It's the law.

Atlas and Guide," in *Guide to Prosthetic Cardiac Valves*.[5] Examples of some of the more common types of mechanical and bioprosthetic valves are illustrated here.

Next, the valve can be cultured, photographed, and x-rayed as indicated. Try out the movement of the valve. Does the valve apparatus open and close fully? Thrombi can form at the junction of the various components of the valve, especially at cloth-metal interfaces. These thrombi are important to identify, because they can be a source of emboli or a nidus for the development of an infection, and they may interfere with valve function. Document the location and size of any thrombi or vegetations, and note whether they interfere with valve function. Some valves incite an intense overgrowth of fibrous tissue, and this fibrous tissue can cause valve dysfunction and even luminal stenosis. Therefore, it is important to note the presence or absence of fibrous tissue. Finally, carefully look for evidence of wear and tear on the various mechanical components of the valve. Is there any evidence of cracking or disk wear? As is true for natural heart valves, the effect of any pathology on valve function should be carefully documented. In most cases, it is not possible to submit any tissue for histologic examination; but if vegetations are present, a section should be submitted for histology. In the United States, the U.S. Safe Medical Devices Act of 1990 (Public Law 101-629) requires you to notify either the manufacturer or the Food and Drug Administration if you discover that a malfunctioning prosthetic valve has contributed to the harm or death of a patient. Finally, as is true for all mechanical devices removed surgically, be sure to save the valve because it may need to be returned to the manufacturer.

Bioprosthetic Heart Valves

A variety of bioprosthetic heart valves are used. These include (1) porcine aortic valves, (2) bovine and pericardial valves, and (3) human aortic homographs. As is true for the native and mechanical heart valves, the first step should be to ask yourself if the valve needs to be cultured, photographed, or x-rayed. Next, carefully inspect the valve leaflets for thrombi, vegetations, calcifications, and evidence of fibrous overgrowth. In particular, look for evidence of tears or perforations in the valve leaflets. Again, make sure to document both the location and size of any lesions and to describe the effect of these lesions on valve function. If a sewing ring is present, be sure to examine it as well.

Left Ventricular Assist Devices

Examination of left ventricular assist devices requires special tools that may need to be provided by the manufacturer. In general, a pump is connected to conduits that contain artificial valves (usually bioprostheses), which in turn connect to the left ventricular apex and the aorta. These devices can become infected, and it is the responsibility of the pathologist to make every attempt to document any sites of infection. One should document the presence or absence of thrombi or vegetations in the diverse parts in contact with blood. The anastomotic sites to the left ventricle and the aorta should be described and sampled for histologic examination. As is true for any prosthetic device, document any identifying numbers or labels and place the device in a "permanent save" area.

Pacemakers and Defibrillators

Recording the serial number of the pacemaker or defibrillator is the first step. These numbers are usually easy to find when the fibrous sac of tissue surrounding the device is incised. On gross examination, the important things to document are the extent of adhesions on the leads and the location of the active interface of these devices (i.e., the electrode tips) within the heart. Rarely, these devices show infected vegetations. Submit representative sections of any adherent fibrous tissue. Again, as was true for left ventricular assist devices, the device should be placed in a "permanent save" area.

Important Issues to Address in Your Surgical Pathology Report on Heart Valves

Native Heart Valves

- How many leaflets are present?
- Do the leaflets show evidence of fusion, myxoid change, fibrosis, calcification, thrombi, or vegetations?

- Do the chordae show evidence of shortening, thickening, stretching, fusion, or rupture?
- Are the papillary muscles infarcted?
- Do any of these changes appear to have an impact on valve function?

Mechanical and Bioprosthetic Valves

- What type of valve is it?
- Is there evidence of thrombi, fibrous tissue overgrowth, wear and tear, or mechanical failure?
- Is the valve function compromised?

Arteries and Veins

The examination of arteries and veins is straightforward, particularly if one remembers the three layers of each: the intima, media, and adventitia. Measure the length and external and internal diameters of the vessel. Examine the lumen for thrombi, examine the intima for evidence of intimal proliferations such as atherosclerosis, and document the percentage of luminal narrowing caused by any lesions. Examine the media for evidence of aneurysm formation or fibromuscular hyperplasia. Take sections that are both longitudinal and perpendicular to the long axis of the vessel. The longitudinal sections will be particularly helpful in demonstrating alterations involving the media, and the perpendicular sections can demonstrate the effect of any lesion on the luminal diameter.

Temporal Artery Biopsies

Biopsies are occasionally taken of the temporal artery in cases for which temporal arteritis is suspected. These biopsies need to be carefully and thoroughly examined, at multiple levels, for focal disease. The average biopsy is about 12 mm long. Cut it into four pieces, each about 3 mm long, and have the laboratory embed each piece on end. We like to get four sets of step sections through the block, each set containing three hematoxylin and eosin stained sections, one elastin stained section (Verhoeff's/van Gieson's), and one unstained section. Thus, one temporal artery biopsy produces at least 16 slides to examine.

20 Lungs

General Comments

Pathologists are routinely called on to process a diverse spectrum of lung specimens, ranging in size and complexity from minute biopsies to pneumonectomies. Despite this diversity, these specimens can be systematically approached by keeping in mind the five basic components of the lung specimen: the airways, the lung parenchyma, the pleura, the vessels, and the lymph nodes.

Before beginning the dissection, be sure to ask yourself two questions: First, does the pathology need to be revealed immediately? For example, if an infection is suspected, cultures may have to be taken from fresh tissues in a sterile fashion. Likewise, in the case of a suspected neoplasm, frozen section evaluation may be required to establish a diagnosis or to assess resection margins, and sampling of fresh tissue may be needed for ancillary diagnostic studies, such as electron microscopy. Next, ask which method of dissection will most effectively reveal the pathologic process and best demonstrate the relationship of the disease to the surrounding lung and pleura. There is more than one way to dissect a lung, and the method of sectioning is often dictated by the type of specimen, the suspected nature of the pathologic process, and the size and location of the pathologic process. Clearly, the more clinical information that is available, including radiographic findings, the more effectively these questions can be answered. Finally, keep in mind that a wealth of information can be obtained simply by palpating the intact specimen. Even small focal lesions can be appreciated by palpation, and this fast and easy method of examination should become a routine part of the initial evaluation of any lung resection.

Limited Pulmonary Resections

Limited pulmonary resections include open lung biopsies and wedge resections for both neoplastic and non-neoplastic diseases. These specimens are generally taken from the periphery of the lung. As illustrated, they usually are wedge-shaped pieces of lung tissue invested by visceral pleura. Because of their small size and peripheral location, lymph nodes and major bronchi are usually not present. Surgical staple lines may be present, and these represent the parenchymal resection margins. Document the dimensions of the specimen and the appearance of the pleural surface. If clinically indicated, fresh tissue can be harvested for microbial cultures and for immunofluorescence. If immediate dissection is not required, however, fix the specimen before proceeding with the dissection. Fixation in distention can be accomplished by gently infusing formalin directly into the lung parenchyma at several sites through a small-gauge needle. Take care not to overdistend the specimen. Submerge the distended specimen in formalin until it is well fixed. Following fixation, trim the staple lines from the specimen. Be careful not to remove too much lung tissue with these staples, because the exposed lung parenchyma immediately adjacent to the staples represents a surgical margin. Dry and ink the exposed parenchymal margin, and then serially section the specimen in a plane perpendicular to that of the parenchymal resection margin.

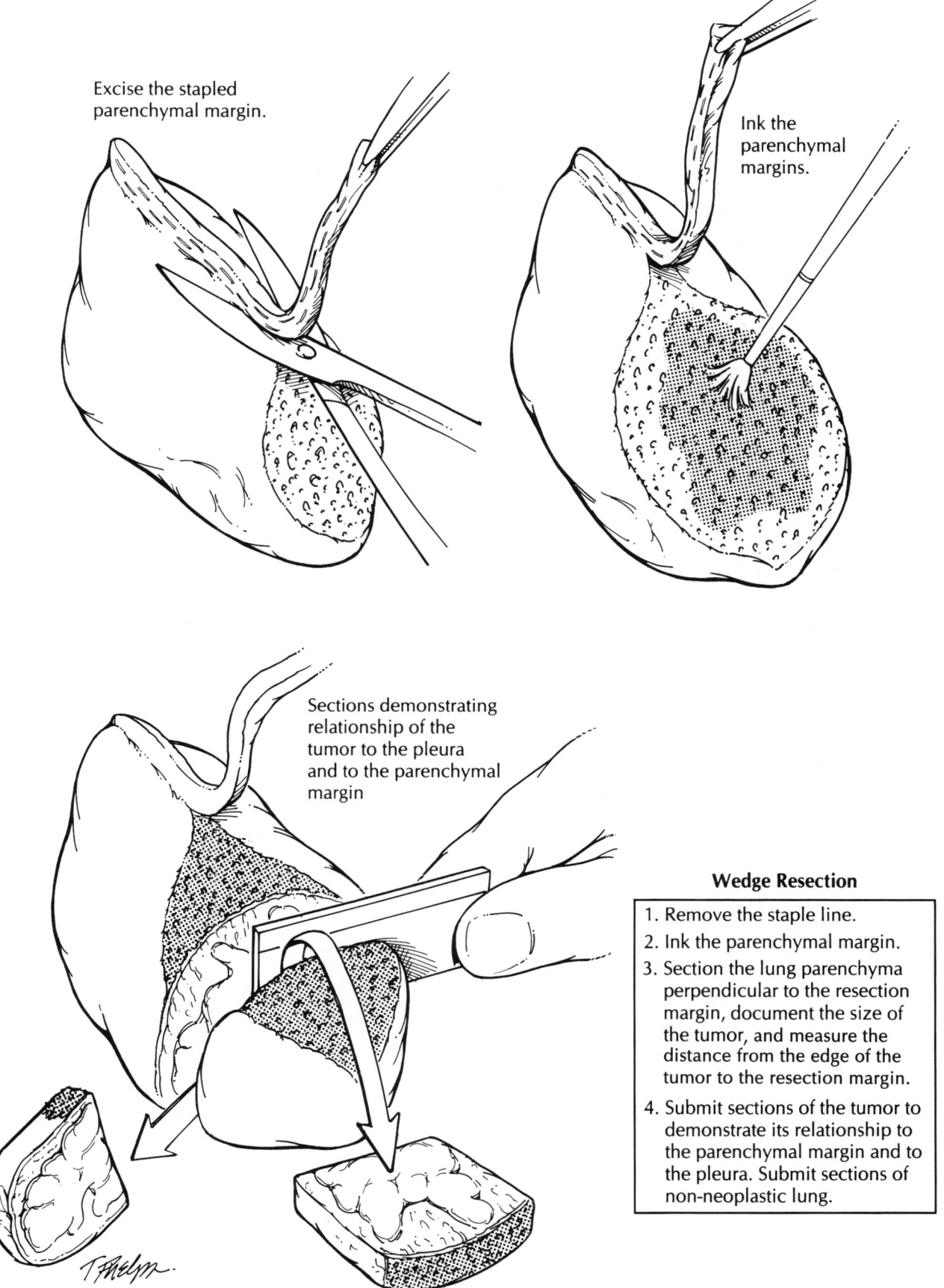

Excise the stapled parenchymal margin.

Ink the parenchymal margins.

Sections demonstrating relationship of the tumor to the pleura and to the parenchymal margin

Wedge Resection

1. Remove the staple line.
2. Ink the parenchymal margin.
3. Section the lung parenchyma perpendicular to the resection margin, document the size of the tumor, and measure the distance from the edge of the tumor to the resection margin.
4. Submit sections of the tumor to demonstrate its relationship to the parenchymal margin and to the pleura. Submit sections of non-neoplastic lung.

After sectioning the specimen, evaluate the lung for focal and diffuse processes, and describe these findings. For neoplasms, note the size of the tumor, the appearance of its cut surface, and the relationship of the tumor to the pleura and to the surrounding lung parenchyma. Note also the distance from the edge of the tumor to the resection margin. Submit one to four sections of the lesion (depending on its size), selecting sections that demonstrate the tumor's relationship to the pleura, to adjacent lung tissue, and to the parenchymal resection margin. Sample the parenchymal margin, using perpendicular sections when the tumor closely approaches the margin. In addition, submit two sections of non-neoplastic lung. Intrapulmonary lymph nodes and bronchi will generally not be present in these peripheral lung biopsies, but if they are present, they should be sampled.

For non-neoplastic lung diseases, submit the vast majority of the specimen for histologic evaluation. In selected instances, a representative section should be fresh-frozen, especially if immunofluorescence studies are needed to establish a diagnosis. Note the size of the airspaces, the patency of any airways that are present, and the crepitance of the parenchyma. Only rarely should intraoperative frozen section consultations be performed for non-neoplastic lung disease.

Lobectomies and Pneumonectomies

The largest lung specimens consist of lobectomies and pneumonectomies. These procedures are usually done to remove neoplasms, although pneumonectomies for non-neoplastic lung disease are encountered in some medical centers performing lung transplantations (see Chapter 21). When a tumor directly invades beyond the pleura, these specimens may also include an en bloc resection of the involved adjacent structures (e.g., chest wall, left atrium, or diaphragm).

Weigh, measure, and anatomically orient the specimen while it is fresh. One quick and easy way to orient the specimen is to inspect the structures at the lung hilum. On the left side the pulmonary artery is situated superior to the airway, while on the right side it is situated anterior to the airway. Also, the right side has three lobes, whereas the left side has two and a prominent lingular segment. Carefully inspect the pleural surfaces. Look for the presence of pleural retraction, because this finding suggests the presence of an underlying neoplasm. Palpate the intact specimen: Is the tumor located centrally or peripherally? Which lobe of the lung appears to be involved? Does the tumor extend across a fissure to involve more than one lobe?

The lung may be processed in either the fresh or the fixed state. If immediate dissection of the specimen is not required, it is best to fix the specimen in distention. Infuse formalin directly into the large airways, and submerge the entire specimen in formalin for overnight fixation. Take care not to overdistend the lung.

If you remember each of the five basic components of the lung (airways, lymph nodes, vessels, parenchyma, and pleura), then your description and dissection can be carried out in a simple and systematic fashion. Many proximal lung tumors arise from the airways, and so we find it most helpful to start the dissection with the airways. Begin by removing the bronchial and vascular margins as shave sections. Next, expose the bronchial mucosa by opening the large airways out to the subsegmental branches with small scissors. Carefully examine the mucosa of the airways, because subtle changes in the appearance of the mucosa may indicate a premalignant lesion. Similarly, open the large pulmonary vessels and evaluate them for invasion by tumor.

By dissecting the larger airways, you have opportunely exposed the regional lymph nodes, and these should be sampled at this time. Direct the search for lymph nodes to the soft tissues at the hilum and to the lung parenchyma immediately surrounding the airways. Lymph nodes are often easily visualized by their black (anthracotic) pigmentation. It is generally not necessary to further designate these peribronchial lymph nodes. The status of the various mediastinal lymph node groups is crucial to the staging of lung tumors. These lymph node groups are usually separately submitted and labeled by the surgeon, although pneumonectomies may be accompanied by attached hilar lymph nodes. Such lymph nodes should be identified by their location in the hilum of the lung and specifically designated "hilar lymph nodes."

Section the lung parenchyma in the plane that best reveals the pathologic process and its relationship to the surrounding structures of the lung. For proximal lung tumors, this relationship can best be demonstrated by sectioning the lung along the plane of the involved airways. As illustrated, this can be accomplished by first placing probes into the airways that have already been partially opened and then using these probes to help guide your knife through the lung parenchyma. In this manner, one can determine the origin and size of proximal tumors and evaluate the lung parenchyma distal to the tumor. The remaining lung parenchyma can then be sectioned at 1-cm intervals. For peripherally located tumors, a site of origin from an airway may not be apparent. In these instances, serial sections through the tumor perpendicular to the closest segmental bronchus may best reveal the relationships of the tumor to the pleura, to the surrounding lung parenchyma, and to the small airways.

For non-neoplastic lung diseases, section the specimen in a manner that best correlates with the radiographic studies. For example, thin serial sections of the fixed specimen in the transverse plane can be used to arrive at a one-to-one correlation between changes identified in computed tomography scans and the pathology. In the description of these large lung specimens, do not lose sight of the systematic approach that includes descriptions of all five basic components of the lung.

For specimens that harbor a neoplasm, the major aims of tissue sampling for histology are to document the tumor type, the origin of the tumor, the extent of the tumor (local and metastatic), and the adequacy of tumor resection. To assess tumor type, submit four sections of tumor, both from the center of the tumor and from the interface of the tumor with the surrounding lung tissue. Make every effort to demonstrate the relationship of the tumor to an associated airway. For more proximal tumors with an apparent endobronchial component, take sections along the involved airway to include both tumor and bronchus. For peripheral lesions, a site of origin from a small airway may not be apparent. In these cases, take sections through the tumor in a plane perpendicular to the airways. Document tumor extension to or through the pleura with sections taken at right angles to the pleura in areas of retraction. Similarly, take sections of tumor extension into the pulmonary vessels, hilar soft tissues, and chest wall. Submit all lymph nodes identified in the hilar and peribronchial regions. If the specimen also contains a portion of chest wall, take sections and margins from all of the attached structures (parietal pleura, skin, soft tissues, and ribs), as if this block were its own specimen. Finally, submit sections of non-neoplastic lung from each lobe, including sections taken distal to the tumor for documentation of an obstructive pneumonic process.

For diffuse non-neoplastic processes, submit representative sections of lung parenchyma from each lobe as well as sections of proximal airways. If a focal lesion is encountered, section it in the manner described above for a neoplasm.

Pleural Resections for Malignant Mesotheliomas

The diagnosis of malignant mesothelioma is usually established on the basis of cytologic material or small incisional biopsies. Rarely, malignant mesotheliomas are resected in an attempt to obtain a surgical cure. For tumors arising in the chest, these specimens generally consist of lung with en bloc removal of any adjacent involved mesothelium-lined structures such as the parietal pleura of the chest wall, the pericardium, and the diaphragm. These specimens can generally be handled using the same principles guiding the dissection of other lung specimens, as detailed above. When it comes to malignant mesotheliomas, however, a few points warrant special emphasis.

1. Immunohistochemistry and electron microscopy have become important adjuncts to routine microscopic evaluation in the diagnosis and classification of malignant mesothelioma. For lung specimens with pleura-based tumors, always consider the possibility of a malignant mesothelioma, and process a small portion of the tumor for electron microscopy should this modality be needed to establish the diagnosis.

2. Because of the variable and sometimes deceptively bland histopathologic appearance of maligant mesotheliomas, the diagnosis and classification are aided by ample sectioning for histologic evaluation. Suspected malignant mesotheliomas should be sampled much more extensively than the conventional lung carcinoma. For smaller lesions, submit the tumor in its entirety. For large lesions, submit at least one section per centimeter of tumor.

3. Depending on the extent of tumor involvement along mesothelium-lined surfaces, these resections may be anatomically complex. Do not

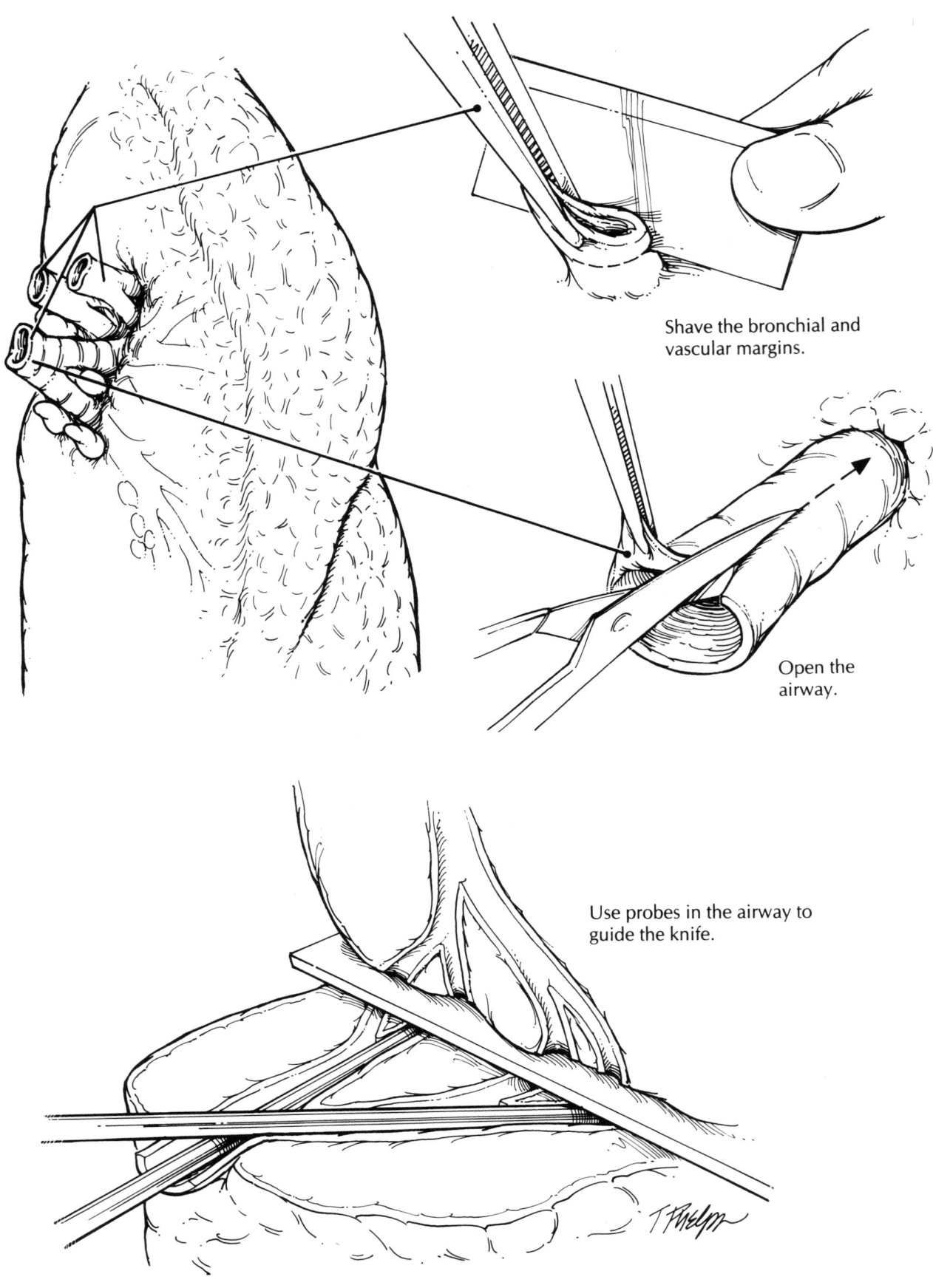

Shave the bronchial and vascular margins.

Open the airway.

Use probes in the airway to guide the knife.

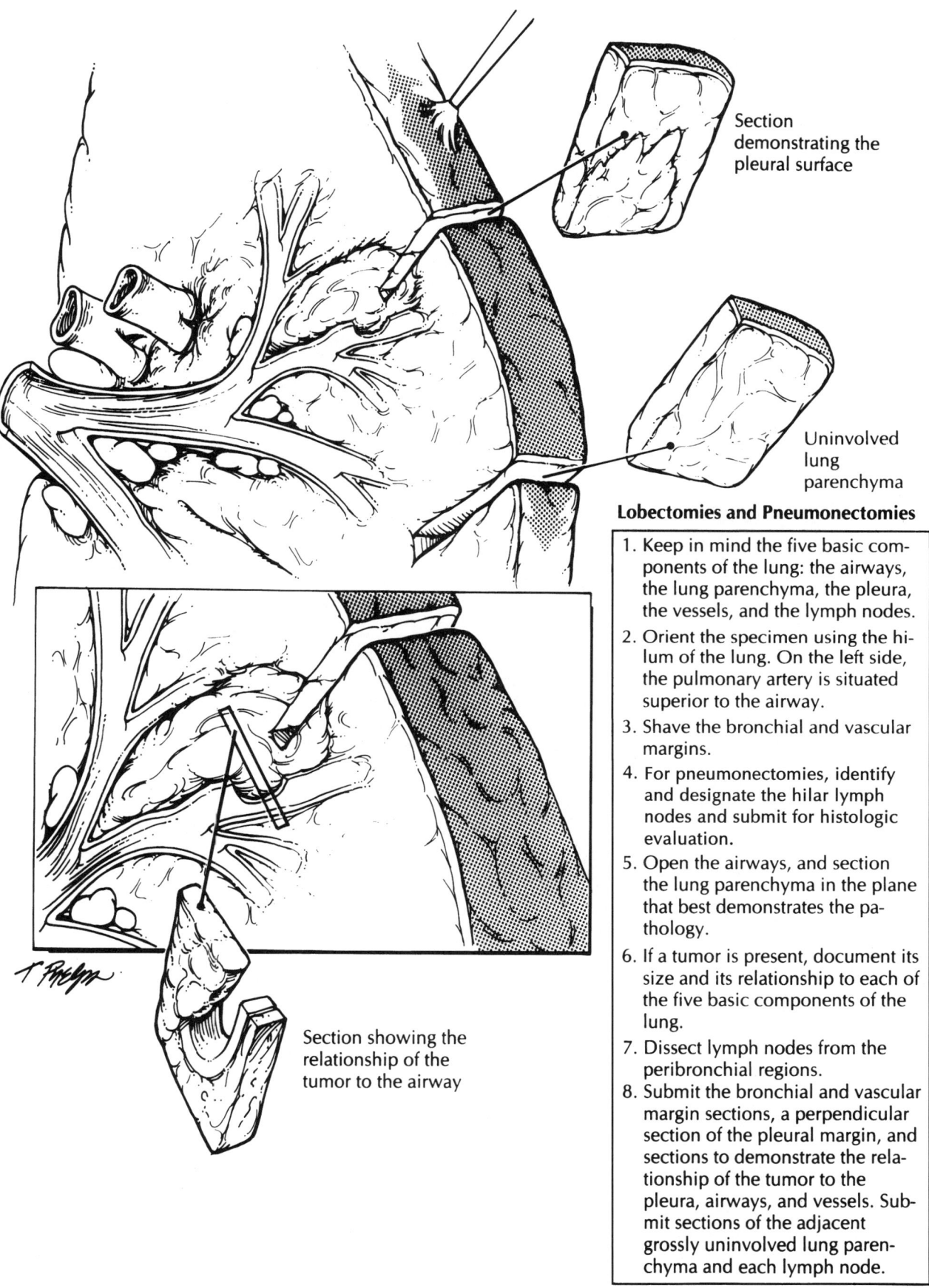

Section demonstrating the pleural surface

Uninvolved lung parenchyma

Section showing the relationship of the tumor to the airway

Lobectomies and Pneumonectomies

1. Keep in mind the five basic components of the lung: the airways, the lung parenchyma, the pleura, the vessels, and the lymph nodes.
2. Orient the specimen using the hilum of the lung. On the left side, the pulmonary artery is situated superior to the airway.
3. Shave the bronchial and vascular margins.
4. For pneumonectomies, identify and designate the hilar lymph nodes and submit for histologic evaluation.
5. Open the airways, and section the lung parenchyma in the plane that best demonstrates the pathology.
6. If a tumor is present, document its size and its relationship to each of the five basic components of the lung.
7. Dissect lymph nodes from the peribronchial regions.
8. Submit the bronchial and vascular margin sections, a perpendicular section of the pleural margin, and sections to demonstrate the relationship of the tumor to the pleura, airways, and vessels. Submit sections of the adjacent grossly uninvolved lung parenchyma and each lymph node.

rush through the dissection. Instead, take the time necessary to orient the specimen, identify all structures present, document the extent of tumor spread, and locate each margin (e.g., bronchus, pulmonary vessels, chest wall, diaphragm) for histologic evaluation.

4. Submit additional sections of uninvolved lung, and evaluate them for the presence of ferruginous bodies, pleural plaques, and interstitial fibrosis.

Important Issues to Address in Your Surgical Pathology Report on Lung Resections

- What procedure was performed, and what structures/organs are present?
- Is a neoplasm present?
- How large is the tumor, and where is it located?
- What are the histologic type and grade of the tumor?
- Does the tumor infiltrate the large airways, pleura, or vessels?
- What is the status of each of the margins (parenchymal, vascular, and bronchial)?
- Does the tumor involve the lobar or mainstem bronchi?
- Is there any evidence of metastatic disease? Record the number of lymph nodes examined and the number of lymph node metastases. If nodal involvement is only by direct extension, this feature should be noted.
- Is there any pathology in the non-neoplastic lung (e.g., granulomas, postobstructive pneumonia)?

21 Transplantation

With the introduction of cyclosporine during the 1980s, transplantation has emerged as an effective therapy for a large number of patients with severe kidney, heart, lung, liver, and hematopoietic diseases. As the transplant population grows, surgical pathologists will encounter an increasing number of specimens from transplant recipients. These surgical pathologists play a pivotal role in the multidisciplinary management of transplant recipients. Although much of the approach to handling specimens from transplant recipients is covered in each chapter on specific organ systems, there are some unique aspects specific to the handling of specimens from transplant recipients that deserve special note.

Handling a specimen from a transplant recipient is in many ways guided by an understanding of the complications associated with transplantation. It is therefore useful to keep in mind the pathology unique to transplantation when handling a biopsy or resection specimen from a transplant recipient. These unique situations include (1) Complications related to the primary disease for which the transplant was performed. Specifically, samples must be handled in a way that allows one to diagnose recurrence of the patient's underlying pathology. For example, although electron microscopy and immunofluorescence are generally not helpful for establishing a diagnosis of acute renal allograft rejection, they can be essential for establishing the diagnosis of a recurrent glomerular disease. (2) Complications of the surgical procedure itself. For example, arterial stenosis in the donor segment of an artery is often due to accelerated graft arteriosclerosis (chronic rejection), whereas stricture at the anastomotic site may be related to the surgery. (3) Complications of acute rejection. Acute rejection can develop rapidly and have a devastating impact on the graft and patient survival. Biopsies from transplant recipients are therefore often rushed. Failure to recognize the urgent nature of most transplant biopsies can result in delayed therapy, which can have a devastating impact on patient management. (4) Infectious complications. Infections in transplant recipients are remarkable for the diversity and multiplicity of the organisms involved. Multiple cultures and the up-front ordering of special stains to detect a variety of infectious agents (fungi, bacteria, viruses) are often indicated. (5) Complications related to the patient's clinical treatment. In addition to a host of immunosuppressive agents, transplant recipients are often treated with a variable pharmacopoeia of drugs. They can cause a host of pathologies that may mimic or be superimposed on rejection. The appropriate management of a specimen from a transplant recipient therefore includes a thorough understanding of the patient's clinical history, including a detailed record of the medications the patient is receiving.

In addition to these five general considerations, there are a number of organ-specific guidelines for handling surgical pathology specimens from transplant recipients. These guidelines are frequently updated; as of January 2003, they included the following.

Heart. The International Society for Heart and Lung Transplantation (ISHLT) established a "working formulation" for grading heart allograft rejection in 1990.[4] This working formulation includes a number of technical considerations. Because acute allograft rejection can be focal, the ISHLT standard grading system requires four to six undivided pieces of myocardium. The individual handling these biopsy specimens should document the number of pieces received. The tissue should be fixed in 10% buffered formalin and paraffin-embedded. Once processed, a minimum of three step levels should be prepared through the block with at least three sections per level. The slides should be stained routinely with hematoxylin and eosin and one slide stained with a connective tissue stain such as a Masson's trichrome. In addition, during the first 6 weeks after transplantation at least one piece should be placed in OCT and fresh-frozen for possible immunofluorescence examination to rule out antibody-mediated rejection.

Kidney. The "Banff" criteria for grading renal allograft rejection were established in 1991.[6] These criteria have been periodically modified, and the current Banff '97 guidelines provide specific recommendations for the handling of biopsy specimens from renal transplant recipients.[7] The recommendation is that seven slides be prepared containing multiple sequential sections. Three of the seven should be stained with hematoxylin and eosin, three with periodic acid–Schiff or silver stains, and one with a trichrome stain. It is also recommended that these sections be prepared at 3 to 4 μm.

Lung. In 1996 the ISHLT presented a revision of the 1990 working formulation for the grading of lung allograft rejection.[8] This revision included the following recommendations for handling transplant lung biopsies from lung transplant recipients. At a minimum, sections of three levels should be stained with hematoxylin and eosin. In addition, one level should be stained with a connective tissue stain to evaluate the biopsy for the presence of submucosal fibrosis associated with the development of bronchiolitis obliterans, and one level should be silver stained for fungi/ *Pneumocystis*. In addition, the ISHLT group emphasized that all biopsy specimens should be studied by pathologists with full knowledge of the native recipient disease and the results of the last biopsy and current bronchioloalveolar lavage.

Liver. The Banff system for grading liver allograft rejection was presented in 1997.[9] Their recommendations included that at least two hematoxylin and eosin-stained sections from at least two levels should be prepared from each needle core biopsy.

The criteria for evaluating transplant biopsy specimens for rejection are beyond the scope of this book, but there are some centralized resources. For example, the University of Pittsburgh's website contains both the current diagnostic criteria and standardized templates for evaluating biopsies from transplant recipients (http://tpis.upmc.edu/).

Important Issues to Address in Your Surgical Pathology Report on Transplant Biopsies

- Evidence of recurrence of a patient's primary or underlying disease
- Any complications related to the transplant procedure itself
- Degree of rejection (both acute and chronic)
- Presence of any infections
- Presence of any neoplasms, particularly post-transplant lymphoproliferative disease
- Presence of any complications related to therapy (drug toxicity)
- When appropriate sampling has not occurred, it is essential to note in the pathology report that the biopsy findings may not be fully representative of the changes in the graft.

VI Bone, Soft Tissue, and Skin

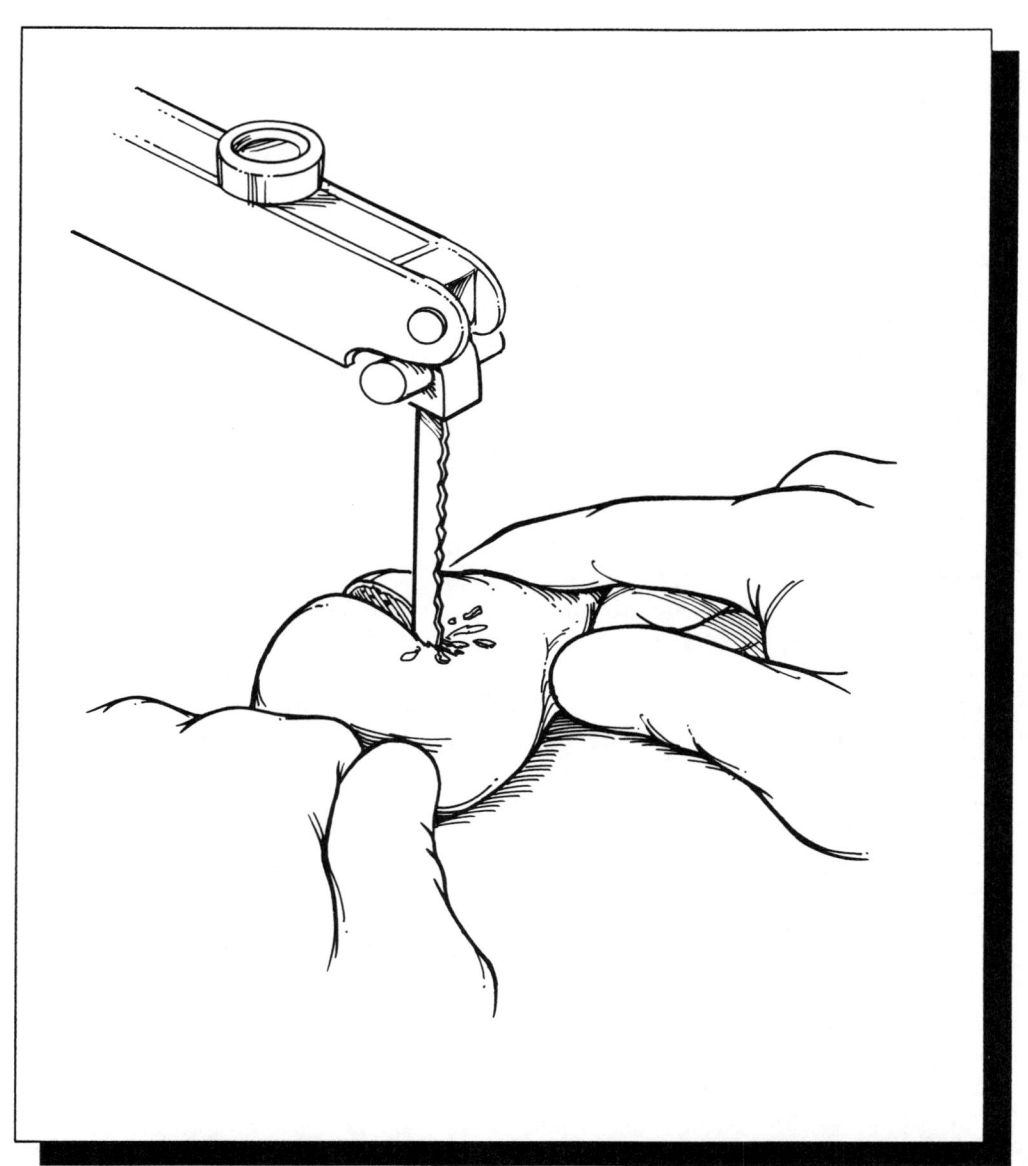

22 Bone

Edward F. McCarthy, Jr., M.D.

General Comments

The hardness of bone introduces three challenges that are unique to the dissection of bone specimens: (1) Many lesions involving bone are not easily appreciated simply by palpating and inspecting the intact specimen. This inability to pinpoint the lesion may frustrate attempts to demonstrate its size and location when cutting the bone specimen. (2) Bone specimens cannot be easily dissected and sampled with standard knives and scalpels. (3) Since the microtome blade also cannot penetrate bone, bone cannot easily be sectioned in the histology laboratory. Fortunately, each of these obstacles can be overcome. Specimen radiographs (Table 22-1) allow one to visualize the extent and location of the pathologic process so that the specimen can be cut in the proper plane; appropriate saws (Table 22-2) allow one to cut bone without destroying the specimen; and finally, special solutions (Table 22-3) can demineralize bone making it easier to section for microscopic evaluation. Thus, the successful dissection of bone specimens requires that the prosector master the use of radiography, special techniques, instruments, and a variety of chemical solutions.

Small Bone Fragments

Whether dealing with bone biopsies, currettings, or the removal of small bones, there is always the danger of overdecalcifying the tissue. Efforts to minimize the time in decalcification solution and to separate out tissue fragments that do not require decalcification will reap great rewards when evaluating these tissues microscopically. When it is necessary to cut a bone fragment before processing, orient and cut the bone to show as much surface as possible. For example, small tubular bones such as metatarsals or ribs should be cut longitudinally rather than in cross section. When articular cartilage is present, sections should be taken to show its relationship to cortical bone. For specimens consisting of multiple pieces of tissue, soft tissues should be separated from bone and processed routinely in formalin without decalcification, while pieces of bone should be grouped in cassettes according to size and density to allow for uniform decalcification.

Large Bone Specimens

Femoral heads are the most common example of large bone specimens. They are usually removed because of either osteoarthritis or a hip fracture. Consequently, it is particularly important to identify, inspect, and sample the articular surface

TABLE 22-1. X-raying specimens.

- An ideal x-ray source is the Faxitron machine—an x-ray machine that is small enough to be kept in the surgical pathology cutting area.
- Take two radiographs of the specimen: one to show the antero-posterior view and the other to show the lateral view.
- Using the findings of the radiograph, cut the specimen in the plane that best demonstrates the lesion. For example, if the lesion is best seen in the antero-posterior view, then cut the specimen in the coronal plane.

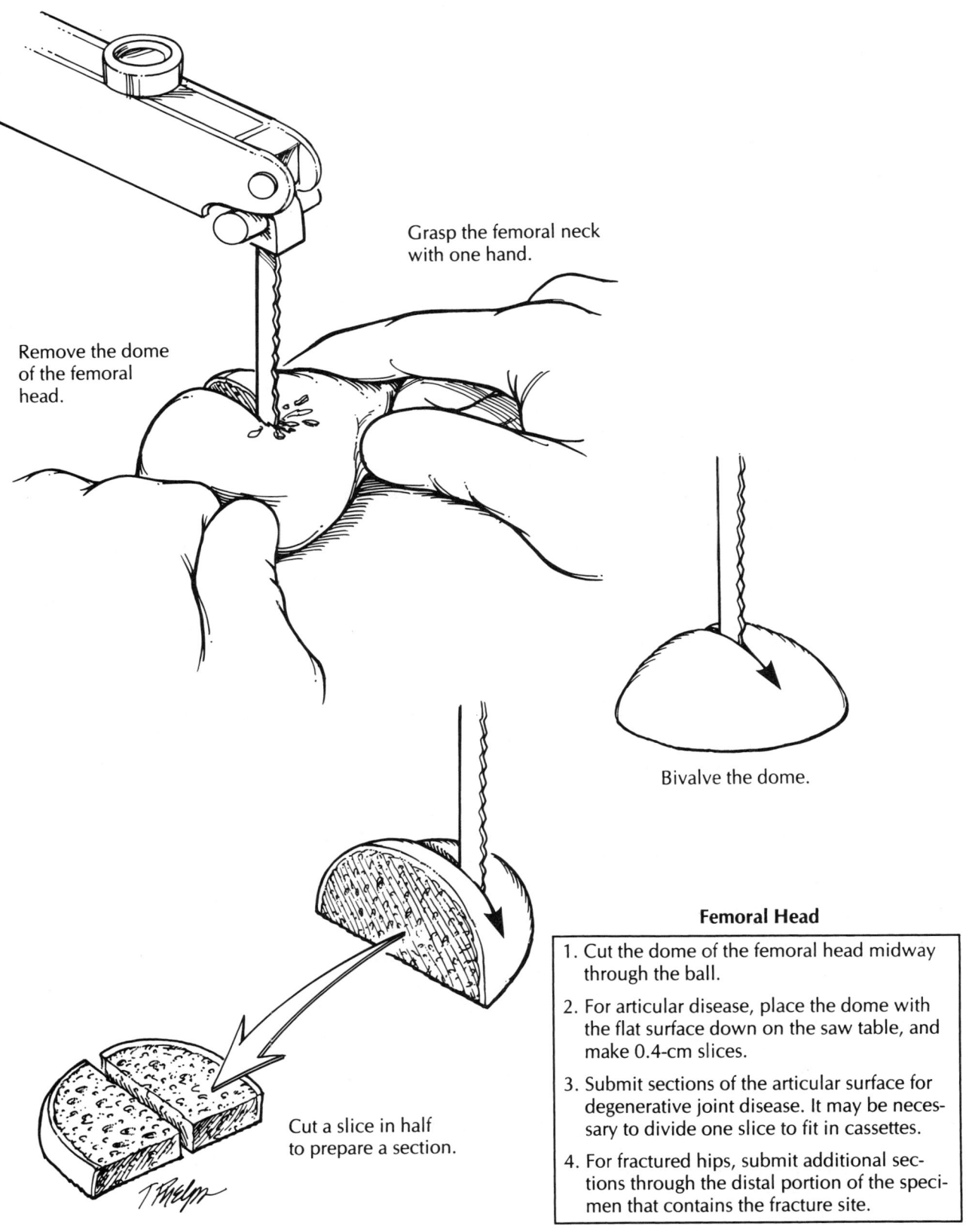

Remove the dome of the femoral head.

Grasp the femoral neck with one hand.

Bivalve the dome.

Cut a slice in half to prepare a section.

Femoral Head

1. Cut the dome of the femoral head midway through the ball.

2. For articular disease, place the dome with the flat surface down on the saw table, and make 0.4-cm slices.

3. Submit sections of the articular surface for degenerative joint disease. It may be necessary to divide one slice to fit in cassettes.

4. For fractured hips, submit additional sections through the distal portion of the specimen that contains the fracture site.

TABLE 22-2. Cutting specimens.

- Always wear eye protection.
- Choose the right saw:

Vibrating table saw	Band saw
Minimizes artifact that is due to bone dust or crushing of the tissue.	Creates bone crush and bone dust artifact.
Relatively safe.	**Dangerous!** (Keep your hands away from the blade.) Have an assistant help hold and guide the specimen.
Inadequate for very large specimens or very dense bone.	Cuts large specimens and dense bone with ease.

- Do not use the band saw to cut through soft tissues (unless the soft tissues are frozen solid).
- Cut the bone longitudinally in the plane that shows the maximum area of diseased bone.
- When serially sectioning bone, the bone slices should be of uniform thickness, not to exceed 3–4 mm.
- Remove bone dust from the cut surfaces of the specimen. Gentle rinsing with saline or water and brushing with a soft toothbrush works quite well.

and any fracture site. Measure the specimen and describe the articular cartilage, noting whether it is eroded, frayed, pitted, or absent. The presence of osteophytes should also be noted. As illustrated, separate the dome of the femoral head from the neck, then place the cut surface of the head on the table saw, and section it into 4-mm slices in a plane perpendicular to the articular cartilage. Note the density of the bone and the thickness of the cartilage. In a similar manner, serially section the femoral neck. Look for the presence of blood clot, marrow hemorrhage, or a neoplasm.

Sampling for histology should be guided by the clinical history and gross findings. For cases of osteoarthritis, sample the femoral head to show cartilage destruction and the reaction of the underlying bone. In cases of fracture, direct your attention to the fracture site; most of the sections should come from this area. Always submit at least one cassette of soft tissue including the synovial membrane and capsule.

TABLE 22-3. Decalcifying specimens.

- Fix tissues in formalin before decalcifying.
- Decalcification obscures cellular detail:
  Never decalcify a specimen over the weekend. Specimen decalcification should be monitored daily.
  If the tissue permits, submit at least one section of tumor without decalcification. This section may be more suitable for histologic evaluation and immunohistochemical analysis.
- Thin sections of uniform thickness permit a faster and more even decalcification process.

Segmental Resections and Amputations for Neoplasms

Segmental Resections

Segmental resections of bone are performed for malignant neoplasms and aggressive benign tumors. Because local recurrence is an important complication, the margins of resection need to be carefully evaluated. The soft tissue margins are best sampled while the specimen is intact and still easy to orient. After inking the soft tissue resection margin, sample the margin using perpendicular sections from those areas for which there is gross or radiologic suspicion of margin involvement (see Chapter 8 for a description of sampling margins from a complex specimen).

After soft tissue margins are sampled, decide which plane of section will best demonstrate the lesion. The radiographic findings will help guide this strategy. For the saw to cleanly pass through the bone, expose the surfaces of the bone as illustrated by cutting through and peeling back the soft tissues in this plane. Next, bisect the bone in the appropriate plane (usually the coronal plane) using a band saw. Inspect the cut surface. The extent of the lesion should then be measured and described. In addition, the presence of cortical penetration and soft tissue extension should be noted. Look for noncontiguous "skip" lesions in the medullary canal, and measure the distance from the edges of the tumor to the bone resection margin. Scoop a small amount of marrow from the end(s) of the bone, and submit this marrow as the bone margin(s).

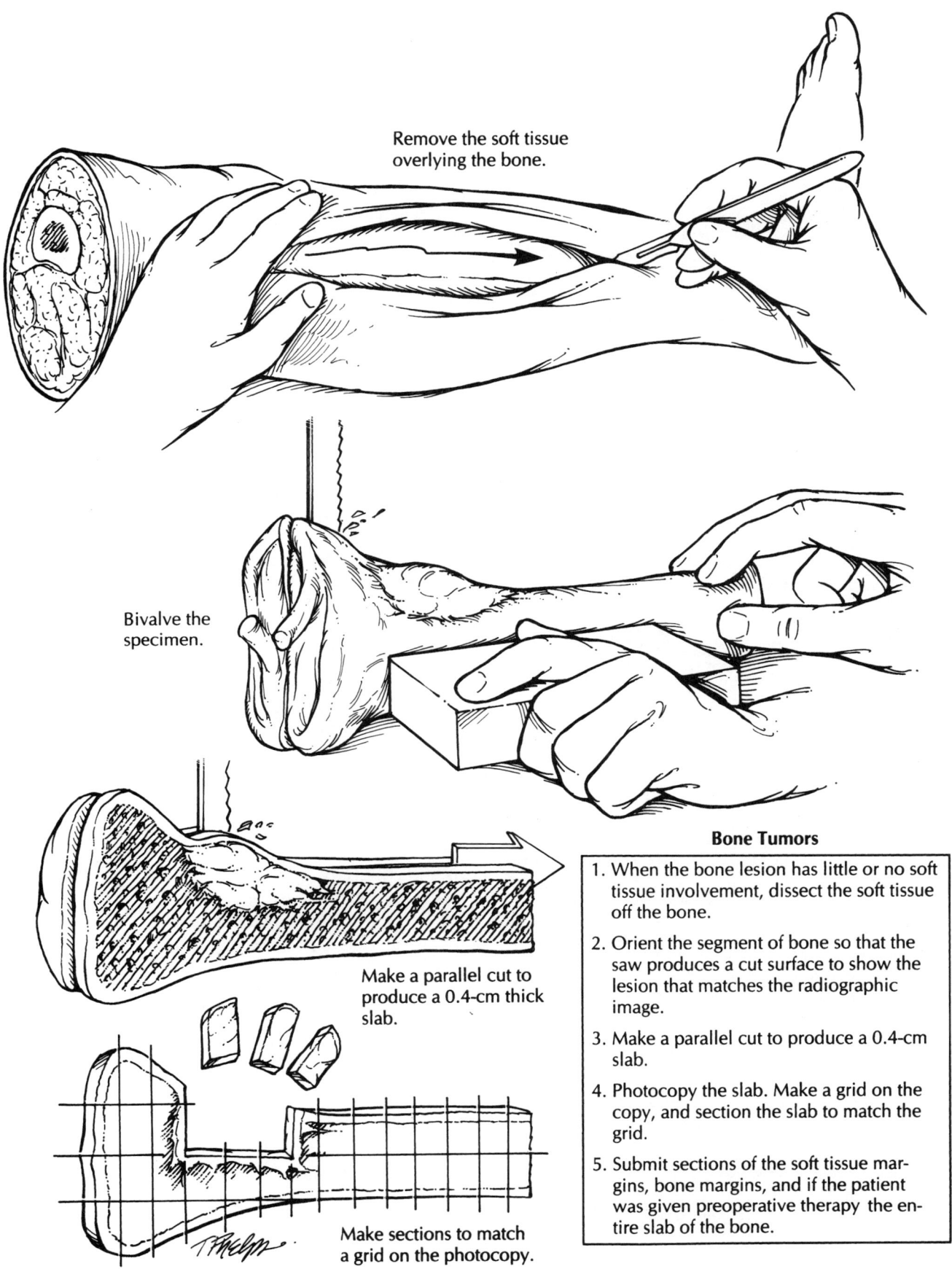

Remove the soft tissue overlying the bone.

Bivalve the specimen.

Make a parallel cut to produce a 0.4-cm thick slab.

Make sections to match a grid on the photocopy.

Bone Tumors

1. When the bone lesion has little or no soft tissue involvement, dissect the soft tissue off the bone.

2. Orient the segment of bone so that the saw produces a cut surface to show the lesion that matches the radiographic image.

3. Make a parallel cut to produce a 0.4-cm slab.

4. Photocopy the slab. Make a grid on the copy, and section the slab to match the grid.

5. Submit sections of the soft tissue margins, bone margins, and if the patient was given preoperative therapy the entire slab of the bone.

An alternative method is to freeze the entire specimen. The frozen specimen does not require removal of the soft tissues before cutting the bone. Thus, the relationship of the bone neoplasm to soft tissue spread is better preserved.

Now you are ready to cut a slab from the face of the bone cut surface. Place one half of the bisected specimen on the band saw, and cut a complete 4-mm-thick slab, then photograph and x-ray the slab. Ideally, this slab should be thin, uniform, and represent the greatest surface area of the tumor. Before sectioning the slab further, make a representation of the slab to map the precise location of each section submitted for histology. One method is to photocopy the slab and then to draw grids slightly smaller than your cassette size on the photocopy. The entire slab can then be blocked out and submitted for microscopic examination according to the grids on the photocopy.

When the patient has received neoadjuvant chemotherapy, the entire face of the slab should be evaluated microscopically to determine the percentage of tumor necrosis. When the patient has not received neoadjuvant chemotherapy, you may be more selective in the sections that you submit for histology. Important areas that should always be sampled include: (1) the intramedullary component of the neoplasm; (2) penetration of the tumor through the cortex; (3) extension of the tumor into soft tissues; (4) the interface of the tumor with normal bone; (5) involvement by the tumor of an articular surface and/or joint space; and (6) the bone margin(s).

Amputation Specimens

Although amputations for tumor appear more complex than segmental resections as a result of their size and bulk, they can be dissected along the same guidelines given for segmental resections. Indeed, after margins are sampled, the portion of the limb containing the bones and joints not involved by the neoplasm can be removed. This, in essence, converts the specimen to one that is similar to the segmental resection.

The dissection of amputations performed because of gangrene is described in Chapter 45.

Important Issues to Address in Your Surgical Pathology Report on Bone Tumors

- What procedure was performed, and what structures/organs are present?
- What type of neoplasm is present?
- What are the size and histologic grade of the neoplasm?
- If the patient received neoadjuvant chemotherapy, what is the percentage of tumor necrosis?
- Is there any cortical penetration or soft tissue invasion?
- What is the status of the soft tissue and bone margins of resection?
- Is a skip lesion present?

23 Soft Tissue, Nerves, and Muscle

Elizabeth Montgomery, M.D.

Soft Tissue

Soft tissue resections are often complex specimens containing soft tissues, skin, and sometimes even bone. The general approach to these specimens is a simple one, and it parallels that outlined for complex head and neck specimens in Chapter 8. First, identify the various components of the specimen (soft tissue, bone, and skin). Second, think of each component as a geometric shape. Third, approach each component separately. Fourth, look for relationships between any lesions and each component.

With the general approach outlined above in mind, start the dissection by orienting the specimen. Do not hesitate to ask the surgeon to help with this step. Large muscle bundles move easily relative to one another. A margin that looks close in fact may have been covered by a large bundle of muscle that has shifted. The only way to be sure that tissue has not shifted is to discuss the specimen with the surgeon. Next, make sure that you know the anatomy. The origin of a sarcoma from a nerve can be missed if one is not familiar with the anatomic location of the major nerves in the specimen. After the specimen has been oriented and the anatomy determined, identify the various components of the specimen (soft tissue, bone, skin, etc.). This step helps ensure that important components of the specimen are not left out of the dissection.

Next, measure the overall dimensions of the specimen, and document the size of each individual component. The external appearance of each component can then be described. In particular, note the size and position of any biopsy sites.

The next step is to sample the margins. The evaluation of the margins of a large complex specimen is simplified by thinking of each component of the specimen as a geometric shape. As illustrated in Chapter 8, the soft tissue can usually be thought of as a cube, the bone as a cylinder, and, if present, the skin as a square sheet. Ink the specimen, and take sections to demonstrate the margins of each of the components. It may be impractical to ink the entire specimen, but the closest margins (identified visually or by palpation) should be inked. There are usually six soft tissue margins (a cube has six sides), and these can be taken as perpendicular margins. These margins usually include the anterior, posterior, medial, lateral, inferior, and superior surfaces. Similarly, there are usually four skin margins (a square has four sides), and these can be taken as perpendicular margins. If a margin consists of a fascial layer, periosteum, or other anatomic barrier such as the diaphragm, this should be specified. The bone (the ends of a cylinder), vascular, and neural margins can be taken as parallel (shave) sections, but perpendicular rather than en face margins are suggested in general.

The specimen can now be sectioned. Determine the location and long axis of the tumor by palpating the specimen and reviewing the preoperative computed tomography (CT) scans. Section the specimen using a long sharp knife in the plane that will demonstrate the largest cross section of the tumor. Carefully document the size (try to give three dimensions), consistency, and color of the tumor. Measure twice, because size is one of the most important predictors of outcome for patients with a soft tissue tumor. It is important to document the epicenter of the tumor

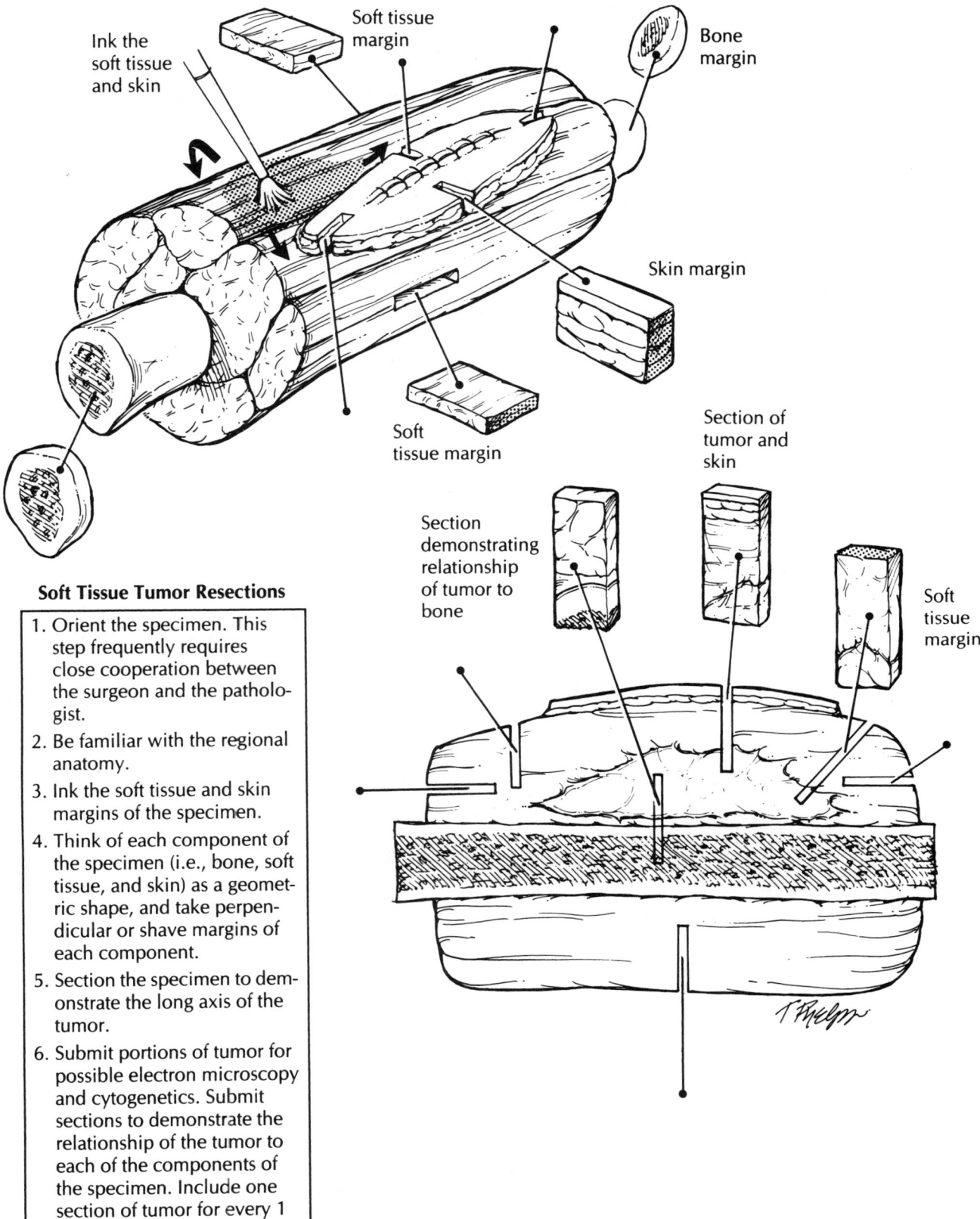

Soft Tissue Tumor Resections

1. Orient the specimen. This step frequently requires close cooperation between the surgeon and the pathologist.
2. Be familiar with the regional anatomy.
3. Ink the soft tissue and skin margins of the specimen.
4. Think of each component of the specimen (i.e., bone, soft tissue, and skin) as a geometric shape, and take perpendicular or shave margins of each component.
5. Section the specimen to demonstrate the long axis of the tumor.
6. Submit portions of tumor for possible electron microscopy and cytogenetics. Submit sections to demonstrate the relationship of the tumor to each of the components of the specimen. Include one section of tumor for every 1 cm of tumor diameter. Submit the indicated margin sections and any lymph nodes.

(e.g., dermal, subcutaneous, fascial, subfascial, intramuscular, visceral, or a combination). Also note whether the tumor is centered on or extends into major vessels, nerves, or joint spaces. These features are important for staging and for identifying the site of origin of the tumor. Also note any cysts and areas of necrosis (estimate the percent if necrosis is identified), hemorrhage, calcification, myxoid change, bone formation, or cartilage, and whether the edge of the tumor is encapsulated, pushing, or infiltrative. It may be helpful to correlate the gross appearance of the tumor with radiographic findings. For example, if calcifications are seen in a particular area of the tumor on CT scan, then that area should be identified grossly.

Next, document the distance of the tumor to each of the margins and the relationship of the tumor to each of the various components of the specimen. It is important to measure margins that are less than 2 cm from the tumor. Areas where the margins are more than 5 cm clear need not be sampled (except in cases of angiosarcoma or epithelioid sarcoma, which are prone to subclinical satellite spread). Document the number of lymph nodes present, and sample each for histology. Lymph nodes may not be included, as only a small number of sarcoma types are likely to have lymph node deposits (e.g., angiosarcoma, epithelioid sarcoma, synovial sarcoma, clear cell sarcoma).

Finally, the tumor itself can be sampled. First, submit a representative piece in glutaraldehyde for possible electron microscopy. Next, as clinically indicated, submit fresh tissue for cytogenetics or other special studies. These studies may be particularly important in the pediatric patient (see Chapter 39). Finally, submit sections for routine histology. These should include sections that demonstrate the relationship of the tumor to each component of the specimen, sections that demonstrate the relationship of the tumor to the closest margins, and sections from any foci within the tumor that look different from other areas of the tumor. A useful rule of thumb is that one section should be submitted for every 1 cm of the maximum diameter of the tumor. As you take these sections, keep in mind that important indications of tumor grade (cellularity, necrosis, mitoses, etc.) and differentiation may be present only focally in large masses.

Important Issues to Address in Your Surgical Pathology Report on Soft Tissue Tumors

- What procedure was performed, and what structures/organs are present?
- What are the size, type, and histologic grade of the neoplasm?
- Does the neoplasm extend into skin, muscle, periosteum, bone, a joint space, major vessels, or major nerves?
- Are any margins involved? List distance from margins closer than 2 cm.
- Are there any satellite lesions?
- Is there evidence of metastatic disease? Record the number of lymph nodes examined and the presence or absence of lymph node metastases.

Nerve and Muscle Biopsies

Nerve and muscle biopsies are subject to a variety of artifacts if they are not properly handled. Furthermore, the interpretation of nerve and muscle pathology frequently requires special studies, including electron microscopy and histochemistry. For these reasons, nerve and muscle biopsies are best handled directly by specialized laboratories. Each laboratory usually has its own protocol for handling these biopsies. A detailed discussion of these specimens is, therefore, beyond the scope of this book. However, you should be aware of a few basics in processing these specimens, in case you do not have access to a specialized neuromuscular laboratory when the biopsy is done.

Muscle biopsies are usually obtained as two strips of muscle approximately 3.0 × 0.5 cm, taken parallel to the direction of the muscle fibers. A portion of tissue should be stretched to its normal *in situ* length, pinned to a card, and placed immediately (in the operating room) in 4% buffered glutaraldehyde. Do *not* mince this piece for electron microscopy. The remainder of the biopsy should be transported in saline-moistened gauze (do not soak) to the pathology laboratory. A portion of the biopsy should then be immediately fresh-frozen and the remainder fixed in formalin. To ensure that the fiber size in the biopsy reflects the *in situ* diameter and to reduce artifacts caused by the extreme contractility of the tissue, this piece of muscle should also be stretched to its normal *in situ* length in the direction of the fibers. This can be accomplished with a special muscle clamp or simply by pinning the stretched biopsy to a stiff index card. Be careful not to overstretch the tissue, as this can cause artifacts as well. Muscle biopsies frozen in liquid nitrogen tend to develop ice crystal artifacts, so it is best to freeze the tissue in 2-methyl-butane (isopentane) cooled to dry ice temperature or below. When submitting muscle biopsies in formalin for histology, remember to submit both longitudinal and cross sections.

Diagnostic nerve biopsies to determine the cause of a neuropathy are usually obtained as 3- to 5-cm-long strips of the sural nerve. As was true for muscle biopsies, these should be processed immediately by a specialized neuromuscular laboratory. You should handle these biopsies only when they cannot be handled by a specialized laboratory. Do not stretch these biopsies! Instead, the biopsy is usually cut into four pieces. One piece should be submitted in 4% glutaraldehyde for electron microscopy, one submitted in formalin for routine microscopy, another fresh-frozen and stored at −70°C, and the fourth saved fresh in saline-moistened gauze for the neuromuscular laboratory. If you have to cut a nerve, be careful not to squash it while cutting. Pressure on the nerve can induce the artifactual appearance of demyelinization. As was true for muscle biopsies, the sections submitted for histology should include both longitudinal and cross sections.

If a nerve biopsy is performed simply to document the transection of a nerve, the specimen should be entirely submitted in formalin for routine paraffin embedding and sectioning.

24 Skin

Thomas D. Horn, M.D.

General Comments

Skin biopsies comprise a large component of the volume of many anatomic pathology laboratories. These biopsies come in many shapes and sizes, both because of the ease with which the cutaneous surface can be sampled and also because biopsies are performed using a wide variety of techniques. Specimens are generally obtained to diagnose tumors, to ensure complete excision of tumors, and to identify or confirm the nature of cutaneous inflammatory diseases. Understanding the suspected diagnosis and purpose of the procedure will help expedite the processing of the tissue and ensure an accurate diagnosis.

Small Biopsies

Specimens obtained to establish the diagnosis of a cutaneous tumor are usually performed by the shave biopsy technique, punch biopsy technique, or curettage. Determining the adequacy of resection in fragmented curettage specimens is not possible. In most other instances, determining resection margins is often not requested, because a second procedure is anticipated by the physician based on the diagnosis. Nonetheless, some physicians may request an estimate of tumor extension to the resection margins, and in fact the occasional tumor is completely removed by deep shave biopsy or by punch biopsy procedures. Embedding the tissue in an orientation such that sections are taken in a plane perpendicular to the epidermis allows easy identification of surgical margins along the exposed dermis. Ink the exposed dermis before sectioning specimens greater than 0.5 cm in largest dimension. In this manner, margins may be reported as free or involved in the planes of section. Bisect any specimen 0.5 cm or greater in largest dimension and at least trisect any shave biopsy specimen 1.0 cm or greater. Tissue bags or similar aids can help confine small pieces of skin.

Elliptical Specimens

Many excisional specimens are submitted as elliptical pieces of tissue because this shape leaves wounds that lie parallel to skin tension lines, allowing easy closure and good cosmesis. That said, excisional specimens can arrive in a variety of other shapes, especially from the face, based on the anticipated closure. Round, triangular, and rhomboid specimens should be expected. Usually, there is some indication of how the specimen was oriented. For example, there can be a suture in one tip indicating the superior margin or ink placed on one or several surfaces of the tissue with an accompanying designation as to orientation. Note such identifiers in your gross description, and ink resection margins, including the deep margin. Use enough colors (generally the same ones used by the surgeon) to allow for accurate determination of precisely which margins are involved or free once the tissue is sectioned. In elliptical and rhomboid specimens, remove the small tips of the tissue fragments and place them in separate cassettes if specimen orientation is provided; one cassette may be used in the absence of anatomic identifiers. Embed the cut surface of the tip (i.e., not the surgical margin) in the block

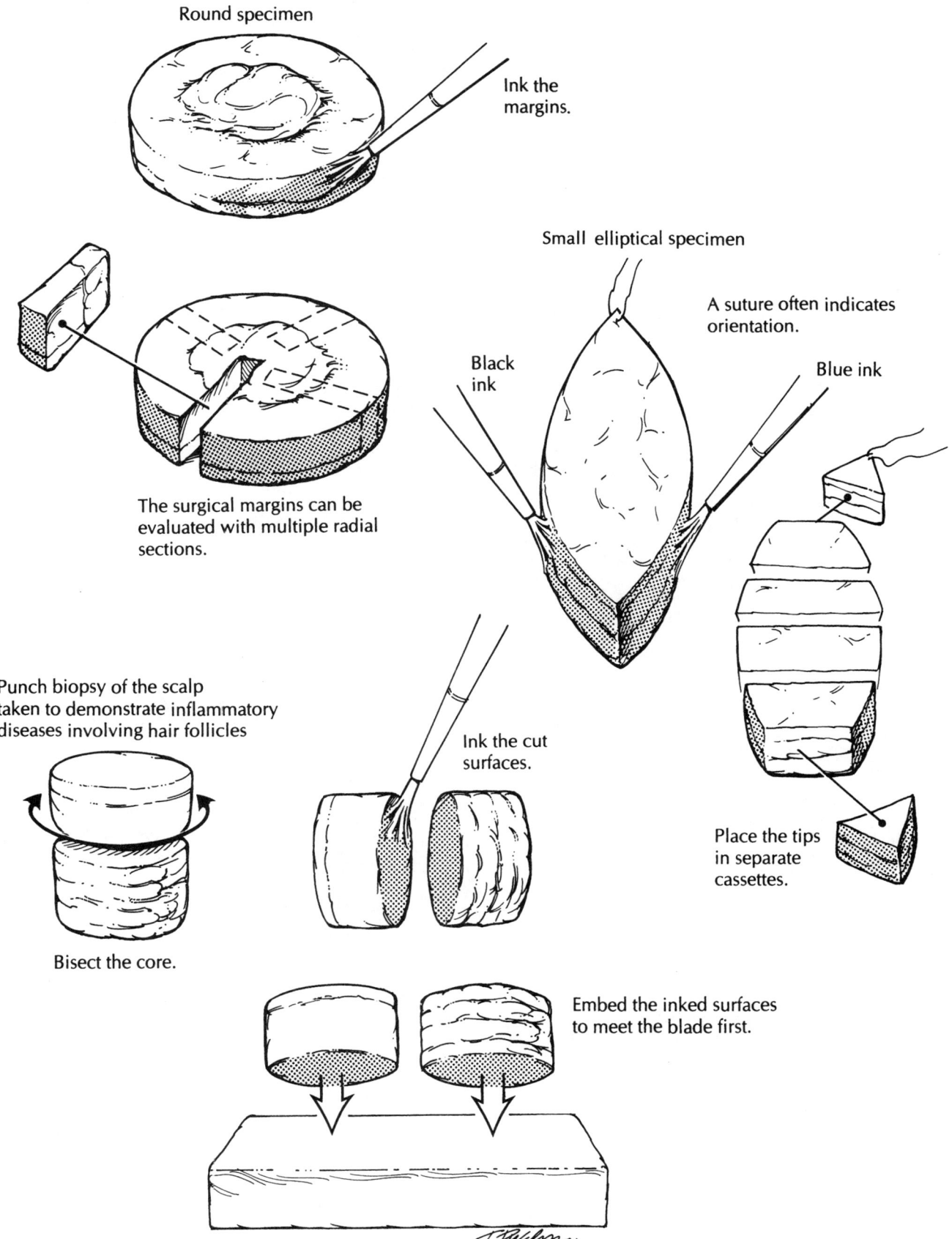

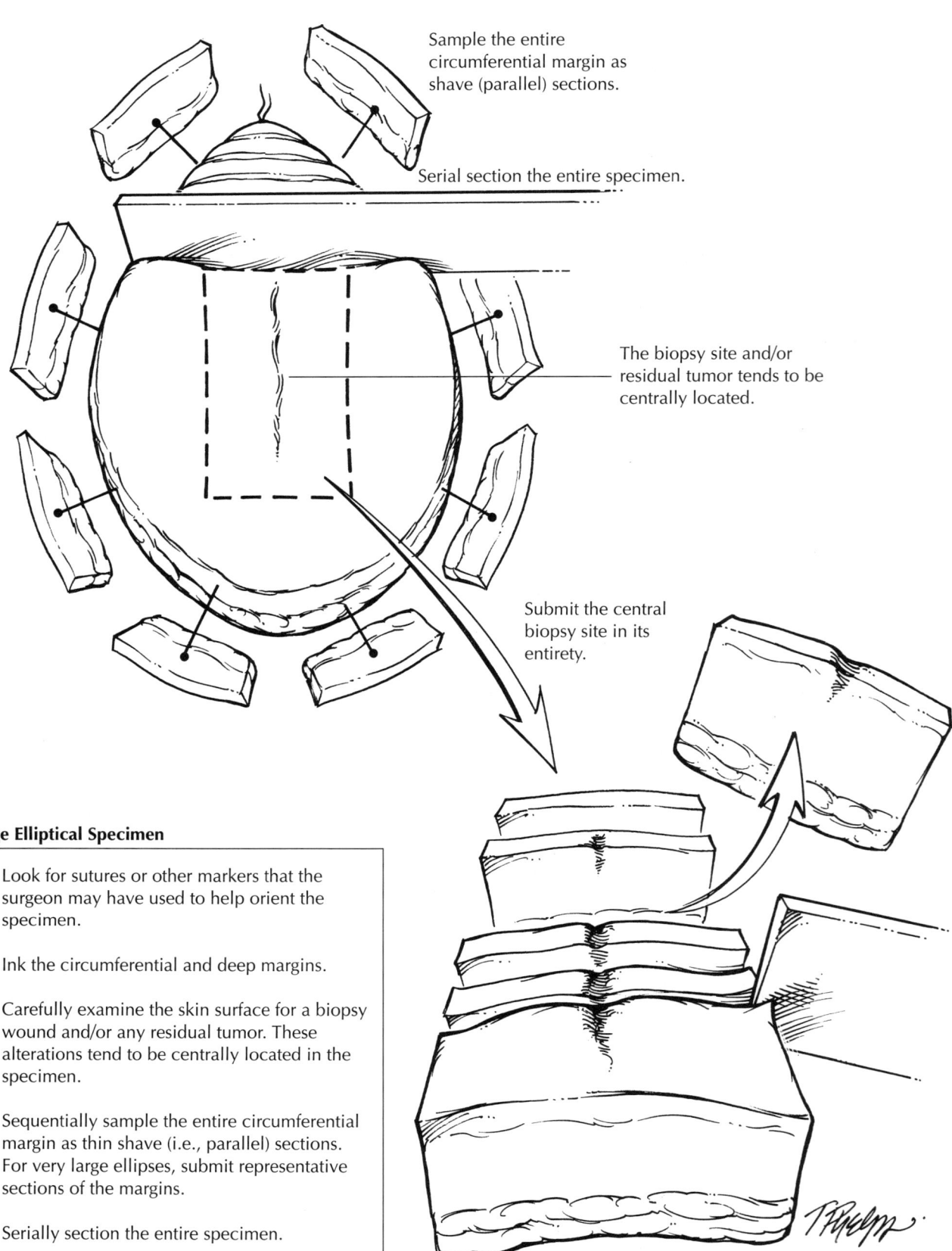

Sample the entire circumferential margin as shave (parallel) sections.

Serial section the entire specimen.

The biopsy site and/or residual tumor tends to be centrally located.

Submit the central biopsy site in its entirety.

Large Elliptical Specimen

1. Look for sutures or other markers that the surgeon may have used to help orient the specimen.

2. Ink the circumferential and deep margins.

3. Carefully examine the skin surface for a biopsy wound and/or any residual tumor. These alterations tend to be centrally located in the specimen.

4. Sequentially sample the entire circumferential margin as thin shave (i.e., parallel) sections. For very large ellipses, submit representative sections of the margins.

5. Serially section the entire specimen.

6. Submit the centrally located lesion and/or biopsy cavity entirely for histologic evaluation. Be sure to include the deep margin.

such that tissue sections progress toward the tip and become smaller over multiple tissue levels. In this way, residual tumor may be traced out into the tip. The body of the specimen can then be serially sectioned perpendicular to the epidermis in sections of roughly a nickel's width. Multiple tissue sections may be placed in single cassettes, but when necessary single slices can be placed in cassettes to allow for more accurate determination of the location of resection margins involved with tumor. Most specimens may be submitted entirely in this fashion. Larger resections for melanoma require sampling of the margins based on visual identification of where the tumor is (was) located. In this instance, multiple samples taken perpendicular to the margin of resection and including the tumor (or biopsy wound) are recommended. The deep subcutaneous margin may have to be sampled separately. Alternatively, sequential sampling of the entire circumference of especially large elliptical specimens may be undertaken as shown in the illustration. The biopsy wound, scar, or residual tumor is generally centrally located and should be submitted in its entirety. In this manner, all critical areas of the specimen are examined, although some tissue is not processed.

Round Specimens

Small, round excisional specimens, generally from the forehead, are a challenge. If the surgeon places an identifier on the tissue, use this information to localize the other resection margins. Because no tips are present to remove, one approach to these specimens is to tangentially shave a small piece of tissue and embed these shaves as described previously for tips from elliptical specimens, with subsequent serial slicing of the remaining tissue. The tips of elliptical specimens are generally separated from the tumor by a reliable amount of uninvolved skin. This safe zone is absent in round specimens where tumor may be close to all margins. An alternative approach is, therefore, to obtain numerous sections in radial configuration, but visualization of all margins is more difficult with this approach.

Irregularly Shaped Specimens

A similar problem arises in determining adequacy of resection margins at the base of triangular specimens. The base of such specimens generally abuts some cosmetically sensitive structure such as the eyebrow or tragus. It is difficult to determine if a margin is clear of tumor in sections taken parallel to the base of the triangle if the tumor is near the resection margin. On the other hand, perpendicular sections may miss a positive margin in the remaining tissue sections. The most reliable approach is to pay scrupulous attention to the gross appearance of the tumor and its relationship to the margins when dissecting round and triangular excisional specimens from the skin.

Punch Biopsy

The most popular method of skin sampling in the evaluation of inflammatory skin conditions is the punch or trephine biopsy. A core of tissue is obtained in this manner. Epidermis, dermis, and subcutis are usually easy to identify, and the specimen should be embedded such that tissue sections are obtained perpendicular to the plane of the epidermis. Punch biopsy specimens greater than 0.4 cm in diameter should generally be bisected. *Read the clinical history carefully!* If the clinician suspects an infectious agent, requesting appropriate special stains at the time tissue is submitted for histology will greatly shorten the time it takes to diagnose a case. Dermatophyte infection is the most commonly overlooked clinical and histologic diagnosis in the skin; obtaining fungal stains prospectively is never a waste of time or money. Certain skin conditions display only subtle or focal histologic findings, and serial sectioning of the block may be required to identify these processes, especially if a 6-mm punch biopsy specimen is submitted from a 1- or 2-mm clinical lesion. Examples include folliculitis, dermatitis herpetiformis, and transient acantholytic dermatosis.

Punch Biopsies of the Scalp

Increasingly, dermatopathologists prefer to interpret punch biopsy specimens from the scalp, taken to diagnose inflammatory conditions, in sections parallel to the plane of the epidermis. Perpendicular sectioning results in the identification of few hair follicles in a given tissue section, and then the hair follicles are only partially seen. Parallel sectioning is performed as follows. Bisect the core of tissue in a plane horizontal to the epidermis at a level approximately 1 mm above (i.e., toward the epidermis) the junction of the dermis and subcutis. Ink and embed the cut surfaces such that the inked surfaces face the microtome blade. The tissue is serially sectioned with all tissue placed on slides. We stain every other slide to reduce the overall number of slides examined as well as to provide unstained slides for fungal stains if indicated after an initial inspection of the tissue. This method allows all follicles at a given depth in the skin to be examined in one tissue section. Examination of serial sections allows the complete assessment of follicles and follicular units contained in the core of tissue. Determination of interface changes at the epidermis (e.g., for lupus erythematosus) is generally still possible despite the horizontal sectioning, but identification of epidermal atrophy is nearly impossible. Embedded as described above, the series of slides provides sections from two pieces of tissue with progression toward the epidermis in one piece and toward the deep margin (hopefully subcutis) in the other.

Other Specimens

Dermatologic surgeons may submit somewhat untraditional specimens. Liposuction specimens consist of a variable volume of fat and serosanguineous fluid. While such specimens may be submitted as a "gross only," always examine a representative amount of fat to reduce the chances of missing the unsuspected superficial liposarcoma. Taking representative sections of certain common benign tumors (e.g., lipomas, cysts, keloids) is acceptable.

Specimens from Moh's Micrographic Surgery

A complete description of Moh's micrographic technique of histologically controlled cutaneous surgery is beyond the scope of this chapter. In brief, after tumor debulking, wafer-thin planes of tissue are obtained from the wound bed in an orientation horizontal to the epidermis. The surgeon then carefully marks the fresh tissue to establish resection margins and to identify the position in the wound bed. A map of the tissue and markings is drawn. The tissue is divided and mounted for frozen sections. The surgeon examines these sections while the patient remains in the operating suite and the wound is still anesthetized. Identification of tumor at a resection margin prompts removal of another plane of tissue only in the involved area(s) and so on until complete removal of tumor is ensured. This technique offers a higher cure rate than conventional procedures and is tissue sparing. Based on the surgeon's routine, frozen tissue sections are placed on the slide such that tissue nearest the resection margin can be identified.

Pathologists can become involved in this procedure in three ways. First, the dermatologic surgeon may seek a second opinion regarding the presence or absence of tumor in a particular frozen section. Second, a review of the frozen section slides may be requested if there is a perceived discrepancy with the biopsy diagnosis. Third, in rural areas, dermatologists will perform a similar modified technique, so-called "slow Moh's." Here, planes of skin are submitted as fixed tissue from a similarly prepared wound bed. The tissue must be processed in horizontal sections, with an effort made to provide anatomic localization of involved margins based on information provided by the clinician. In the face of positive margins, the clinician will reanesthetize the (now granulating) wound base and obtain another plane of tissue. Success in this endeavor requires exceptionally good communication between the clinician, pathologist, and laboratory personnel. Occasionally, closure is delayed while immunohistochemistry is performed on putatively negative margins to ensure removal, particularly for melanoma, using S-100 protein.

Important Issues to Address in Your Surgical Pathology Report on Melanomas

- What procedure was performed, and what structures/organs are present? Specifically, record the components present (e.g., skin, subcutaneous tissue, and other soft tissue such as muscle or nerve).
- What is the histologic type of the tumor?
- What is the growth phase?

- What is the deepest level of penetration of the tumor (confined to the epidermis, into the papillary dermis, filling the papillary dermis, into the reticular dermis, into the subcutaneous tissue)?
- What is the maximum tumor thickness? (Measure from the top of the granular layer to the deepest extent of the tumor.)
- Are any margins involved by tumor?
- Is the tumor ulcerated?
- How many mitotic figures are identified per square millimeter?
- Are any precursor lesions identified?
- Is any evidence of regression of the lesion present?
- Is any host inflammatory response to the tumor present?
- Is there evidence of vascular or neural invasion?

VII   The Breast

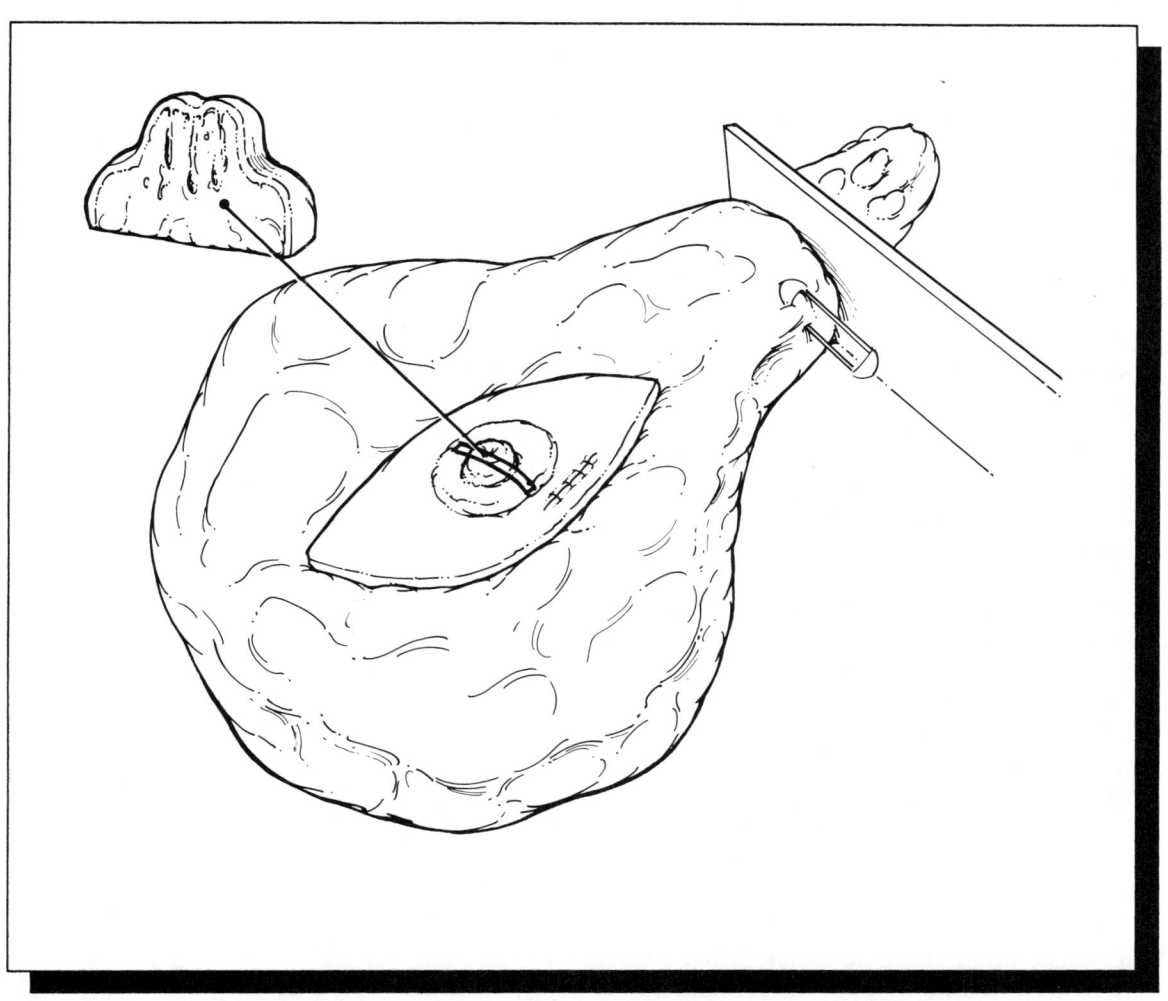

25 Breast

Pedram Argani, M.D.

General Comments

A wide variety of surgical techniques are employed to biopsy or resect breast tissue. In general, these specimens can be divided into several groups: (1) needle core biopsies performed by radiologists; (2) small biopsies performed for mammographic abnormalities; (3) "lumpectomies" for grossly benign palpable tumors and grossly malignant palpable tumors; (4) mastectomies with or without a lymph node dissection, performed for carcinoma; and (5) reduction mammoplasties.

The processing of these specimens can be difficult and labor-intensive for a number of reasons. Breast specimens are fatty tissues that require meticulous attention to proper fixation to ensure adequate microscopic and immunohistochemical evaluation. Breast specimens often harbor subtle mammographic abnormalities that may not be apparent on gross examination. Detection of these lesions relies on careful dissection coupled with ample tissue sectioning. Breast specimens usually do not contain useful anatomic landmarks, yet important treatment decisions ultimately rest on your ability to assess the status of the specimen margins accurately. Detailed attention to specimen orientation and margin designation is therefore critical. Chapter 1 covers many of the fundamental issues of tissue processing and sampling; but when it comes to handling breast specimens, a few points warrant special emphasis.

Examination of the Specimen

All breast tissue, even if removed for cosmetic reasons, should be examined fresh. It is much easier to appreciate subtle scirrhous areas that could correspond to small invasive carcinomas in the background of fresh tissue. After formalin fixation, all of the tissue is firm, making this distinction more difficult.

Inking

Breast specimens (with the exception of needle core biopsies) should be inked prior to immersion in formalin. Before the ink is applied, blot the surface of the specimen dry so the ink better adheres to the surface of the specimen. After the ink is applied, again blot the surface of the specimen dry. This step helps prevent the ink from penetrating the tissues as the specimen is sectioned. Immersion for 20 seconds in Bouin's fixative immediately after inking may help fix the ink to the specimen, but remember to rinse the Bouin's solution from the specimen before sectioning. Always be certain that the ink is completely dry before cutting into the specimen. Be patient; you may have to wait 5 to 10 minutes or so for the ink to dry completely.

Sometimes the surgeon designates (e.g., using sutures) the anatomic orientation of a specimen. The easiest way to maintain this orientation is to use inks of different colors to designate each of the six specimen margins (superior, inferior, medial, lateral, anterior, posterior). If only one color is used, you must keep track of and dictate which inked surfaces are represented in each of the cassettes. Also, if the specimen is not submitted in its entirety, it must be stored so one can go "back to the bucket" and take more sections from a specific area as needed.

Fixation

Breast tissue that has not been properly fixed compromises the ability of the histopathology laboratory to cut high quality sections for microscopic examination, limits the ability of the pathologist to interpret difficult "borderline" lesions (e.g., atypical duct hyperplasia), and diminishes the reliability of immunohistochemical assays (e.g., Ki-67 proliferation index, estrogen and progesterone receptors) for predicting tumor behavior. If the specimen is to be fixed prior to complete processing and sampling, take the time to "bread-loaf" the specimen at 1-cm intervals before submerging it in formalin. This step allows the formalin to penetrate all of the tissue. Keep in mind that formalin penetrates tissue at a rate of approximately 4 mm in 24 hours. If the specimen is not bread-loafed prior to submersion in formalin, much of the tissue will remain unfixed, particularly in the center of the specimen. If you are not sure that the specimen is adequately fixed when it is time to submit it for processing at the end of the day, it is better *not* to submit it that day. Allow the specimen cassettes to fix overnight in formalin; then submit them for processing the next day.

Needle Core Biopsy

Record the number, size, and color of the tissue cores. All of the cores should be entirely submitted to the histopathology laboratory for further processing. Each tissue block should be sectioned at three levels.

As part of the microscopic evaluation of these specimens, the histopathologic findings must be correlated with the clinical and mammographic findings. For example, if the biopsy specimen is from a mass lesion, your report should indicate whether the microscopic findings account for a breast mass. If, on the other hand, the biopsy was performed because of worrisome calcifications, your report should document the presence of these calcifications when they are found. Discrepancies between the microscopic findings and the clinical/mammographic findings may necessitate additional work on your part. If you cannot find calcifications when they were seen by mammography, additional levels of the tissue block should be cut. It may be necessary to confirm the presence of calcifications by obtaining radiographs of the paraffin blocks. However, you should be aware that calcifications that were present in the tissue submitted to pathology (as documented in radiology by specimen radiographs) sometimes chip out of the block when it is sectioned by the histotechnologist. The presence of tissue tears in the hematoxylin and eosin (H&E) section is a good clue that this has occurred.

Biopsies for Mammographic Abnormalities

Nonpalpable lesions detected mammographically are often biopsied by the surgeon and the specimen then sent to radiology, where a specimen radiograph is obtained to confirm that the surgeon has indeed biopsied or excised the lesion detected on the clinical mammogram. In these cases the radiologist frequently marks the lesion with a needle or dye, and both the biopsy and the specimen mammogram are then sent to the surgical pathology laboratory.

Once received in pathology, the specimen should be measured, inked, and serially sectioned (Figure 25-1). Take care to slice the breast thinly (2 mm). Take advantage of the specimen radiograph; the gross findings can be correlated with the lesion seen radiographically. If a lesion is seen, note the largest dimension of the lesion and carefully note the relationship of the lesion to the inked margins as well as the circumscription and nature of the border of the lesion.

Sequentially submit the entire specimen, up to 20 blocks of tissue, for histologic examination. Sequential sectioning allows one to better reconstruct the distribution of the lesion from the slides. When taking these sections, be sure that the sections demonstrate the relation of the lesion to the closest inked margin. Be sure also to designate which block contains the area marked by the radiologist's needle as containing calcification.

For large biopsy specimens that cannot be completely submitted in 20 or fewer sections, the extent of tissue sampling is not clear. Owings et al.[10] suggested a method for selective tissue sampling in these large specimens. According to their method, initial sampling should include the submission of all tissue corresponding to radiographic calcifications and all surrounding fibrous tissue. If carcinoma or atypical duct hyperplasia is identified in these initial sections, the remaining tissue should be submitted in its entirety to determine the extent of the lesion and the status of the margins and to exclude invasion in cases of ductal carcinoma *in situ*.

Lumpectomy

Lumpectomy for a Grossly Benign Palpable Mass

A lumpectomy specimen from a palpable mass that is grossly benign should be measured, inked, and serially sectioned perpendicular to the closest palpable margin. Inspect the cut surface and record the size and appearance of the lesion as well as its distance from the margins. Sequentially submit the entire lumpectomy specimen in up to 10 cassettes. Be sure that your sections show the border of the lesion with the surrounding breast tissue (important for distinguishing fibroadenoma from phyllodes tumors), and take perpendicular sections from the lesion to the margins. If the margins are designated, be sure to obtain a section perpendicular to each of the six margins. Cost-effective strategies for handling large lumpectomy specimens have also been proposed. Schnitt et al.[11,12] suggested submitting a maximum of 10 initial sections of the fibrous tissue in these cases, as carcinoma and atypical hyperplasia are unlikely to be found in the fatty tissue alone.

Lumpectomy for Grossly Identifiable Cancers

Lumpectomy biopsies for grossly identifiable cancers are usually brought to the surgical pathology laboratory with some indication of orientation provided by the surgeon. Frequently, but not universally, a short stitch is used to designate the superior aspect of the specimen and a long stitch to designate the lateral aspect of the specimen. From these two landmarks you can then determine the inferior, medial, anterior, and posterior margins. As illustrated, these margins are easier to conceptualize if you think of the specimen as a cube. After orienting the specimen, measure it, ink it, and obtain one or two perpendicular sections from each of the six margins (superior, inferior, medial, lateral, superficial, deep). Serially section the specimen at 2- to 3-mm intervals. Note the size of the tumor and the distance to each of the margins. Obtain two to five sections of the tumor. If a portion of skin is present, it should also be sampled for histologic examination. If the lumpectomy specimen is relatively small, submit it entirely (Figure 25-2). For large lumpectomy specimens, where the entire specimen cannot be submitted in 20 cassettes, submit representative sections (Figure 25-3).

Additional (Revised) Margins Submitted by the Surgeon

Sometimes the surgeon separately submits additional (revised) margins for one or all six of the lumpectomy surfaces. Usually these specimens appear as a strip of tissue with a stitch on one face marking the new margin. The opposite surface, which would face the lumpectomy specimen, often contains fresh blood and is not a true margin. Ink the surface containing the stitch, obtain serial sections perpendicular to the ink, and submit all of the sections for microscopic examination (Figure 25-4). Do not ink the opposite surface; otherwise, it may be impossible to tell which is the true margin.

Re-excision Lumpectomy

Re-excision lumpectomies are generally performed because a positive margin was identified during a prior excision. Therefore, specimen sampling should focus on the biopsy cavity to document the presence of residual disease and on the new specimen margins to ensure the adequacy of tumor removal during the re-excision. Try to submit re-excision specimens in their entirety if they can be submitted in fewer than 10 cassettes. If the biopsy cavity appears grossly benign, two sections per centimeter of greatest specimen diameter is probably adequate.

Mastectomy

True radical mastectomies are seldom performed anymore. The procedure includes complete axillary dissection including removal of the

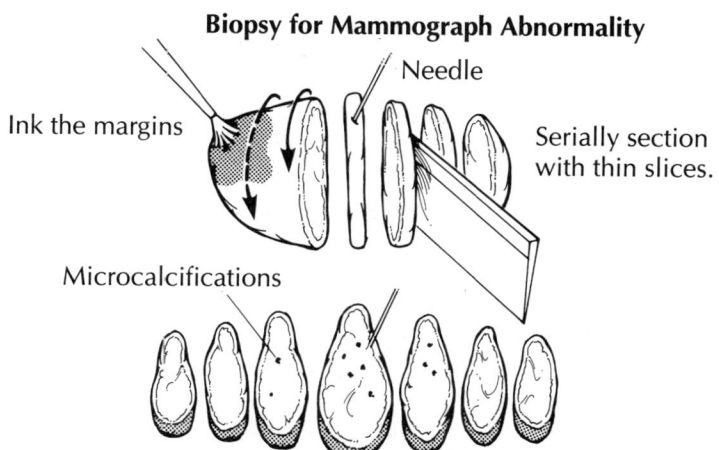

Fig. 25-1. Biopsy for Mammographic Abnormality

1. Ink the specimen in different colors to main orientation (if provided).
2. Serially section the specimen into thin slices.
3. Describe any lesions and distance to the margins.
4. Submit entire specimen sequentially (if under 20 cassettes); indicate which cassettes contain the lesion and the site of the needle.

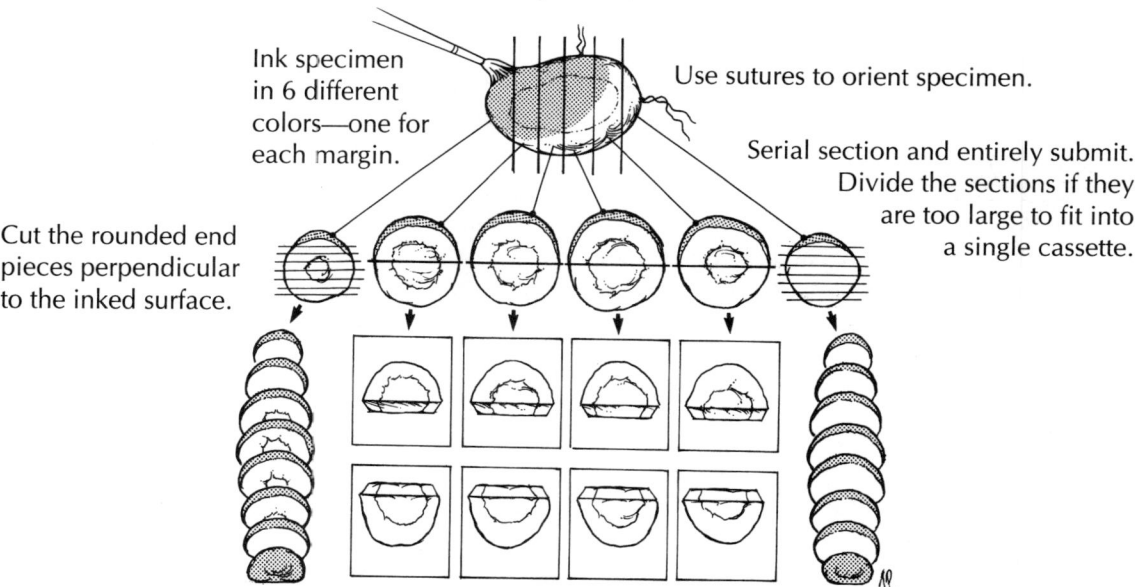

Fig. 25-2. Small Lumpectomy for Breast Cancer

1. Orient the specimen using the attached sutures, and record its dimensions.
2. Ink the specimen borders using 6 ink colors, one for each specific margin.
3. Serially section the specimen perpendicular to the largest dimension. Record the size of the tumor and its distance to each margin.
4. Serially section the round end pieces perpendicular to demonstrate their margins.
5. Submit the specimen in entirety in sequential cassettes. Some slices may be too large to fit comfortably in one cassette, and should be bisected.

Large Lumpectomy for Cancer

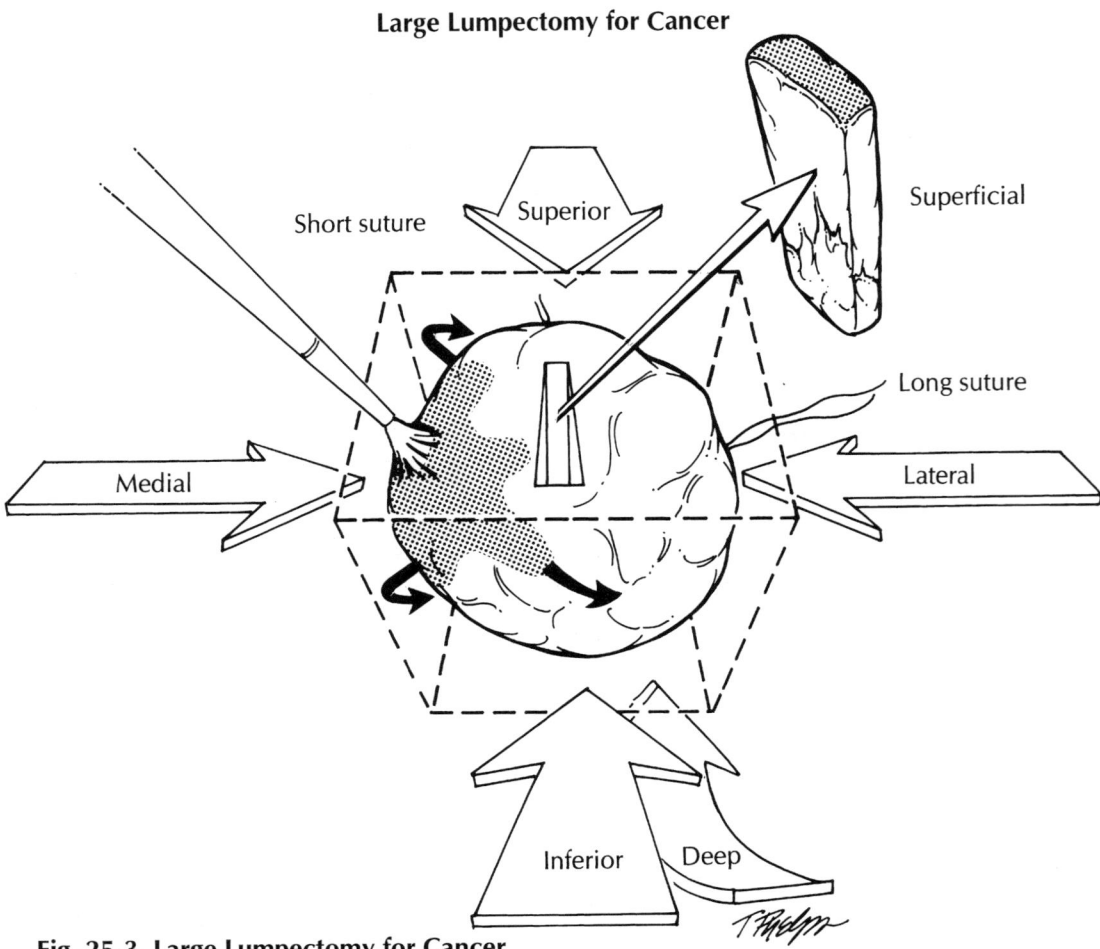

Fig. 25-3. Large Lumpectomy for Cancer

1. Ink the specimen in different colors to maintain orientation.
2. Serially section the specimen into thin slices.
3. Describe the size of the tumor, and distance to the margins.
4. Submit 1–2 perpendicular sections from each of the six margins.
5. Submit sections from tumor (2–5 sections).

Additional (Revised) Margin of Lumpectomy

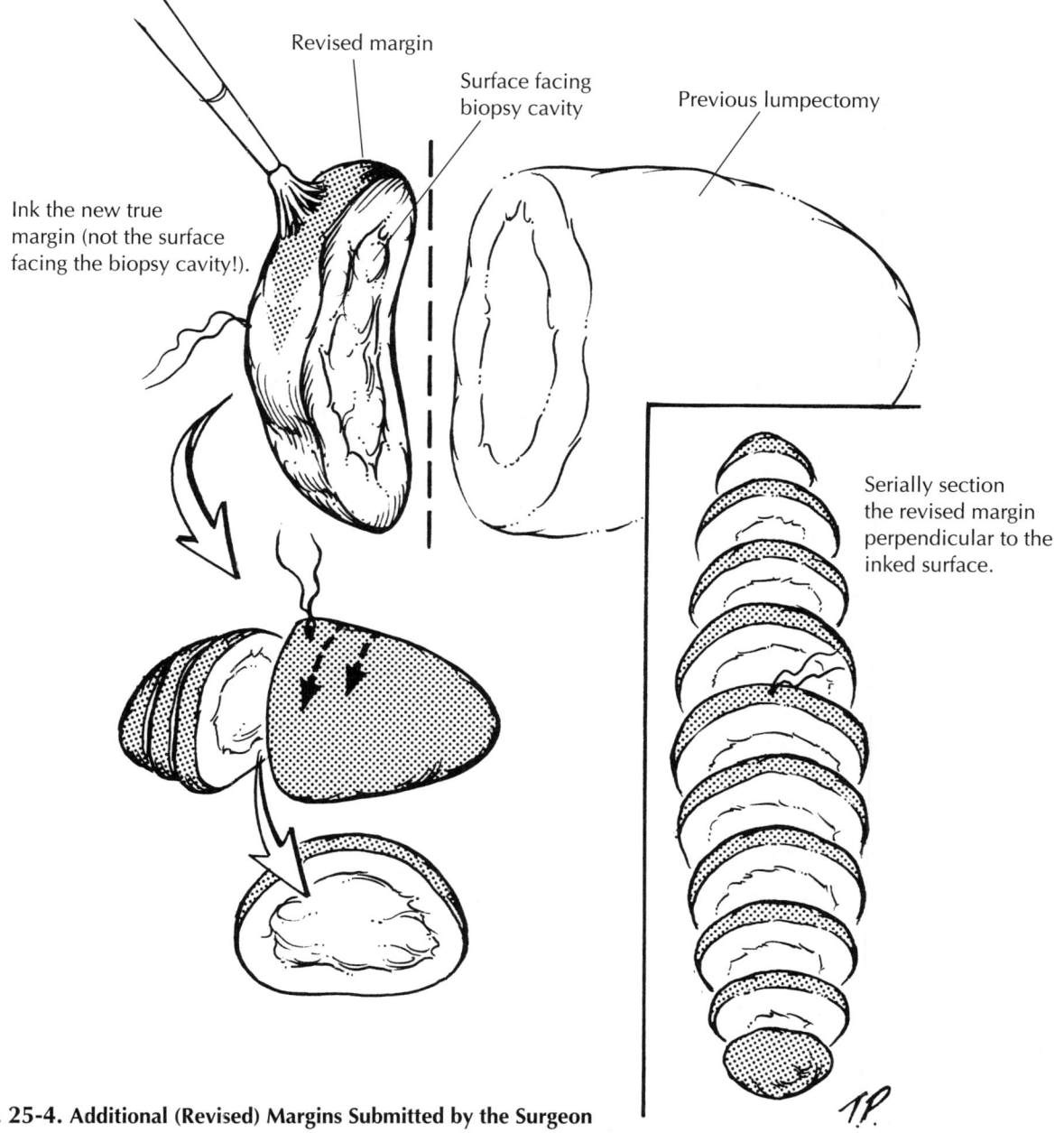

Fig. 25-4. Additional (Revised) Margins Submitted by the Surgeon

1. Measure the specimen, and orient it by identifying the new true margin (usually designated by a suture) and the opposite surface, which faces the biopsy cavity from the earlier lumpectomy specimen.
2. Place the specimen on the cutting board so that the true margin (designated by the suture) is facing up.
3. Ink only the true margin (not the surface facing the biopsy cavity!)
4. Serially section the specimen perpendicular to the inked surface and submit it in entirety.

modified radical mastectomy is more common. With this procedure the undersurface of the specimen is composed only of fascial planes with occasional shreds of pectoralis major muscles attached. The anterior surface usually contains an island of skin and nipple with the subcutaneous tissue extending beyond it. Nevertheless, complete axillary dissection typically is included within the specimen, forming an elongated tail at one end of the otherwise elliptical specimen. Most mastectomies are performed after a core needle biopsy has established a diagnosis of invasive carcinoma or after a lumpectomy has not been successful in completely removing an *in situ* and/or invasive carcinoma.

First, orient the specimen to localize the four quadrants of the breast correctly. This step should not be difficult if you use the axillary contents, the sidedness of the breast, and the surgeon's description of the location of the tumor. Once the specimen has been oriented, place a safety pin in the corner of the upper outer quadrant. This practice helps you to reorient the specimen quickly in case you have to return to the specimen. Weigh and measure the specimen; then describe the skin, nipple, and any biopsy sites seen. The axillary tail can be removed now for later examination. Next, take the time to palpate the specimen. Localize the biopsy scar, the biopsy cavity, and any masses. Examine the deep surface of the specimen for attached fragments of skeletal muscle, and ink it so perpendicular sections can be obtained to evaluate the deep soft tissue margin. Also ink the exposed breast tissue lateral to the skin ellipse on the anterior surface of the specimen (preferably with ink of a different color). These constitute the anterior margins. Hence, all surfaces except for the skin and axillary tail should be inked.

The breast can then be placed skin surface down on a cutting board and sectioned. As illustrated (Figure 25-5), use the nipple to center the specimen; then with two long perpendicular cuts section the breast into four quadrants. Each quadrant can be further sectioned, each in its own direction. These cuts should not go all the way through the specimen but, instead, should leave the pieces attached together by a rim of unsectioned breast or skin. This procedure not only helps orient the specimen in a clinically relevant way, it helps remind you to document in which quadrant(s) the lesion lies.

The gross dictation should include (1) the overall dimensions and the weight of the specimen; (2) the overall dimensions of the skin surface; (3) the presence or absence of a biopsy scar and biopsy cavity and their relation to the nipple; (4) the presence of any retraction or ulceration of the nipple and/or surrounding skin; (5) the presence or absence of muscle on the undersurface of the specimen; (6) *the size and gross appearance of the tumor including the quadrant of the breast in which it is localized*; and (7) the distance of the tumor to the deep and anterior margins. At least two and ideally five sections of the primary lesion should be submitted for histologic examination. Two sections can then be submitted from each of the remaining breast quadrants. If the mastectomy was performed as a prophylactic procedure in a patient with an *in situ* carcinoma, submit at least three sections from each quadrant; also submit any suspicious lesions in their entirety. Submit a section of the nipple and one of the skin in the area of the prior biopsy site.

Finally, dissect all lymph nodes from the axillary contents. If lymph nodes are separated into levels I, II, and III by their relationship to the pectoralis minor muscle (lateral, below, and medial to it, respectively), maintain this orientation. Chapter 5 details the procedures for processing sentinel and nonsentinel lymph nodes for metastatic tumors. When dealing with axillary lymph nodes in patients with carcinoma of the breast, it is particularly important to identify and evaluate each lymph node and to submit lymph nodes that are grossly negative for tumor in their entirety. Grossly positive nodes do not need to be submitted in their entirety. The size of the tumor in the grossly involved lymph node should be documented in your gross report.

Reduction Mammoplasty

There are no rigid criteria that dictate the number of sections to submit from reduction mammoplasty. In the absence of such criteria, a few considerations provide some helpful guidelines for specimen sampling. First, thorough gross examination of the thinly sliced specimen is the key to identifying clinically significant lesions. Second, because the risk of breast cancer increases with age, submit relatively more sections from specimens removed from older patients.

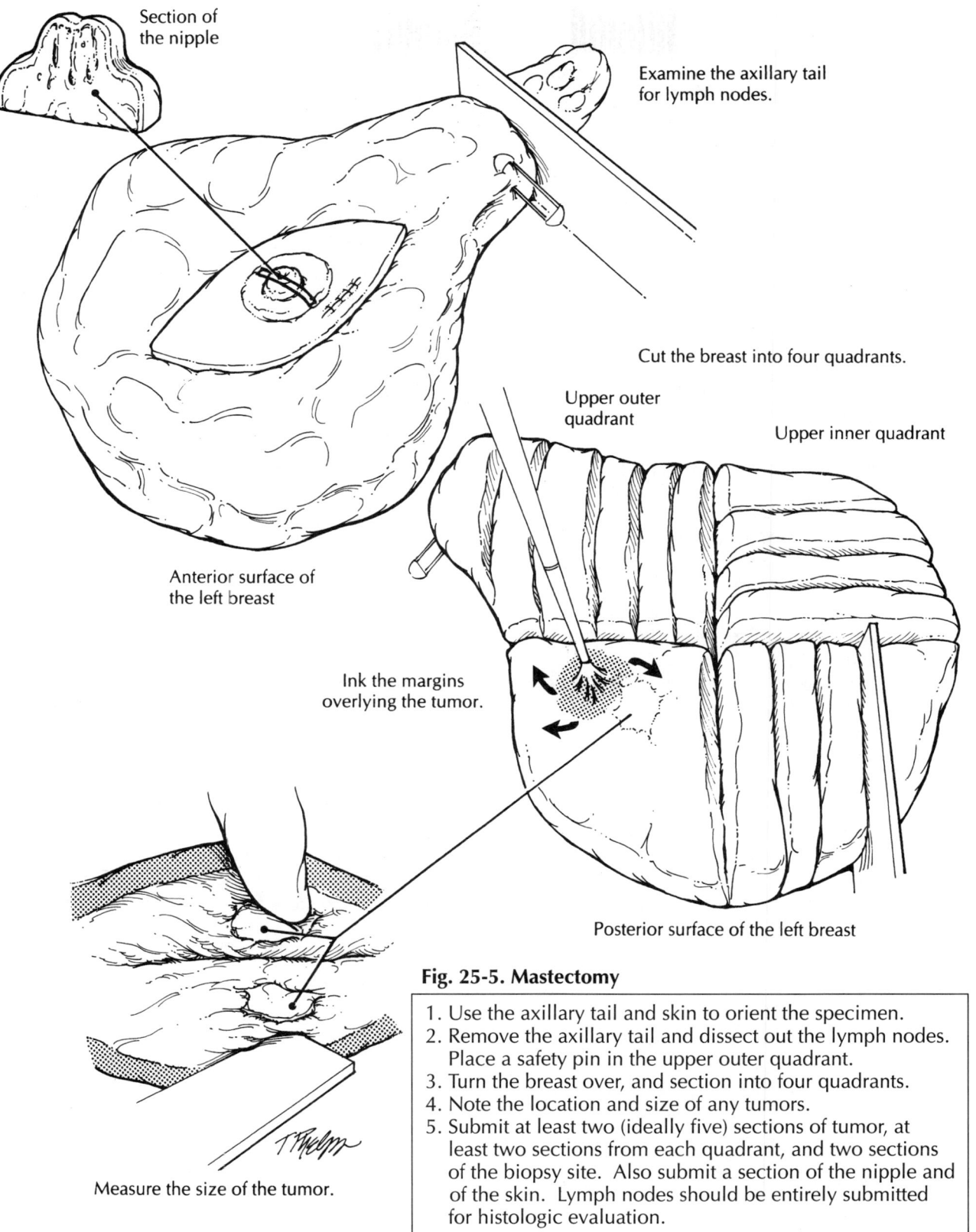

Fig. 25-5. Mastectomy

1. Use the axillary tail and skin to orient the specimen.
2. Remove the axillary tail and dissect out the lymph nodes. Place a safety pin in the upper outer quadrant.
3. Turn the breast over, and section into four quadrants.
4. Note the location and size of any tumors.
5. Submit at least two (ideally five) sections of tumor, at least two sections from each quadrant, and two sections of the biopsy site. Also submit a section of the nipple and of the skin. Lymph nodes should be entirely submitted for histologic evaluation.

We suggest submitting three sections from patients under 30 years of age and five sections from patients over 50 years of age. Third, because carcinomas and atypical hyperplasias are much more likely to involve fibrous breast tissue than fatty breast tissue, sections should selectively target dense and fibrotic breast parenchyma. The identification of atypical lesions or carcinoma on these initial sections indicates the need to go back to the specimen to obtain additional sections.

Important Issues to Address in Your Microscopic Surgical Pathology Report

- What procedure was performed and what structures/organs are present?
- What are the gross size and location (nipple, central portion, upper inner quadrant, upper outer quadrant, lower inner quadrant, lower outer quadrant, axillary tail) of any tumors identified? What is the microscopic size of the tumor? Are these measurements concordant?
- Are the tumors *in situ* or infiltrating? If the lesion contains both *in situ* and infiltrating carcinoma, what proportion of the lesion is *in situ*, and what proportion is infiltrating? Does *in situ* carcinoma extend away from the main tumor mass?
- What are the histologic type and grade of the *in situ* or infiltrating carcinoma?
- Is vascular/lymphatic invasion present?
- Is there skin or nipple involvement?
- Does the tumor involve the margins of resection? If it is close to a margin (i.e., less than 10 mm), record in millimeters the exact distance of the tumor from each of the margins.
- Does the tumor directly extend into the chest wall or the skin?
- Are microcalcifications present?
- Record the location and number of nodes examined and the presence or absence of metastatic carcinoma in these nodes. What is the size of the largest metastasis? Does the metastasis extend beyond the lymph node capsule into the surrounding perinodal fat?

Breast Implants

The handling of prosthetic breast implants deserves a special note. We suggest that you follow The College of American Pathologists (CAP) recommendations.[13] Briefly, they suggest that you first weigh the implant and describe its external surface (e.g., smooth, textured), its contents (clear gel, oil, watery fluid), and its condition (intact or ruptured). Next, document any inscriptions printed on the implant and *photograph the implant*, particularly if it is ruptured. You can then turn your attention to the tissue capsule—the wall of fibroconnective tissue that forms around the breast implant. Weigh and measure the capsule, describe its inner surface, and submit one or two tissue cassettes of the capsule for histologic examination. If any nodules are present in the capsule, they should be sampled more extensively. Finally, store the implants. With the current flood of litigation, the implants should probably be stored indefinitely.

VIII   The Female Genital System

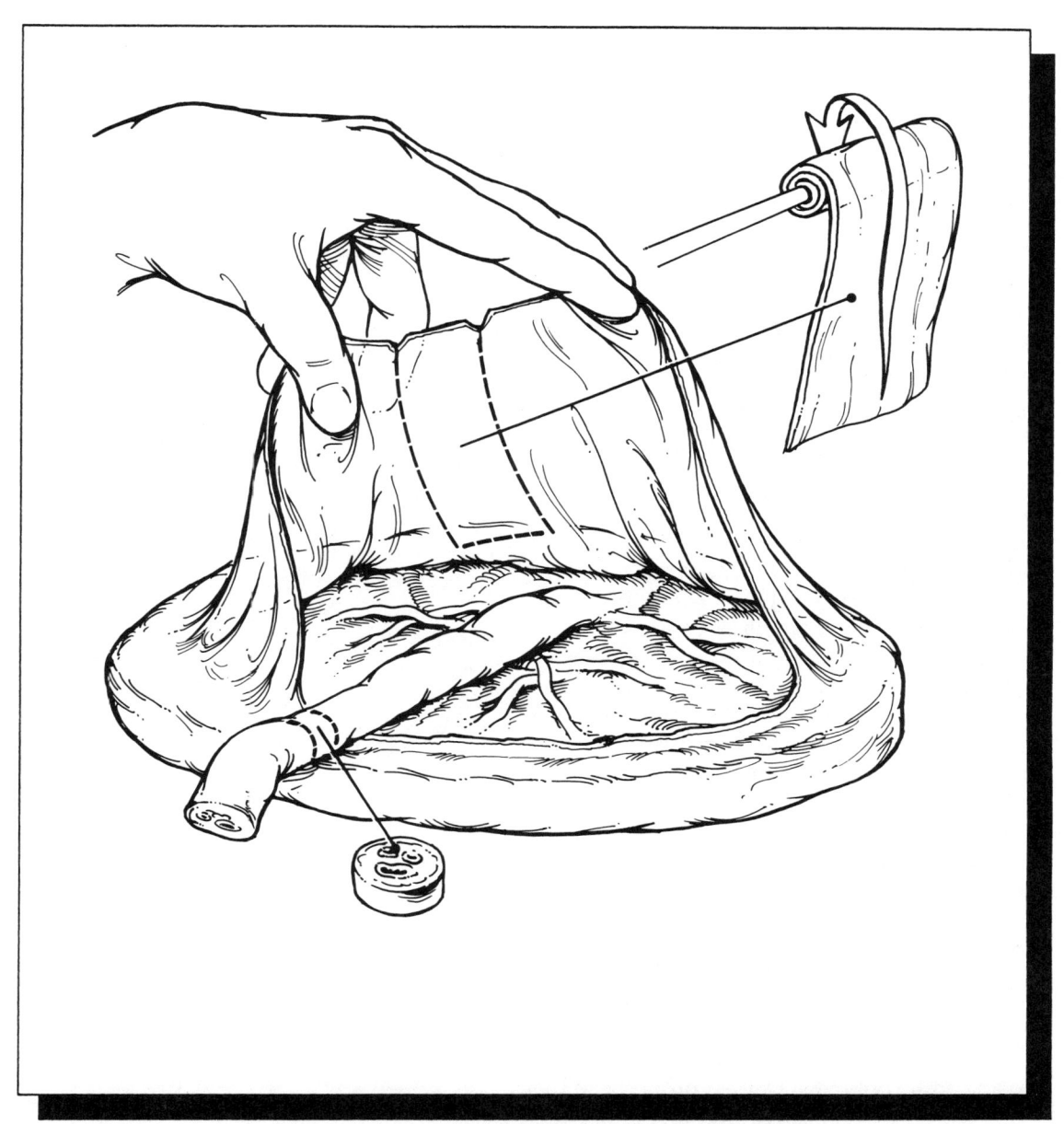

26 Vulva

General Comments

The *vulva* collectively refers to the external female genitalia. It includes the mons pubis, labia majora and minora, clitoris, vestibule with the urethral and vaginal orifices, posterior fourchette and perineum. The epithelial covering is predominantly skin (keratinized, stratified squamous epithelium), except for the vestibule, which is mucosa (nonkeratinized). Vulvar diseases are primarily epithelial in origin and usually can be seen externally. Therefore, most vulvar specimens can be handled in a manner similar to other skin specimens with emphasis on proper orientation and an evaluation of surgical margins.

Small Biopsies

Diagnostic punch biopsies are usually performed for lesions that appear as unusual discolorations or thickenings of the vulva. The most important tasks are to orient the specimen so that sections will be taken perpendicular to the epithelial surface and to secure the specimen properly so that small pieces are not lost in processing. When multiple sites have been biopsied to map out the extent of a lesion, be sure to clearly designate each separate location in the diagnosis.

Cavitronic Ultrasonic Surgical Aspirator (CUSA) Biopsies

A CUSA can be used for the treatment of condyloma acuminata and vulvar intraepithelial neoplasia (VIN). This technique simultaneously disrupts tissue by ultrasound and aspirates tissue. Numerous small fragments of epithelium with little or no underlying stroma are generated. Due to the size and quantity of the fragments, orientation of the epithelial surface is not possible. The best approach is to handle these tissues like a curettage specimen. First, collect all the tissue fragments by pouring the contents of the specimen container through a filter. Next, submit the tissue as an aggregate either within a fine-mesh biopsy bag or wrapped in tissue paper. Multiple levels can then be ordered on each tissue block to assist with the three-dimensional orientation of the lesion.

Excisional Biopsies

Excisional biopsies of the vulva range from simple excisions of inclusion cysts to wide local excisions of premalignant lesions or minimally invasive cancers. The tissue submitted usually consists of an ellipse of skin with a variable amount of underlying soft tissue, and it often lacks any identifiable anatomic landmarks. Look for a stitch or diagram provided by the gynecologist for orientation. It is crucial not to proceed with the dissection until you understand the *in situ* configuration of the specimen. These specimens can be handled in the same way as other excisional biopsies of skin (see Chapter 24). Ink all the margins (both cutaneous and deep) and take sections perpendicular to the epithelial surface. The separate cutaneous margins should be clearly designated. Be prepared to submit the entire specimen in order to rule out or confirm

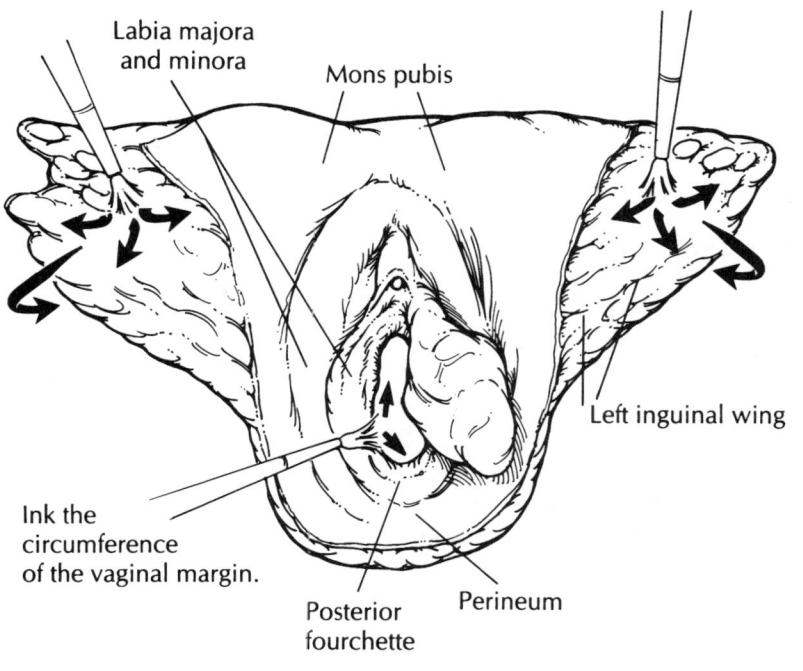

Total Vulvectomy

1. Orient the specimen as if viewed in situ with the inguinal wings superior and lateral.

2. Ink all cutaneous and soft tissue margins, including the deep margin. Ink the vaginal margin with a separate color.

3. Document the size of all lesions, and section with full-thickness incisions perpendicular to the epithelial surface.

4. Dissect the inguinal wings for lymph nodes and maintain their right and left orientation.

5. Submit sections of tumor to demonstrate maximum tumor thickness; nearest margins (vaginal, cutaneous, and deep); any other skin lesions; all lymph nodes; and uninvolved skin including clitoris, fourchette, perineum, and contralateral labia majora and minora.

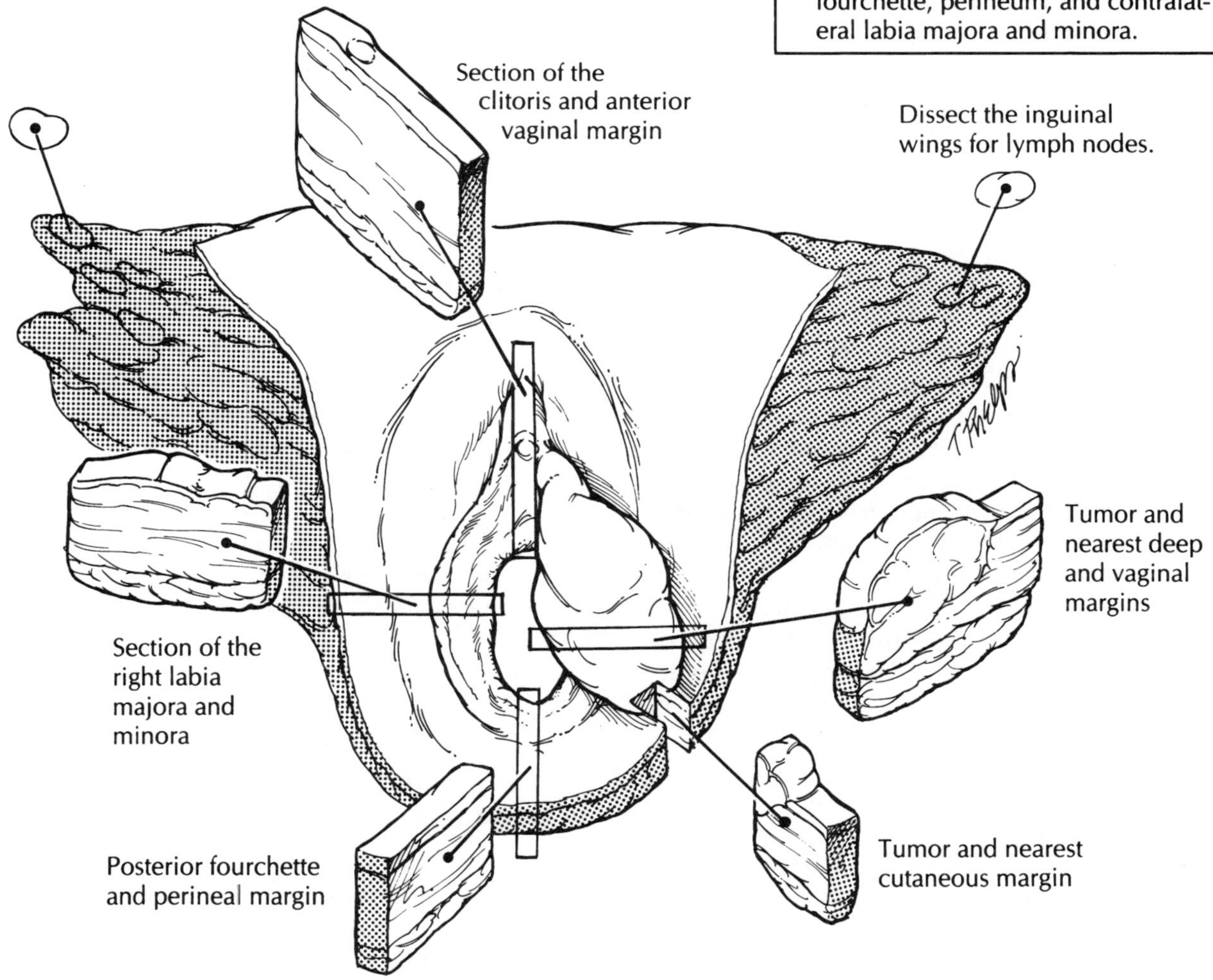

invasive disease and to document the adequacy of the resection margins.

Vulvectomies

The majority of vulvectomies are performed for the treatment of invasive squamous carcinoma. Most squamous carcinomas arise on the labia (usually the labia majora), with the remainder primarily located on either the clitoris or posterior fourchette. Vulvectomy specimens can be either partial—when only a portion of the vulva is removed—or total—when the whole vulvar region is removed. A portion of the vagina and extensions of perineum around the anus may also be included. The depth of the resection is variable. A *superficial vulvectomy* refers to removal of the epidermis with a variable amount of dermis and subcutaneous tissue. A *deep vulvectomy* refers to removal of the vulva to the superficial aponeurosis of the urogenital diaphragm and/or pubic periosteum. Inguinal node dissections can either be attached to the vulvectomy specimen as superolateral wings or submitted separately.

The initial evaluation includes orientation and documentation of the tissues received. Begin by orienting the specimen as if viewed *in situ*. With a total vulvectomy, this is easily accomplished by placing the inguinal fat superiorly and laterally. If the inguinal region is not present, use the clitoris to define the superior and midline position. In partial vulvectomies, orient the specimen using the hair-bearing labia majora, which represents the lateral extent of the resection. If there is any doubt, ask the surgeon to help with orientation. Document the type of specimen received and the anatomic structures present. Measure the width of the specimen, the length from the superior to inferior limits, and the depth from the epithelial surface to the deep soft tissue margin. It may be helpful to have photographs, line drawings, or preprinted diagrams to demonstrate the margins of resection and extent of the lesion. Ink all the exposed epithelial and soft tissue margins. The vaginal margin should be painted with a different color ink than the other cutaneous margins. The specimen can then be pinned to a cork or wax board for fixation.

After fixation, examine the epithelial surface for ulcerative, exophytic, and flat lesions. Evaluate all lesions with full-thickness incisions perpendicular to the epithelial surface. Record their location, size, and distance to the nearest skin and vaginal margins. For invasive tumors, also measure the maximal tumor thickness and the distance from the deepest tumor edge to the nearest deep margin. Submit sections of the tumor in such a way as to include the nearest deep and epithelial (both vaginal and cutaneous) margins as well as adjacent normal-appearing skin. Preneoplastic lesions such as vulvar intraepithelial neoplasia (VIN) may be found adjacent to tumors. Margins should be evaluated with sections that are perpendicular rather than parallel to the surgical margin. Representative epithelial margins distant to the tumor do not need to be submitted. Judiciously sample any other skin lesions, especially those within 0.5 cm of any margin. Include sections of non-neoplastic skin so that it can be evaluated for the presence of lichen sclerosus, squamous hyperplasia, and condylomata.

In vulvectomy specimens with attached inguinal regions, the lymph nodes can be dissected either before or after obtaining the appropriate epithelial sections. Turn the specimen over so that the epithelial surface is face down and the subcutaneous tissue is exposed. Beginning at the superior tip of one inguinal wing, and progressing medially, make parallel 0.3- to 0.4-cm-wide sections through the fatty tissue. Examine the cut fat carefully for lymph nodes. Although the lymphatic drainage of the vulva can be divided into superficial and deep node groups, this is usually not necessary and important nodes, such as Cloquet's node, must be separately designated by the surgeon. All the lymph nodes should be entirely submitted unless grossly positive, in which case a representative section will suffice. Be sure to clearly designate and submit the right and left inguinal node groups separately. Lymph nodes may also be received as separate specimens designated by the surgeon. State the location (inguinal-femoral or pelvic); specify right side, left side, or both; and submit all lymph nodes in their entirety.

Important Issues to Address in Your Surgical Pathology Report on Vulvectomies

- What type of vulvectomy was performed (partial vs. total, superficial vs. deep), and what structures are present?

- Where is the tumor located? Is it unifocal or multifocal?
- What is the size of the tumor (in centimeters; 2 cm is a cutoff point for TNM staging)?
- What are the histologic type and grade of the neoplasm?
- What is the "maximum tumor thickness" (in millimeters)? (Measure from the granular layer if keratinized or surface if nonkeratinized.)
- What is the "maximum depth of invasion" (in millimeters)? (For carcinomas, measure from the epithelial stromal junction of the adjacent most superficial dermal papillae. For melanomas, measure from the deep border of the granular layer.)
- Does the tumor involve any of the margins? (vaginal, cutaneous, or deep)? Give the distance of the tumor from closest margin (in centimeters).
- Does the tumor extend into any adjacent tissues (lower urethra, upper urethra, vagina, anus, bladder, or rectum)?
- Is there evidence of lymphatic, vascular, or perineural invasion?
- Does the adjacent skin show any precancerous lesions (VIN or dysplastic nevi)?
- Does the tumor involve any lymph nodes? (Include the location, number of nodes involved, and the number of nodes examined separately for each site. Also, note the presence or absence of extranodal extension.)
- Does the non-neoplastic portion of the vulva show any pathology (e.g., squamous hyperplasia, lichen sclerosus, condyloma acuminatum, or other)?

27 Uterus, Cervix, and Vagina

Biopsies

Cervical and vaginal biopsies consist of an epithelial surface and varying amounts of underlying stroma. Usually, no grossly identifiable lesion can be seen. The most important objectives are to orient the specimen so that perpendicular sections will be taken through the surface and to secure the specimen properly to ensure that small pieces are not lost. These tasks can be accomplished in several ways. If the specimen is large enough (i.e., greater than 0.4 cm), the tissue can be bisected perpendicular to the surface and marked with either mercurochrome or tattoo powder to indicate the surface to be cut. If the specimen is small, it can be secured between Gelfoam sponges, within fine-mesh biopsy bags, or it can be wrapped in tissue paper. The gynecologist may also submit the biopsy oriented mucosal side up on a mounting surface such as filter paper. In this case, instruct your histotechnologist to embed and cut the biopsy specimen perpendicular to the mounting surface. All biopsy specimens should be entirely submitted, and it is often useful to routinely request that multiple levels be examined by the histology laboratory.

Endometrial biopsies should be handled similarly to curettage specimens.

Curettings

Endocervical and endometrial curettings consist of multiple small fragments of epithelium, which are often admixed with blood and mucus. The surgeon may put the curettings on Telfa pads or directly into fixative. Scrape the Telfa pad carefully on both sides, and filter the fluid of the specimen container into a tissue bag to obtain all tissue fragments. Record the aggregate dimension, and note the percentage of tissue versus the percentage of blood and mucus. The entire specimen should be submitted either wrapped in tissue paper or within a fine-mesh biopsy bag. Even if no tissue is visible, the blood and mucus should still be submitted for histologic evaluation, as they may contain entrapped small epithelial fragments. Multiple levels are often useful in evaluating these specimens. For endometrial specimens, if the tissue obtained is not representative of functioning endometrium (e.g., endocervix, lower uterine segment, or surface endometrial epithelium only), this fact should be specified. If endometrial cancer is identified, estimate the percentage of the specimen involved by tumor.

Cervix

Loop Electrocautery Excisions

The loop electrosurgical excision procedure (LEEP) and large loop excision of the transformation zone (LLETZ) are electrocautery excisions of the cervical transformation zone that excise less tissue than the traditional cone biopsy. Their use is increasing in the treatment of squamous intraepithelial lesions. Depending on the type of loop used and on the depth of the excision, the specimen may be large enough to allow one to orient, open, and process it like a conventional

Loop Electrocautery Excisions of the Cervix

1. Orient the specimen by identifying the ectocervical and endocervical margins.
2. Ink the endocervical margin and the stromal/ectocervical margins with separate colors.
3. For small cylindrical specimens, divide in half and section longitudinally.
4. For shallow, saucer-shaped specimens, section radially—like a pie.
5. Submit the entire specimen.

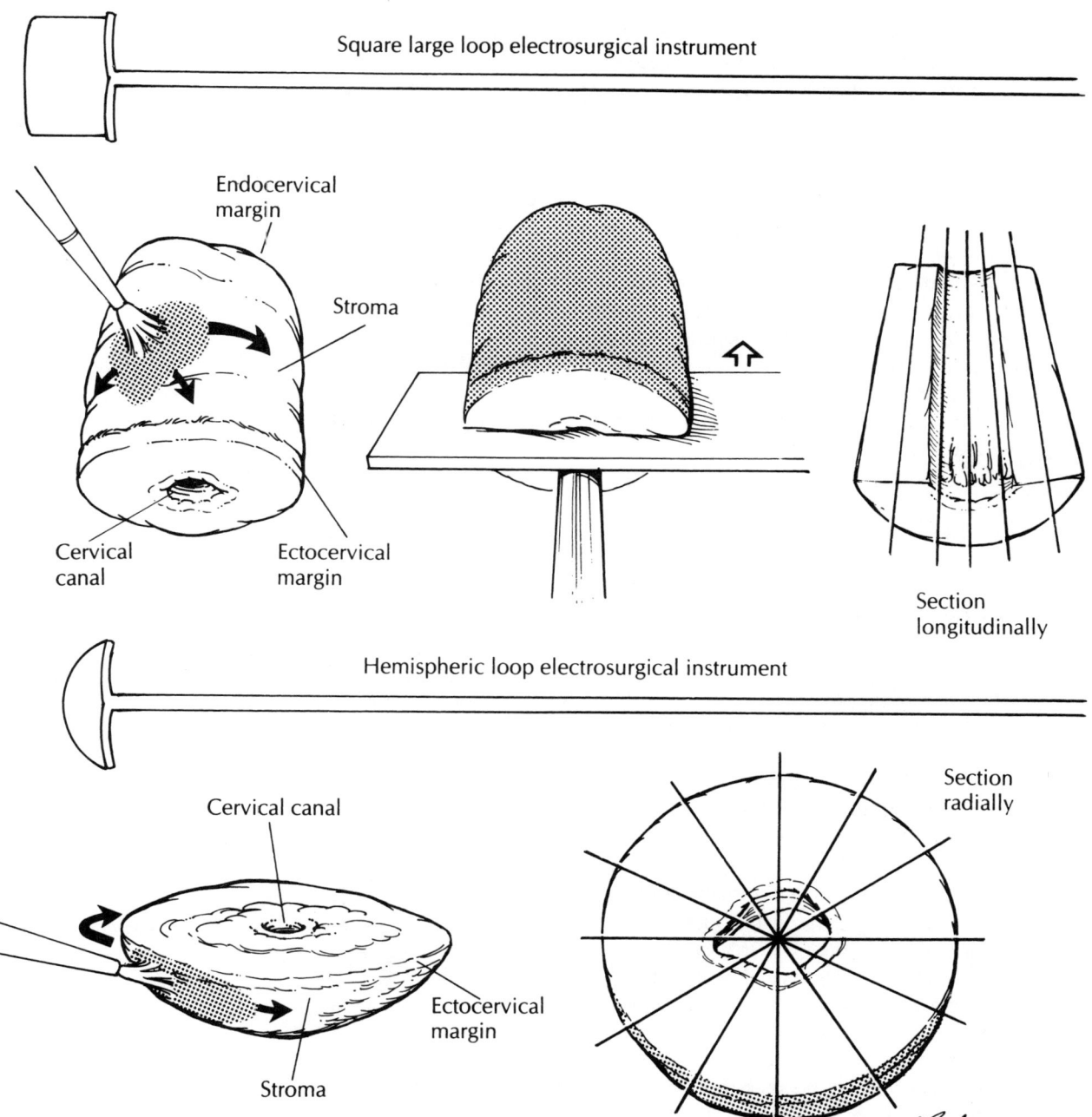

cone biopsy, as described later. However, many of these specimens arrive in the surgical pathology laboratory already fixed in formalin and/or in several pieces. The endocervical margin will sometimes be submitted separately, and an overall orientation may or may not be provided. If multiple fragments are submitted, identify the mucosal surface, and try to distinguish the smooth, gray squamous mucosa from the rugated, mucoid, tan endocervical mucosa. Divide the fragments into strips with sections perpendicular to the squamocolumnar junction. For shallow, saucer-shaped specimens, divide the specimen radially as illustrated. This is similar to slicing a pie. For small conical specimens that are already well fixed, divide the specimen into anterior and posterior halves, and section each half longitudinally as shown. Conceptually, cutting the biopsy this way is similar to the handling of the perpendicular sections of the distal urethral margins in a radical prostatectomy specimen. Note that in contrast to large cone biopsies, not all sections will demonstrate the cervical canal mucosa. Although cautery artifact may make the limits of resection of these specimens difficult to evaluate, it is always best to ink the mucosal margins and exposed stroma for histologic evaluation.

Cone Biopsy

A cervical cone biopsy is a conical excision of the cervical canal performed with either a laser or a surgical blade (cold knife excision). The wider part of the cone is the outer ectocervix, and the tapered end is the endocervical margin. Measure the length of the cone biopsy corresponding to the endocervical canal, the diameter at the ectocervical margin, and the diameter at the endocervical margin. By convention, the ectocervix is described as a clock face with the most superior midpoint of the anterior lip designated as 12 o'clock. This point is usually marked with a stitch by the gynecologist. After orienting the cone biopsy as if viewed *in situ*, ink the exposed fibrous stroma and the ectocervical mucosal margin. Use a different color to ink the endocervical mucosal margin. Make a longitudinal incision through the outer stroma to the inner canal at the 3-o'clock position, and open the specimen so that the inner mucosal surface is exposed. The convention of incising the cervix at either 3 or 9 o'clock is based on the fact that most cervical lesions arise on the anterior and posterior surfaces, rather than laterally. Pin the specimen to either a wax or cork board with the epithelial surface upward, using pins placed through the stroma on both sides. Examine the mucosal surface, and look for any lesions, especially along the squamocolumnar junction.

After fixation, cut serial full-thickness sections perpendicular to the mucosal surface in the plane of the endocervical canal. Use the endocervical apex as a pivot, and angle the cuts to provide a continuous line from the endocervical mucosa to the ectocervical mucosa. These cuts will encompass the squamocolumnar junction and will demonstrate the extent of the transformation zone. The sections should be 0.2 to 0.3 cm wide and will end up being slightly wedge-shaped. All sections should be submitted sequentially and designated as to their clock-face orientation. As with other biopsies, multiple levels are often routinely requested.

Important Issues to Address in Your Surgical Pathology Report on the Cervix

- What procedure was performed, and what structures/organs are present?
- What grade of squamous intraepithelial lesion is identified?
- Is adenocarcinoma *in situ* present?
- Is the lesion focal, multifocal, or extensive? State the percentage or quadrants of tissue involved.
- Are the resection margins involved (endocervical, ectocervical or stromal)?
- Is evidence of invasion present? If so, what is the depth of invasion from the base of the epithelium, either surface or glandular, from which it arises (in millimeters)? What is the horizontal spread (in millimeters)? Is there any evidence of capillary–lymphatic space invasion?
- If no precursor lesion or invasive tumor is identified, what is the adequacy of the specimen (i.e., state the presence or absence of the squamocolumnar junction)?

Uterus

The uterus is removed for a wide variety of reasons. Common indications for hysterectomy

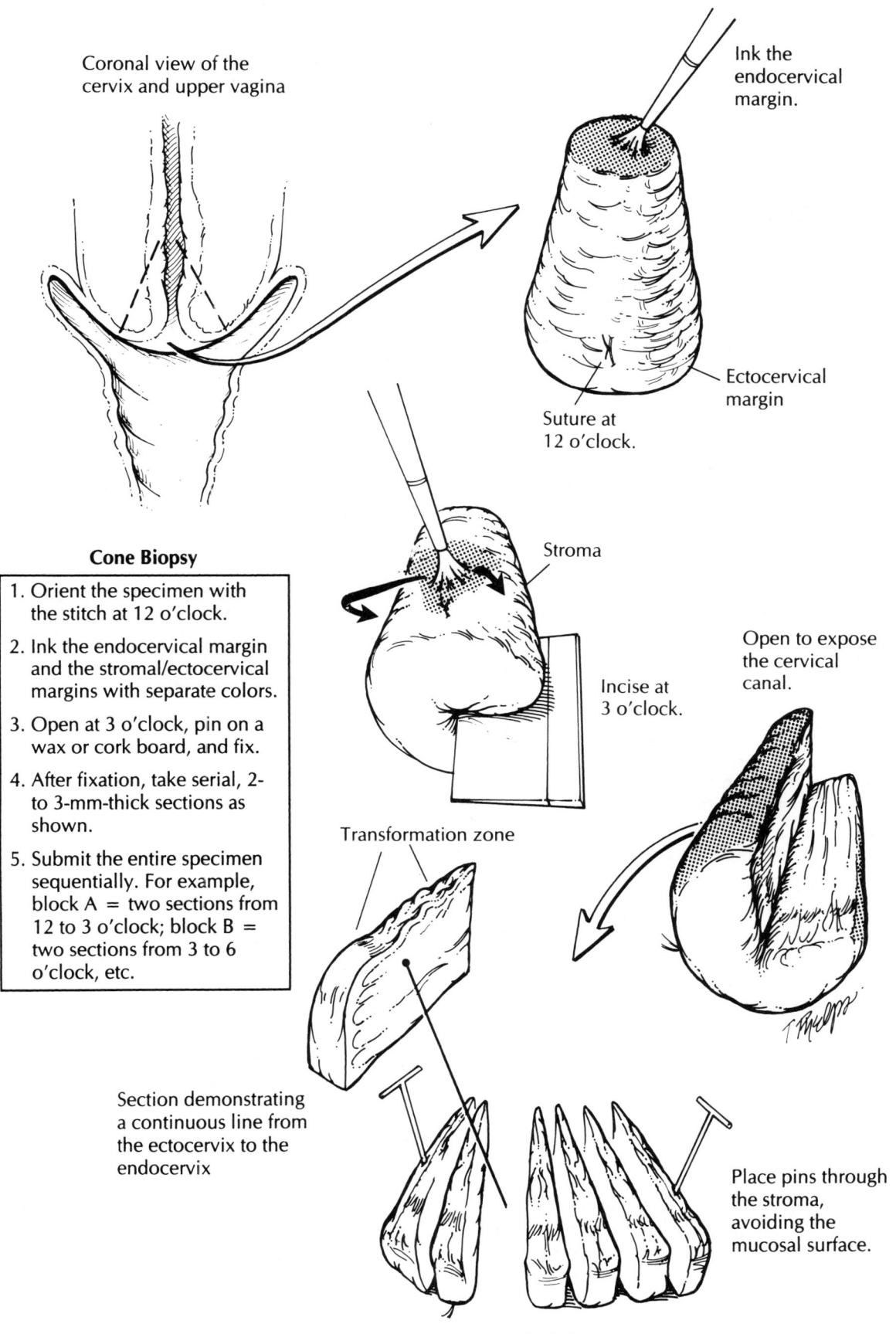

include uterine prolapse, leiomyomas, endometrial hyperplasia, cervical cancer, and endometrial cancer. Given the diverse nature of these processes and the variation in the appearance of the uterus due to the hormonal environment, it is important to know both the clinical indication for the surgery and the patient's reproductive status when evaluating a hysterectomy specimen.

The uterus is traditionally divided into two components: (1) the uterine corpus and (2) the uterine cervix. The uterine corpus (or body) extends from the superiorly located fundus to the point of maximal narrowing which corresponds to the location of the internal os. The right and left cornual regions are located superolaterally, at the insertion of the fallopian tubes. The inferior 1 to 2 cm of the corpus is referred to as the isthmus or lower uterine segment (LUS). This region is a "bridge" between the cervix and the uterus and demonstrates a gradual transition from endocervical to endometrial mucosa. The cervix encompasses the lower portion of the uterus, beginning at the internal os. The cervix is composed of an inner endocervical canal lined by columnar epithelium and a rounded outer ectocervix covered by squamous epithelium. The location of the squamocolumnar junction moves in and out of the cervical canal with age and parity. It is within this region that most intraepithelial lesions arise. Although the exact limits of this region are not visible grossly, the term "transformation zone" encompasses this entire transition area including the squamocolumnar junction.

This section provides an approach to the evaluation of hysterectomy specimens in four categories: (1) hysterectomies for nonmalignant disease, (2) hysterectomies for endometrial cancer, (3) radical hysterectomies for cervical cancer, and (4) pelvic exenterations with vaginectomies for vaginal cancer or recurrent cervical cancer.

Hysterectomy for Nonmalignant Disease

zpThe category of hysterectomy of nonmalignant disease includes hysterectomies for uterine prolapse, persistent abnormal bleeding, intractable pelvic pain, leiomyomas, and endometrial hyperplasia. The procedure can be performed either vaginally or abdominally. The fallopian tubes and ovaries may also be present.

Orient the uterus by identifying the stubs of the round ligaments that insert anterior to the fallopian tubes. The ovaries should lie posteriorly. In addition, because the anterior peritoneum reflects onto the bladder, the anterior peritoneum does not extend as far inferiorly along the uterus as does the posterior peritoneum. Vaginal and abdominal hysterectomies may be distinguished by examining the peritoneal surface in the region of the posterior cul-de-sac. The peritoneum appears V-shaped in a vaginal and U-shaped in an abdominal hysterectomy specimen.

If the adnexa are present, remove them from the right and left cornual regions, and examine them separately (see Chapter 28). Weigh the uterus, and record the following measurements: fundus to ectocervix, cornu to cornu, and anterior to posterior. Measure the length of the cervix from the level of the internal os to the ectocervix and the diameter of the cervix from side to side and from anterior to posterior.

The uterus can now be evaluated with a systematic examination of each of its main components. Begin by examining the uterine serosa. Look for and describe any adhesions or small "powder burn" spots, which may signify endometriosis. These may be seen more frequently on the posterior aspect.

Next, evaluate the cervix. Note the shape of the external os, which is usually circular in nulliparous women and slit-like in parous women. Examine the ectocervix for any lacerations, scars, masses, ulcers, or cysts. Place a probe through the cervical canal and into the endometrial cavity. Beginning at the cervix, incise the uterus with a large blade using the probe as a guide to divide it into anterior and posterior halves. Another method for bivalving the uterus is to use a pair of scissors to cut along the lateral margins from the ectocervix to the cornu. Gently remove the excess mucus from the endocervical canal, and examine it for the presence of polyps. At this point, the uterus may be photographed and then pinned to a wax tablet for fixation. Be sure to avoid placing pins through the mucosal surfaces. After fixation, longitudinally section the cervix at 0.2- to 0.3-cm intervals, and evaluate the transformation zone and stroma.

Now, measure the thickness of the endometrium, and look for any unusual thickenings or polyps. Keep in mind the age and reproductive status of the patient. If the woman is postmenopausal, an endometrial thickness greater than

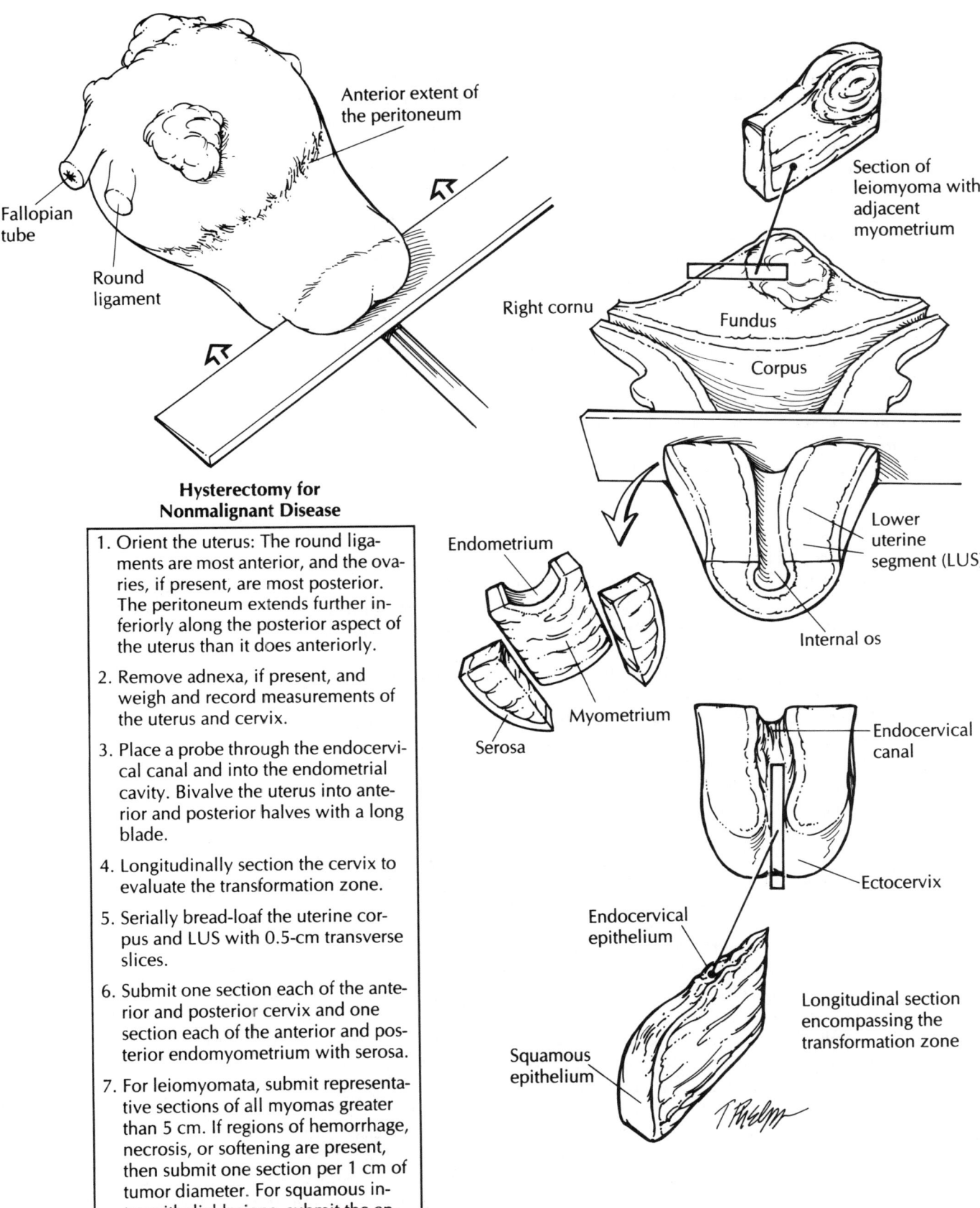

Hysterectomy for Nonmalignant Disease

1. Orient the uterus: The round ligaments are most anterior, and the ovaries, if present, are most posterior. The peritoneum extends further inferiorly along the posterior aspect of the uterus than it does anteriorly.

2. Remove adnexa, if present, and weigh and record measurements of the uterus and cervix.

3. Place a probe through the endocervical canal and into the endometrial cavity. Bivalve the uterus into anterior and posterior halves with a long blade.

4. Longitudinally section the cervix to evaluate the transformation zone.

5. Serially bread-loaf the uterine corpus and LUS with 0.5-cm transverse slices.

6. Submit one section each of the anterior and posterior cervix and one section each of the anterior and posterior endomyometrium with serosa.

7. For leiomyomata, submit representative sections of all myomas greater than 5 cm. If regions of hemorrhage, necrosis, or softening are present, then submit one section per 1 cm of tumor diameter. For squamous intraepithelial lesions, submit the entire cervix as in a cone biopsy. For endometrial hyperplasia, submit the entire endometrium.

2 mm may signify a hyperplastic process. Conversely, a thick endometrium in a premenopausal woman may reflect only the normal secretory phase.

The myometrium is examined last. Make serial 0.5-cm-thick transverse cuts through the uterine corpus and lower uterine segment, and record the maximum myometrial thickness. Look for intramural leiomyomas or evidence of adenomyosis. Adenomyosis is usually more extensive in the posterior wall and may be recognized by a thickened wall with trabeculations and small hemorrhagic or cystic foci.

If no lesions are identified, standard sections of the uterus include longitudinal sections of the anterior and posterior cervix (including the transformation zone) and full-thickness sections of the anterior and posterior walls of the uterus to include endometrium, myometrium, and serosa. At our institution, sections of the anterior and posterior lower uterine segment regions are routinely submitted as well.

Additional sampling may also be required if the standard sections reveal either endometrial hyperplasia or a cervical intraepithelial lesion. In the case of endometrial hyperplasia, the entire endometrium may need to be evaluated to rule out an invasive process. Multiple thin strips of endometrium with only a small amount of underlying myometrium can be submitted in a limited number of tissue cassettes. If a high-grade squamous intraepithelial lesion is identified, the cervix should be processed and submitted as described for cone biopsies. For low-grade squamous intraepithelial lesions, a section from each quadrant may suffice.

The evaluation of a uterus with multiple leiomyomas deserves special mention. A leiomyomatous uterus is one of the most frequently encountered specimens, and the gross examination of these specimens is the key to their proper handling. Orient, weigh, measure, and section the uterus as described above. Record the number of nodules present and their size. Specifically state whether they are submucosal, intramural, or subserosal in location. All nodules should be sectioned at 1- to 2-cm intervals and examined grossly but not necessarily microscopically. Benign leiomyomas are firm and white with a whorled cut surface. Their border with the surrounding myometrium is smooth and well-circumscribed. If these criteria are met, representative sampling of each leiomyoma is sufficient. Always include sections demonstrating the border between the leiomyoma and the surrounding myometrium or overlying endometrium. Any leiomyomas with areas of hemorrhage, necrosis, or softening need to be sampled more extensively. In these cases, the general rule of one section per 1 cm of tumor diameter should be followed. Smooth muscle tumors less than 5 cm do not need to be sampled, as they rarely metastasize, regardless of their microscopic appearance.

Important Issues to Address in Your Surgical Pathology Report on Hysterectomies for Non-Malignant Disease

- What procedure was performed, and what structures/organs are present?
- Cervix: Are any preinvasive or invasive lesions identified?
- Endometrium: Is the endometrium hyperplastic, atrophic, or functional? If functional, specify whether it is in the proliferative or secretory phase. Are any polyps present?
- Myometrium: Are any leiomyomas or regions of adenomyosis identified? Specify whether the leiomyomas are submucosal, intramural, or subserosal.
- Serosa: Are any adhesions or regions of endometriosis identified?

Hysterectomy for Endometrial Cancer

The approach to hysterectomies performed for endometrial cancer parallels the approach to hysterectomies for benign disease. Additional steps include inking the paracervical and parametrial soft tissue margins and evaluating the extent of the tumor.

Orient, weigh, and measure the uterus as described in the section on hysterectomies for benign disease, and ink the soft tissue resection margins around the cervical canal. Also, ink the parametrial tissue, which extends along the body of the uterus and into the broad ligament. Carefully examine the serosal surfaces for evidence of tumor extension. Ink these areas a different color

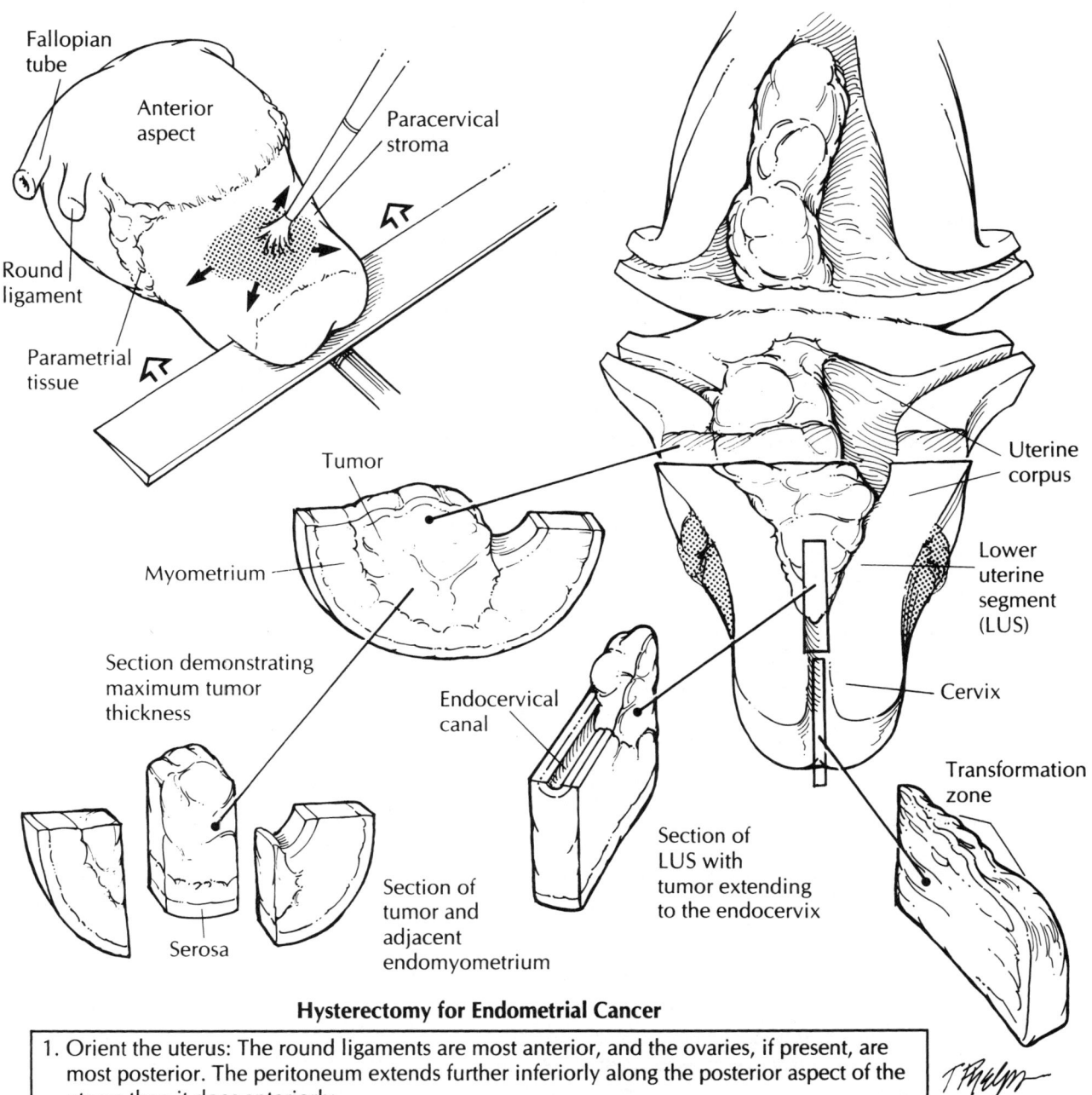

Hysterectomy for Endometrial Cancer

1. Orient the uterus: The round ligaments are most anterior, and the ovaries, if present, are most posterior. The peritoneum extends further inferiorly along the posterior aspect of the uterus than it does anteriorly.

2. Weigh and measure the uterus and cervix. Ink the paracervical and parametrial soft tissue margins.

3. Place a probe in the endocervical and endometrial canal. Bivalve the uterus into anterior and posterior halves with a long blade.

4. Longitudinally section the cervix, extending the incision upward through the LUS. Serially bread-loaf the uterine corpus with 0.5-cm transverse slices.

5. Describe the size, appearance, and location of the tumor.

6. Submit sections of tumor to demonstrate the maximum tumor thickness, anterior and posterior LUS sections, uninvolved endometrium, and anterior and posterior cervix. If the adnexa are present, submit sections of the ovary and fallopian tube with adjacent soft tissue.

for orientation. If the adnexa are present, remove them at their lateral insertions along the uterus. Make multiple transverse cuts through the ovary and fallopian tube, looking for evidence of either direct tumor extension or metastatic spread. Submit at least one section from each side to demonstrate the ovary and fallopian tube with adjacent soft tissue.

Bivalve the uterus by using a long, sharp knife guided by a probe placed through the cervical canal. Closely examine the endometrial cavity. Endometrial carcinomas can be shaggy, sessile tumors or polypoid masses arising from the surface of the endometrium. They may be either focal or diffuse. The sounding depth of the uterus from the external cervical os to the superior limit of the endometrial cavity may be measured, but it is no longer used in the staging of endometrial cancers. While the tumor is fresh, remove a portion to freeze for future molecular diagnostic tests if desired. The bivalved uterus may now be photographed and pinned to a wax tablet for fixation.

The dissection begins with longitudinal sectioning of the cervix. Extend these incisions through the lower uterine segment to include both endometrial and endocervical mucosal surfaces. Note whether or not the tumor grossly involves the endocervical mucosa and/or stroma. Submit a section of this region from the anterior and posterior halves to evaluate for tumor extension into the cervix, an important factor in determining the stage of the cancer. This step may also be accomplished by taking transverse sections of the upper endocervix and lower uterine segment. Next, serially bread-loaf the uterine corpus and lower uterine segment with transverse sections. Record the size, location, and appearance of the tumor. Describe the pattern of invasion. Does the tumor have a broad pushing front, an infiltrating finger-like pattern, or is it discontinuous? Measure the greatest depth of tumor invasion into the myometrium starting from the normal junction of the endometrium and the myometrium. In addition, measure the total myometrial thickness at this point, and specify the uninvolved distance from the deep tumor/myometrial junction to the serosa. When selecting sections for histologic analysis, include the deepest point of tumor invasion as well as the interface with grossly uninvolved endometrium. The best sections are those that show the full thickness from the endometrium to the serosa. Sometimes, however, the myometrium may be too thick to fit in a standard-size tissue cassette. In these situations, divide the section into endometrial and serosal halves. Be sure to designate their relationship clearly in your summary of sections.

Lymph nodes from the pelvic and para-aortic regions may also be included as separate specimens. They can be handled in a routine manner for evaluation of metastatic disease.

Important Issues to Address in Your Surgical Pathology Report on Hysterectomies for Endometrial Cancer

- What procedure was performed, and what structures/organs are present?
- What is the size of the tumor?
- What are the histologic type and grade of neoplasm present?
- What is the maximum depth of tumor invasion (in millimeters)? (Measure from the normal endometrial/myometrial junction.)
- What is the total myometrial thickness at the deepest point of invasion (in millimeters)?
- What is the distance from the deepest tumor/myometrial junction to the serosa (in millimeters)?
- Does the tumor extend through the serosa?
- Does the tumor involve the endocervix? (Specify surface glandular and/or stromal involvement.)
- Is capillary–lymphatic space invasion seen?
- Does the tumor involve the adjacent adnexa?
- Does the tumor involve any margins (cervical/vaginal, right paracervical/parametrial, left paracervical/parametrial)? Give the distance of the tumor from closest margin (in centimeters).
- Does the tumor involve any lymph nodes? (Include the number of nodes involved and the number of nodes examined at each specified site.)

Radical Hysterectomy for Cervical Cancer

Radical hysterectomies are performed for early stage invasive squamous carcinomas and adenocarcinomas of the cervix. In addition to the

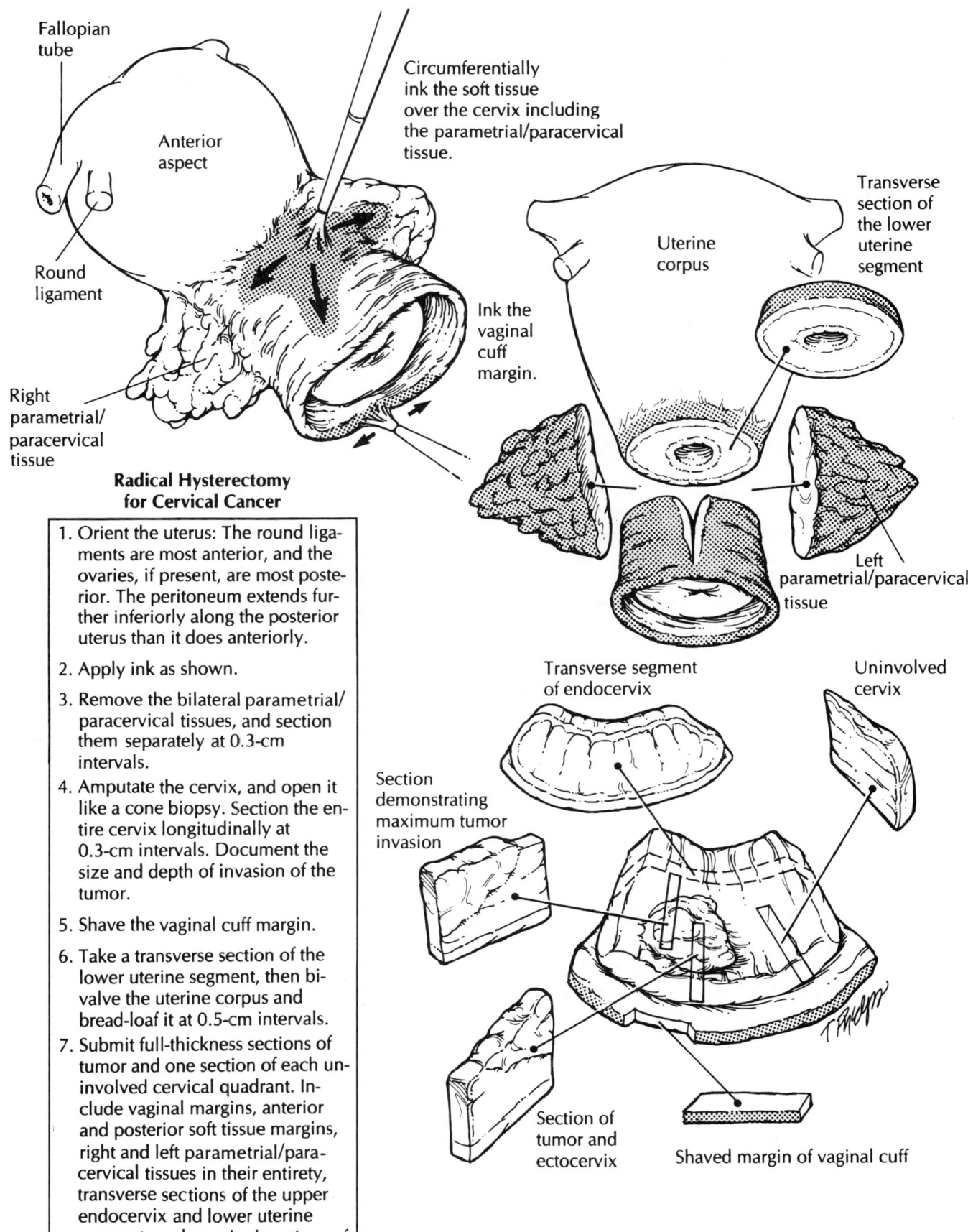

Radical Hysterectomy for Cervical Cancer

1. Orient the uterus: The round ligaments are most anterior, and the ovaries, if present, are most posterior. The peritoneum extends further inferiorly along the posterior uterus than it does anteriorly.

2. Apply ink as shown.

3. Remove the bilateral parametrial/paracervical tissues, and section them separately at 0.3-cm intervals.

4. Amputate the cervix, and open it like a cone biopsy. Section the entire cervix longitudinally at 0.3-cm intervals. Document the size and depth of invasion of the tumor.

5. Shave the vaginal cuff margin.

6. Take a transverse section of the lower uterine segment, then bivalve the uterine corpus and bread-loaf it at 0.5-cm intervals.

7. Submit full-thickness sections of tumor and one section of each uninvolved cervical quadrant. Include vaginal margins, anterior and posterior soft tissue margins, right and left parametrial/paracervical tissues in their entirety, transverse sections of the upper endocervix and lower uterine segment, and standard sections of anterior and posterior endomyometrium.

uterus and cervix, the specimen has attached parametrial/paracervical soft tissue and a vaginal cuff.

Begin by orienting, measuring, and weighing the uterus and cervix as described in the section on hysterectomies for benign disease. Also, measure the size of the attached parametrial/paracervical tissue and the length of the attached vaginal cuff. Note whether the shape of the cervix is rounded or barrel shaped. Ink the right and left parametrial/paracervical tissues, the anterior/posterior soft tissue margins of the cervical canal, and the vaginal cuff margin. Remove the parametrial/paracervical tissue by shaving each side close to its lateral attachment on the cervix. Section this tissue at 0.3-cm intervals, and submit the entire tissue for histologic examination. Any identifiable lymph nodes may be dissected and separately designated.

Next, amputate the cervix at the level of the internal os, and open the canal with a longitudinal incision opposite the tumor. Pin it open, and fix it as you would a cone biopsy. Measure the maximum tumor width and length as well as the distance to the nearest vaginal margin. Examine the vaginal cuff. Unless the tumor is close to the vaginal margin, the margin may be removed with a 0.3-cm parallel shave and submitted as four designated quadrants. If the tumor closely approaches the vaginal margin, leave the vaginal cuff intact and take perpendicular margins to demonstrate the relationship of the tumor to the margin. Serially section the cervix at 0.3-cm intervals, and measure the maximum tumor thickness as well as the thickness of the cervical wall at that site. Occasionally, a cervical tumor may not be easily discernible as a result of prior surgery or therapy.

Now turn your attention to the uterine corpus. Take a transverse section of the lower uterine segment and bivalve the uterus into anterior and posterior halves. Examine the corpus with serial transverse sections as you would in any hysterectomy specimen.

Sections for microscopic analysis should be chosen to demonstrate the maximum thickness of the tumor and its interface with any normal-appearing mucosa. If the tumor is not visible, the cervix with attached vaginal cuff should be entirely submitted as in a cone biopsy. The superior extent of the tumor can be documented by taking transverse sections of the upper endocervix and lower uterine segment. The inferior extent of the tumor is documented by taking sections of the cervical tumor that include the adjacent vaginal tissue. Margins to be evaluated include the left and right parametrial/paracervical tissues, submitted in their entirety, and the vaginal cuff. The anterior and posterior cervical soft tissue margins should be submitted to delineate the extent of the tumor in relationship to the bladder and rectum.

Lymph nodes are usually submitted separately by the surgeon from the right and left internal iliac, external iliac, obturator, pelvic, and para-aortic node groups. They can be handled in a routine manner for evaluation of metastatic disease.

Important Issues to Address in Your Surgical Pathology Report on Radical Hysterectomies for Cervical Cancer

- What procedure was performed, and what structures/organs are present?
- What are the histologic type and grade of the tumor?
- Are any associated precursor lesions present [cervical intraepithelial neoplasia (CIN) or adenocarcinoma in situ (AIS)]?
- What is the tumor size? Give horizontal spread (in millimeters) for microinvasive tumors and overall size (in centimeters) for gross tumors. State which quadrants of the cervix are involved.
- What is the maximum depth of invasion (in millimeters)? Measure from the base of the squamous or glandular epithelium from which it originates.
- What is the thickness of the cervical wall at the point of deepest tumor invasion (in millimeters)?
- Does the tumor involve capillary–lymphatic spaces?
- Does the tumor extend into the vagina, parametrial/paracervical tissue, uterus, or adnexa? Specify the extent of involvement and depth of invasion.
- Does the tumor involve any resection margins (vaginal, anterior and posterior cervical, and bilateral parametrial/paracervical)? If the tumor is close to but does not involve a resection

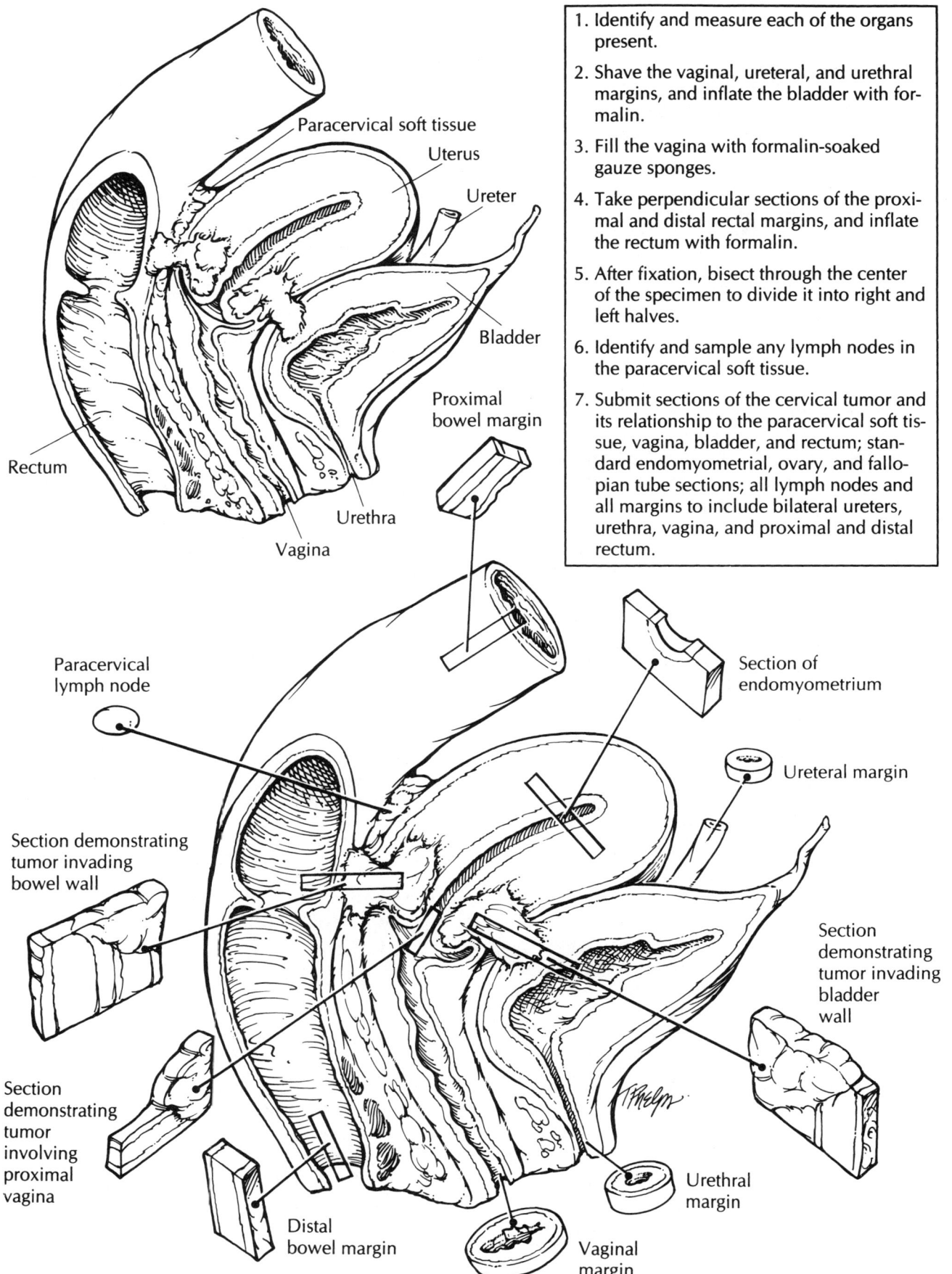

Total Pelvic Exenteration

1. Identify and measure each of the organs present.
2. Shave the vaginal, ureteral, and urethral margins, and inflate the bladder with formalin.
3. Fill the vagina with formalin-soaked gauze sponges.
4. Take perpendicular sections of the proximal and distal rectal margins, and inflate the rectum with formalin.
5. After fixation, bisect through the center of the specimen to divide it into right and left halves.
6. Identify and sample any lymph nodes in the paracervical soft tissue.
7. Submit sections of the cervical tumor and its relationship to the paracervical soft tissue, vagina, bladder, and rectum; standard endomyometrial, ovary, and fallopian tube sections; all lymph nodes and all margins to include bilateral ureters, urethra, vagina, and proximal and distal rectum.

margin, give the distance between the tumor and the margin (in millimeters).
- Is metastatic disease present? Record the number of lymph nodes with metastases and the number of lymph nodes identified by site.

Pelvic Exenterations Including Vaginectomies

Vaginectomies for vaginal cancer include a portion of vagina attached to the uterus and cervix. These specimens can be handled in the same manner as radical hysterectomies for cervical cancer, although the paracervical soft tissues may not be present. Note that a clinical history of prenatal diethylstilbestrol (DES) exposure is related to the presence of vaginal adenosis and clear cell adenocarcinoma of the vagina and cervix. Adenosis appears as a red, granular change on the normally smooth, white vaginal mucosa. Also look for structural abnormalities of the cervix and fallopian tubes associated with DES exposure. Important observations include the size of the tumor and the distance of the tumor to the vaginal margin. If the uterus has been previously removed, the resulting vaginal pouch can be opened along one side and handled in the same manner as a large skin excision. Sections should be taken so as to demonstrate the greatest depth of tumor invasion, the tumor with adjacent normal-appearing mucosa, and the relationship of the tumor to the cervix. If the bladder is included with the uterus the resection is termed an *anterior exenteration*, and if the rectum is included the resection is termed a *posterior exenteration*. With these added structures, additional sections include documentation of the extent of tumor involvement of the bladder or rectal wall, and an evaluation of their respective surgical margins. Specifically, these include the urethral and ureteral margins for the bladder, and the proximal and distal bowel margins for the rectum.

Exenterations are also performed for centrally recurrent cervical cancer. Perhaps the most daunting specimen received in the surgical pathology laboratory is a total pelvic exenteration, which includes the bladder, uterus with attached adnexa, vagina, and rectum. The evaluation of these specimens uses both a separate and an integrated approach, as described in Chapter 8. Resection margins are best handled if each of the four main components (i.e., bladder, vagina, uterus, and rectum) is thought of separately. Appropriate examination of the central tumor involves demonstrating its *in situ* relationship to these surrounding organs.

When a total pelvic exenteration specimen is received for recurrent cervical cancer, do not panic. Instead, calmly note the organs present and their dimensions. Specifically, look for the ureters, urethra, bladder, uterus, fallopian tubes, ovaries, vagina, and rectum. Take shave sections of the vaginal, ureteral, and urethral margins. Take perpendicular sections from the proximal and distal rectal margins, providing ink for margin orientation. Next, ink all the exposed soft tissue that surrounds the cervix and tumor.

Fill the vagina with formalin-soaked gauze pads, and distend the bladder and rectum with formalin. Submerge the entire specimen in formalin, and fix it overnight. The fixed specimen may then be bisected in a sagittal plane to demonstrate the tumor and its relationship to surrounding structures. This is best accomplished by using probes in the urethra and uterine canal as midline guides. After the specimen has been sectioned, a diagram can facilitate the description of the tumor, including its extension. Take sections of the tumor to demonstrate invasion of the bladder, rectum, vagina, and/or paracervical tissue. Document the vaginal and paracervical soft tissue margins with perpendicular or shave sections. Last, dissect the soft tissue surrounding the cervix, and submit for histology a section of any lymph nodes found.

Important Issues to Address in Your Surgical Pathology Report on Pelvic Exenterations

- What procedure was performed, and what structures/organs are present?
- What is the site of origin of the tumor?
- What are the histologic type and grade of the tumor?
- What is the size of the tumor?
- What other organs are involved by the tumor? Specify the extent of tumor involvement into these structures. That is, does it reach the muscular wall, submucosa, or mucosa?

- Does the tumor infiltrate the capillary–lymphatic spaces?
- Does the tumor involve any resection margins? Give the distance of the tumor from the closest margin (in centimeters).
- Does the tumor involve any lymph nodes? Include the number of nodes involved and the number of nodes examined at each specified site.
- Are any radiation effects present?

28 Ovary and Fallopian Tube

Ovarian Biopsies and Wedge Resections

Biopsies and wedge resections of the ovary are infrequently performed procedures that are used primarily for the evaluation of infertility. Biopsies should be measured, briefly described as to color and texture, and submitted in their entirety. Wedge resections should also be weighed and evaluated for capsule thickening, "powder burns" of endometriosis, subcortical cysts, and yellow stromal nodularity indicating hyperthecosis. Sections should be taken perpendicular to the ovarian surface to demonstrate the relationship of the capsule, cortex, and medulla.

Salpingectomies

Fallopian tubes can be removed in part or in total. Partial salpingectomies are commonly performed for tubal sterilization. Total salpingectomies are performed for ectopic pregnancies, in conjunction with an oophorectomy, or as part of a hysterectomy specimen. Salpingectomies for primary neoplasms of the fallopian tube are uncommon.

The evaluation of the incidental salpingectomy specimen is straightforward. The gross appearance of the tube is usually unremarkable. Record the length, diameter, and color of the tube. Describe any features in relationship to the different portions of the fallopian tube. The intramural portion lies within the uterus and is not seen in separate salpingectomies. The isthmic portion is the first 2 to 3 cm external to the uterus. The ampullary portion is the next 5 to 8 cm, and the infundibulum starts where the tube begins to widen and encompasses the fimbriated end. The patency of the lumen may be tested with a blunt-tipped probe. Serially section the fallopian tube at 0.5-cm intervals, and examine it for nodularity, cysts, or masses. Submit one transverse section from each region.

Small segments of intervening fallopian tube are usually submitted in tubal sterilizaton procedures. For legal purposes, a *complete* cross section of each fallopian tube must be microscopically documented.

Salpingectomies for ectopic pregnancy should be examined for signs of rupture. Serially section the fallopian tube, and submit any tissue with the gross appearance of products of conception. Be sure to include the adjacent wall. If no products of conception are grossly identified, submit several sections from the wall in regions of hemorrhage as well as several from the intraluminal clot. In contrast to uterine products of conception, in which villi are seldom seen within the blood clots, villi are often identified in the clots from ectopic pregnancies. Sections of uninvolved fallopian tube should also be submitted to look for evidence of tubal disease contributing to the occurrence of an ectopic pregnancy (e.g., chronic salpingitis, endometriosis, or salpingitis isthmica nodosa).

A salpingectomy for tubal carcinoma should be evaluated in the same manner as an incidental salpingectomy. In addition, the size, location, and extent of the tumor should be documented. The maximum depth of tumor penetration can be evaluated with full-thickness transverse sections of the tube. Margins include the cut edge of the broad ligament and the proximal fallopian tube end, if not submitted with the uterus. In the case of a fused tubo-ovarian mass, the primary site is almost always assumed to be the ovary.

Ovarian Cystectomies and Oophorectomies

Ovarian cystectomies and oophorectomies are evaluated in a similar manner. Oophorectomies may be accompanied by the fallopian tube or may be part of a total hysterectomy specimen. A portion of broad ligament may also be present as the ovary attaches to the posterior surface of the broad ligament and lies inferior to the fallopian tube.

Incidental oophorectomies are easily handled. Record the weight and dimensions of the ovary. Examine the outer surface for cysts, nodules, or adhesions. Bivalve the ovary with a cut through its longest dimension and midhilum. Evaluate the sectioned surface for any cysts or nodules, and designate their location as either cortical, medullary, or hilar. Keep in mind that the appearance of the ovary will vary considerably with the age and the reproductive status of the woman. The normal ovary in the reproductive years can measure up to 4 cm, whereas an ovary this size in a postmenopausal woman warrants close evaluation. Submit one section for every 2 cm of non-neoplastic ovary. If the ovary and fallopian tube were removed as a prophylactic procedure in a woman with a family history of ovarian or breast carcinoma, the entire ovary and fallopian tube should be submitted.

Cystectomies are usually performed for benign lesions or in women with ovarian masses who wish to preserve their fertility. The most common indication is for the removal of a dermoid cyst. After weighing and measuring the cyst, examine the external surface for evidence of rupture. Place the cyst in a container, and carefully make a small incision in the wall to allow its contents to be drained. Note the color and consistency of the cyst fluid. Continue the incision with a pair of scissors to expose the entire inner surface. The thick sebaceous fluid within a dermoid cyst may have to be removed by rinsing briefly with hot water. Examine the cyst lining, and look for any regions of granularity or papillary projections. In dermoid cysts, look for Rokitansky's tubercle, which appears as a firm, nodular excrescence. This region and any other thickened areas should be submitted in their entirety to look for evidence of immature elements. Large, unilocular cysts with a smooth inner lining may be cut in strips and submitted like placental membrane rolls to get a maximum view of the cyst wall. Cystectomies for lesions other than unilocular smooth-walled cysts or dermoid cysts should be handled as described next.

Oophorectomies for ovarian tumors can be quite large and heavy. Often, the only recognizable structure is the fallopian tube, which may be attenuated and stretched over the ovarian surface. Begin by weighing and measuring the specimen. Closely examine the surface for evidence of rupture, adhesions, or nodular tumor excrescences. Ink these regions for orientation. Section the ovarian mass at 1-cm intervals through its longest axis. If the mass is cystic, you may want to perform this in a pan or on a work station that allows for easy drainage of fluid. Remember to document the color and consistency of the cyst fluid. Is the fluid serous, mucinous, or hemorrhagic? Note whether the mass is solid, cystic, or both. If both, document the percentage of each region. Examine the surfaces of the cysts for evidence of granularity, nodules, or papillary projections. The thickness of the cyst walls should also be recorded. Describe any regions of hemorrhage or necrosis. Try to find any residual ovarian parenchyma. This is commonly found in the region immediately adjacent to the fallopian tube. If a stromal or steroid cell tumor is suspected, tissue should be saved frozen in case fat stains are needed. Consider saving frozen tissue for any small, blue, round-cell tumor, particularly if the tumor is in a pediatric patient or is predominantly intra-abdominal. Photographs of the cut surface can aid in documentation of the mass and for designating where sections were taken. At this point, it may be helpful to fix the 1-cm slices in formalin before further manipulation.

Historically, ovarian tumors are submitted with a minimum of one section per 1 to 2 cm of the greatest tumor dimension. This rule is especially useful in the case of mucinous tumors, which tend to have only focal regions demonstrating atypical or frankly invasive elements. If the tumor is uniform throughout, as many serous tumors are, fewer sections may be prudent. In general, sections should be submitted from regions that are solid, hemorrhagic, or necrotic. Cysts that show granular, nodular, or papillary excrescences should be thoroughly sampled. Also

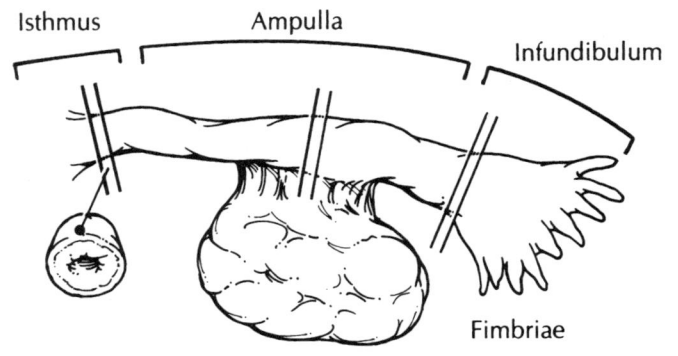

Incidental Salpingo-oophorectomy

1. Identify the fimbriated end of the fallopian tube. Record the length and diameter of the tube.
2. Probe the lumen for patency.
3. Serially section the fallopian tube at 0.5-cm intervals. Submit one transverse section from each of the isthmic, ampullary, and infundibular regions.
4. Weigh and measure the ovary.
5. Section the ovary through its longest dimension and hilum. Submit one section for every 2 cm of non-neoplastic ovary.

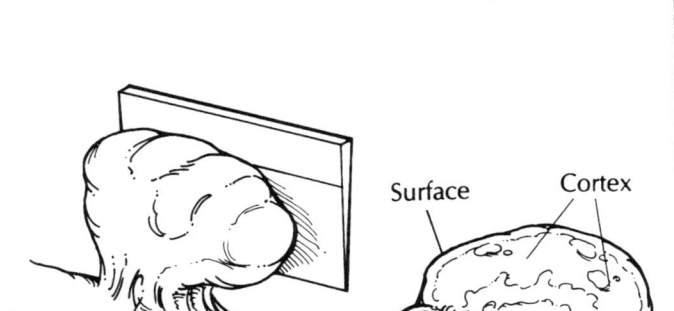

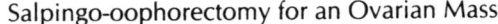

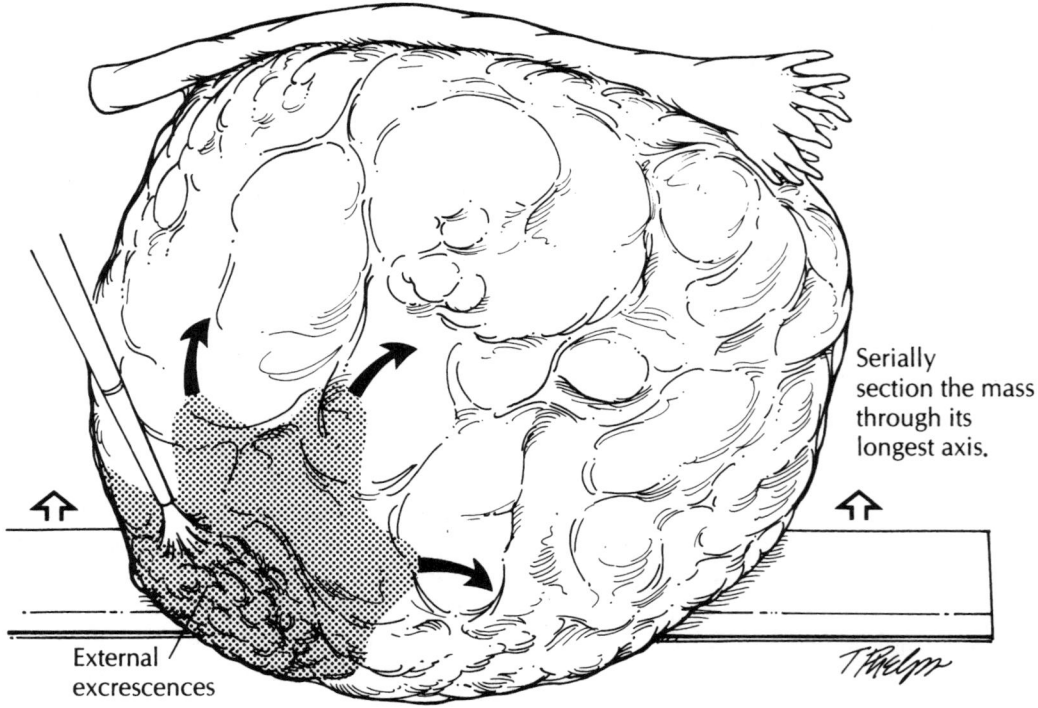

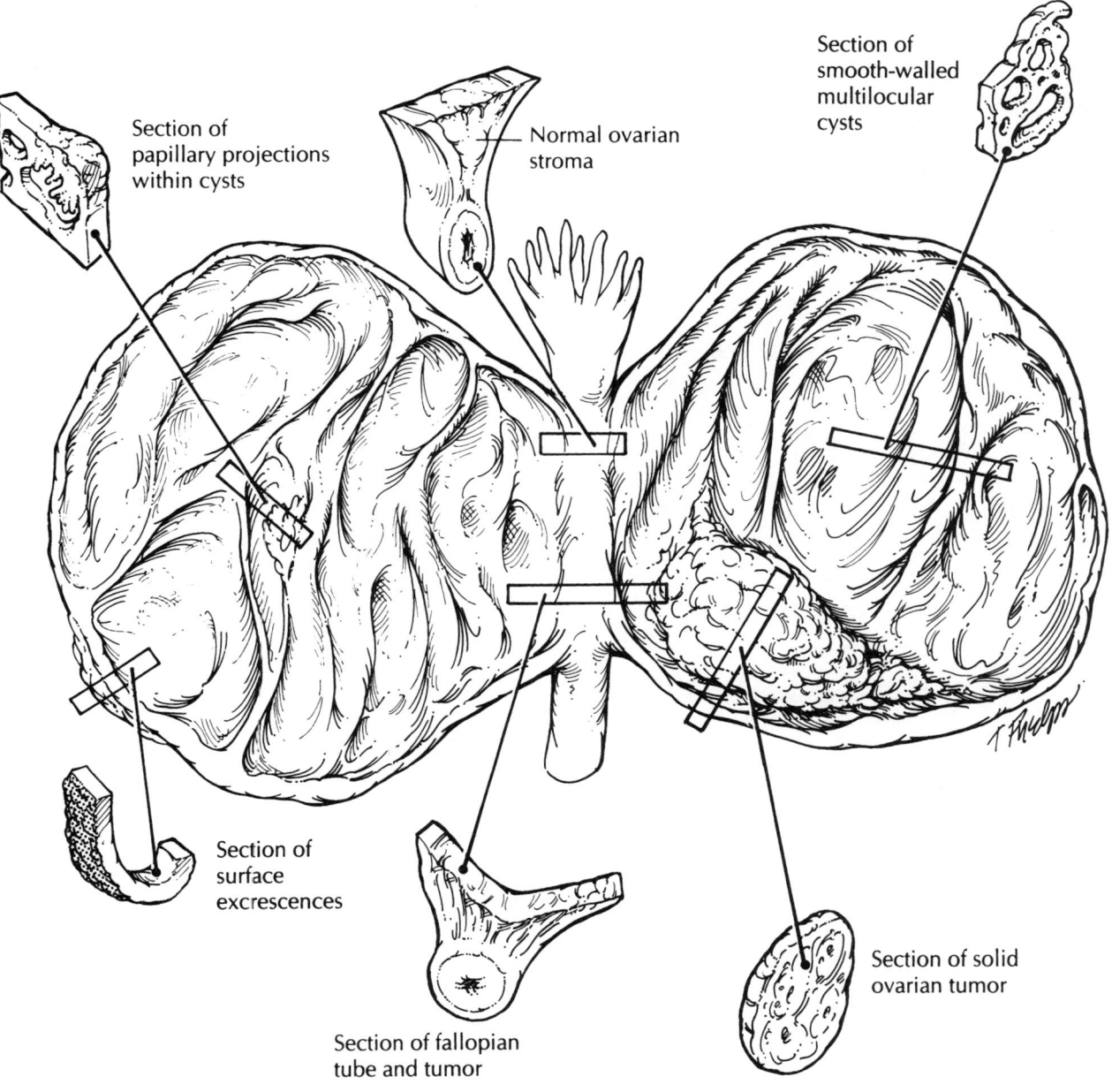

Salpingo-oophorectomy for an Ovarian Mass

1. Weigh and measure the mass. Identify the fallopian tube, if present.
2. Carefully inspect the ovarian surface for evidence of rupture, adhesions, or tumor excrescences.
3. Ink any external surface excrescences, and section the ovarian mass at 1- to 2-cm intervals through its longest axis. If the mass is cystic, note the color and consistency of the cyst contents.
4. Submit one section per 1 to 2 cm of tumor diameter. Sample to emphasize solid, papillary, necrotic, and hemorrhagic regions. Include any surface excrescences, extension to the fallopian tube, and any residual ovary.

include any regions that appear sieve-like or honeycombed. Multiple large unilocular cysts may be more judiciously sampled. Sections that demonstrate the junction between the ovary and adjacent fallopian tube, as well as any residual ovary, should also be submitted.

Specimens for Ovarian Tumor Staging

The staging procedure for an ovarian tumor can include an omentectomy, multiple biopsies of the peritoneum, and lymph node dissections.

Omentectomy specimens should be weighed, measured, and serially sectioned at 0.5-cm intervals to look for gross tumor nodules. Measure the size of the gross tumor and specifically indicate if it is 2 cm or less or more than 2 cm for staging purposes. Palpate the fat for areas of induration or small miliary nodules. For grossly visible tumor involvement, one to three representative sections should be submitted for histology. If the tumor is not grossly visible, take multiple sections from the firmest regions in the omental fat. Five representative sections are usually sufficient, although some authorities recommend up to ten sections.

Peritoneal small biopsies should be routinely processed and submitted in their entirety. If the tumor extensively involves the pelvic peritoneum, a cavitronic ultrasonic surgical aspirator may be used to remove the implants. Tissue removed this way can be handled like a curettage specimen.

A predominant mass in the omentum or peritoneum, with no ovarian involvement and no tumor in the ovary invading to a depth of 5 mm or more, is generally considered to be a primary peritoneal carcinoma.

Lymph nodes are received separately and designated by location. They can be handled in a routine manner for evaluation of metastatic disease, as detailed in chapter 5.

Important Issues to Address in Your Surgical Pathology Report on Ovarian Tumors

- What procedure was performed, and what structures/organs are present?
- Is a neoplasm present? Is it of epithelial, sex-cord/stromal, germ cell, or metastatic origin? Metastatic involvement is suggested by the presence of multiple tumor nodules, surface implants, and vascular space involvement.
- What are the size, histologic type, and grade of the neoplasm?
- Was the ovarian capsule ruptured?
- Does the tumor involve the ovarian capsule?
- Does the tumor involve the adjacent fallopian tube or broad ligament?
- Is there capillary–lymphatic space invasion?
- If submitted, does the tumor involve the contralateral ovary and/or the serosa or parenchyma of the uterus? When identical tumors involve both the ovary and endometrium, consider independent primary sites of origin.
- Does the tumor involve the omentum? Is the tumor microscopic, 2 cm or less, or more than 2 cm? Consider a primary peritoneal origin if there is no or minimal ovarian involvement.
- Does the tumor involve any lymph nodes? Include the number of nodes involved and the number of nodes examined at each specified site.
- Do the soft tissue staging biopsies show tumor implants? If so, specify whether they are invasive or noninvasive.

29 Products of Conception and Placentas

Products of Conception

Products of conception is the term used for intrauterine tissue that is either passed spontaneously or removed surgically in early gestation. These specimens are usually sent for diagnostic or therapeutic purposes. The major goal is to verify that a gestation was present. This requires the identification of either fetal parts, chorionic villi, or trophoblastic cells. The presence of decidua alone is not sufficent for diagnosis. Molar pregnancies and placental neoplasia may also be identified, although these are much less common. Always be familiar with the patient's clinical history, as this will help guide your examination.

Specimens from first trimester gestations are usually composed of irregularly shaped small tissue fragments and blood clots suspended within a fluid-filled container. Strain the entire contents of the container, and give an estimate of the amount of the specimen by volume (in cubic centimeters) or as an aggregate measurement. Spread the specimen across your work bench, and separate the blood clots from the tissue. Carefully inspect the tissue for fetal parts and villous tissue. Villous tissue is soft and spongy, whereas decidua is more likely to be firmer and membranous. Another method of examination is to suspend the tissue fragments in saline. The delicate villous fronds will then become readily apparent. Also, look for evidence of swollen or hydropic villi, which appear as small, grape-like vesicles.

If fetal parts are identified, measure them separately, and submit several pieces along with representative villous tissue in one or two tissue cassettes. If no fetal parts are identified and you are confident of your identification of villi, submit representative sections in two or three tissue cassettes. However, because the confirmation of an intrauterine pregnancy is often needed immediately, it may be wise to use the following guideline: Submit the entire specimen if it is small or as much as can be included in five tissue cassettes. Always specify the percentage of the specimen that was submitted, and include only tissue fragments. We have found that the microscopic evaluation of blood clots from intrauterine pregnancies often does not reveal entrapped villi. If no villi are identified after your initial microscopic evaluation, the entire specimen may need to be submitted.

In the case of a clinically suspected molar pregnancy or the presence of hydropic villi, the submission of at least eight tissue cassettes is recommended to assess the degree of trophoblast proliferation. Any large tissue fragments, that is, fragments greater than 3 to 4 cm, should be sectioned and entirely submitted if they are firm, indurated, or necrotic. Consider sending fresh tissue for flow cytometric ploidy analysis or tissue culture cytogenetic analysis. Partial moles are triploid, whereas complete moles are diploid or tetraploid. Uterine resection specimens for gestational trophoblastic malignancies should be handled as for hysterectomies for endometrial or cervical cancer depending on the site of the tumor.

Second trimester therapeutic or elective abortion specimens may have intact placentas and fetuses. These specimens may be handled in the routine surgical pathology laboratory if the fetus is less than 500 g and/or less than 20 to 21 weeks' gestation. A description of a full neonatal autopsy is beyond the scope of this chapter;

however, most cases can be appropriately handled with a limited approach. Briefly, weigh the fetus, and measure the crown–rump, crown–heel, and foot length. Examine the external appearance for skin slippage and any gross abnormalities of structure such as missing limbs or extra digits. Open the thorax and abdomen with a vertical midline incision. Confirm the appropriate position of the internal organs, and take a piece of liver, lung, and gonads for microscopic evaluation. For the examination of a fetus with either chromosomal or congenital abnormalities, the reader is referred to Wigglesworth and Singer.[14] The placenta can be routinely handled, as described in the next section.

Placentas

Placentas are submitted for evaluation because of maternal conditions, fetal/neonatal conditions, or gross anomalies of the placenta and in all multiple gestations. Many abnormalities can be recognized with a thorough gross examination. Approach each placenta by systematically evaluating the three main components: the fetal membranes, the umbilical cord, and the placental disk.

Placentas should initially be examined in the fresh, unfixed state. Choose a work area that allows for the drainage of blood and fluid, which is copiously expressed from the placental bed on sectioning. Always be aware of the clinical history before proceeding, and check the contents of the container in which the placenta was received for any separate blood clots. Orient the placenta by placing the spongy, red maternal surface face down and the shiny, membranous fetal surface with umbilical cord face up. Invert the membranes, if necessary, so that they are draped around the fetal surface.

Begin your examination with the fetal membranes, noting their color, lucency, and insertion. Normal membranes should be shiny and clear and should insert at the edge of the placental disk. Look for any opacities, which may indicate inflammation; small white nodules, which indicate amnion nodosum; and meconium staining, which may indicate intrauterine fetal hypoxia. As illustrated, membrane insertion within the circumference of the fetal surface is called *placenta extrachorialis* and can be subdivided into either circummarginate (a smooth chorionic surface at the insertion) or circumvallate (a grooved or ridged chorionic surface at the insertion). Both may reflect previous bleeding from earlier placental separation. Next, re-create the gestational sac by gently lifting the membranes, and cut a 2- to 3-cm-wide strip of membrane from the ruptured margin to the placental margin. Beginning at the ruptured end, roll the membrane strip with the amnion inward around a small probe. Remove the probe, and cut the newly created "membrane roll" transversely for histologic examination. The membranes can now be removed by trimming them along the placental margin.

The umbilical cord is examined next. Record its length and site of insertion. Although the length provided may be artificially shortened if a segment was removed in the delivery room, excessively short (less than 30 cm) or long (more than 70 cm) cords are significant because of their association with abnormal fetal development and activity. Insertions at the edge of the placenta or in the membranes may be associated with exposed vessels, which should be examined carefully for any tears or thrombi. Remove the umbilical cord at its insertion, and examine the entire length of the cord for thinning, thrombi, or knots. True knots can be undone when the umbilical cord ends are freed, whereas false knots cannot. Make several transverse cuts along the cord, and examine the vessels. There should be two small thick-walled arteries and one large thin-walled vein. At the insertion site, many vessels join together and they may not be fused into their terminal vessel until just above this point. Also, twisted regions of the umbilical cord can give the artificial appearance of an increased number of vessels on cross section. Therefore, for an accurate documentation of the number of vessels, it is best to submit a transverse section of the umbilical cord for examination from an area that is not excessively twisted and at least 1 cm above the insertion site.

The placenta should now be a solitary disk. Record its weight and three-dimensional measurement. Any unusual shapes or extra lobes should be noted. Examine the membranes on the fetal surface first, and look for nodules within or just below the amnion/chorion layer. Superficial white nodules or fine granularity may represent amnion nodosum, whereas firm, yellowish nodules beneath the membranes may represent subchorionic fibrin deposition. If present, these

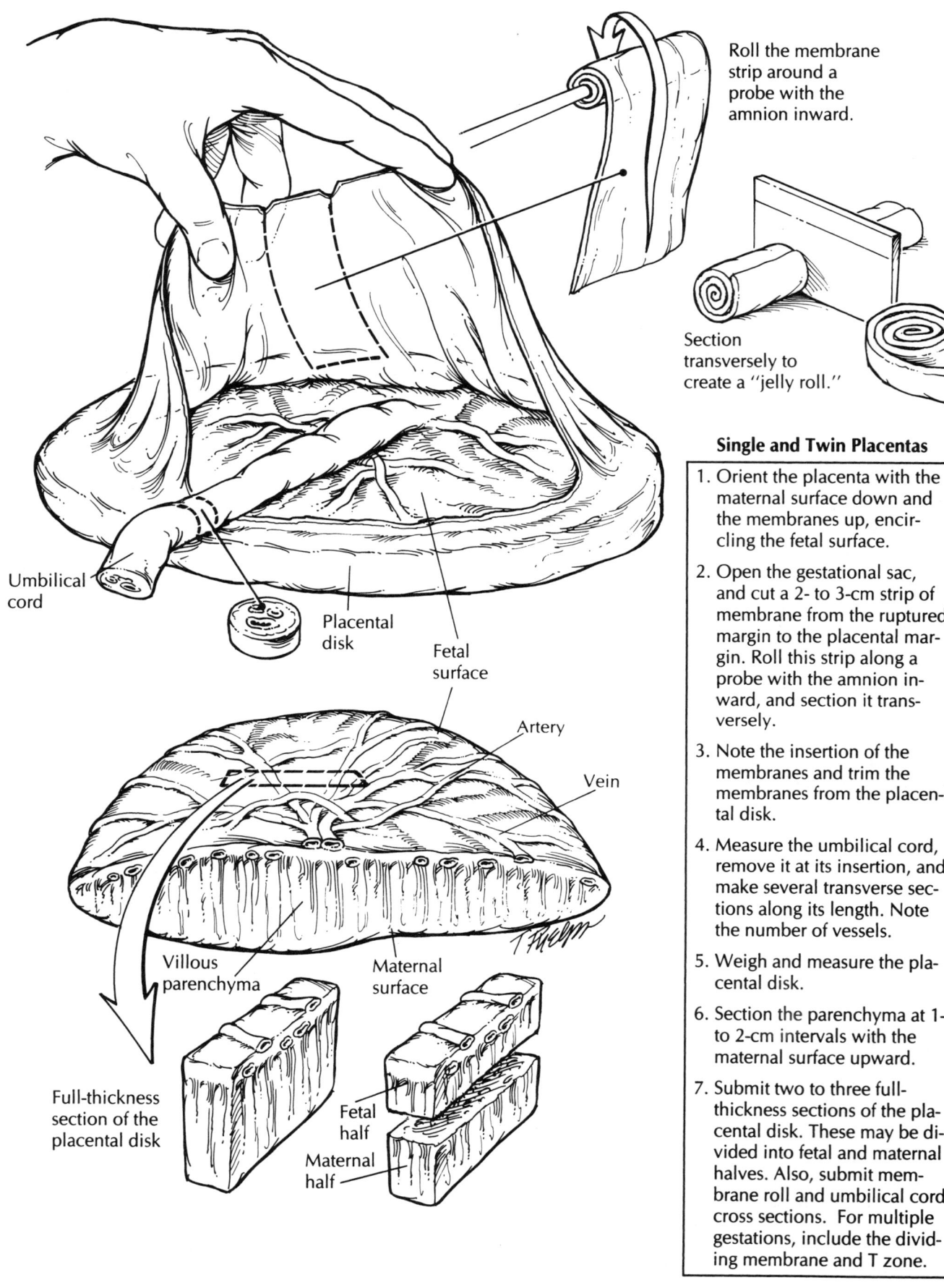

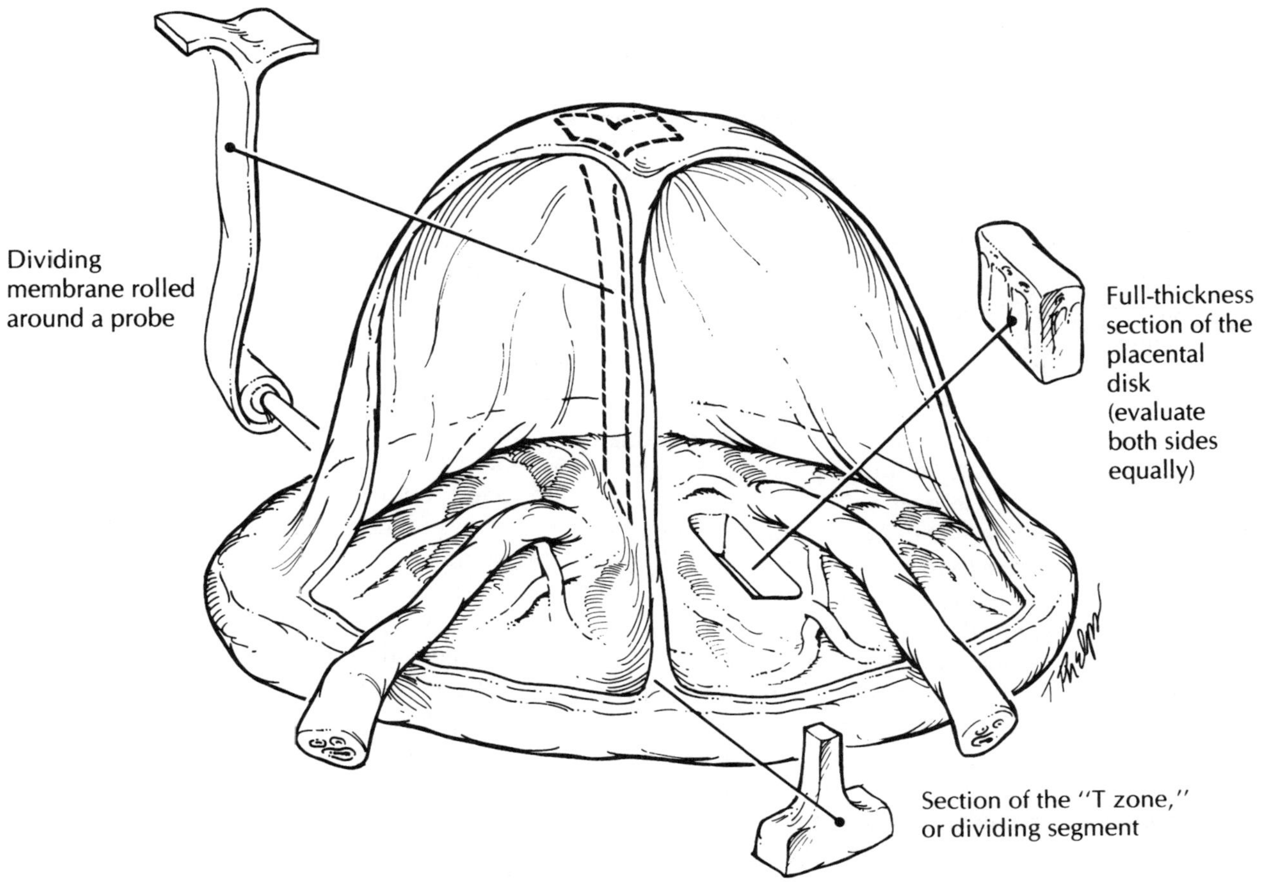

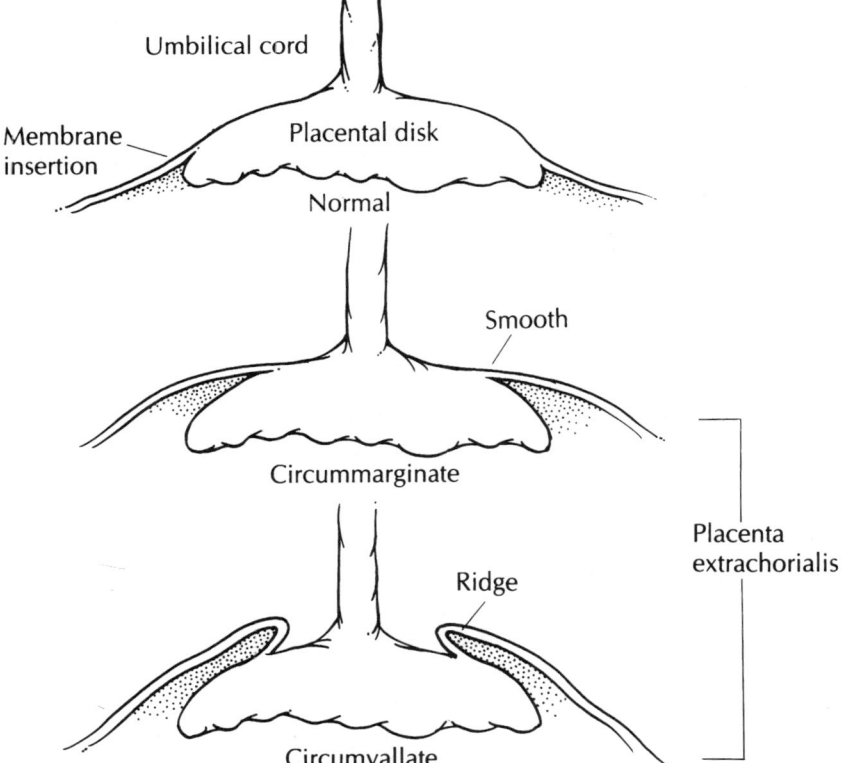

Fetal Membrane Insertion

1. Before removing the fetal membranes, examine their insertion at the edge of the placental disk.

2. Normally, the membranes insert at the margins of the fetal surface.

3. In placenta extrachorialis, the membranes insert <u>within</u> the circumference of the placental disk.

4. Circummarginate insertions have a smooth chorionic surface at their insertion site, whereas circumvallate insertions are grooved or ridged in this region.

should be sampled for histology. Next, examine the vessels that radiate toward the umbilical cord, and look for tears or thrombi. Turn the placenta over, and examine the maternal surface. The cotyledons should be relatively uniform and intact. Look for any evidence of disruption or indentation of the parenchyma. Adherent clots without underlying compression do not necessarily signify a placental abruption. Serially section the placenta at 1- to 2-cm intervals with the maternal surface upward, and examine the parenchyma. The greatest thickness of the placenta from the fetal to the maternal surface should be measured. Look for infarcts, intervillous thrombi, or tumors. Both infarcts and intervillous thrombi can appear yellow or white. Intervillous thrombi are usually smooth and displace the villous parenchyma, whereas infarcts involve the villous tissue and appear more granular. If an infarct is identified, be sure to specify the percentage of parenchyma that is involved. Tumors are rare in the placenta, but hemangiomas, choriocarcinomas, and metastatic cancers can be found.

Sections should include the full thickness of the placenta from the central regions, rather than from the margins. If the section is too thick to fit into one tissue cassette, it may be divided into maternal and fetal halves. Standard sections include two central sections from different cotyledons and any focal lesions.

Fused placentas from multiple gestations can be evaluated in a similar manner to single gestations. Additional handling includes an examination of the dividing membranes and the identification of any vascular anastomoses. Dividing membranes are composed of two outer amnions and either one or two intervening chorions. All monochorionic placentas come from monozygotic (identical) twins, whereas dichorionic placentas may belong to either monozygotic or dizygotic (fraternal) twins. The dividing membrane can be easily peeled apart in monochorionic placentas. Dichorionic placentas are moreopaque and difficult to separate. Although you can perform this separation yourself, histologic verification is necessary, and a membrane roll should be submitted from a region that has not been separated. A section from the "T zone," where the membranes attach to the fetal surface, may also be submitted. Look for any vascular anastomoses between the two sides. Note whether these are artery-to-artery (AA), vein-to-vein (VV), or artery-to-vein (AV). Arteries can be readily recognized by the fact that they lie on top of the veins. Abnormal anastomoses may be reflected by one side being severely congested and large, with the other being pale and small.

Additional Studies

You may be requested to send cultures or cytogenetic studies on obstetric specimens. For aerobic and anaerobic cultures of the placenta, it is best to sear a small region of the membranes over the placental disk with a heated scalpel and then sample the underlying subchorionic zone. This technique reduces surface contamination. For cytogenetic studies, small fragments of villous tissue, skin, or pericardium from a fetus can be submitted in sterile media containers provided by the cytogenetics laboratory. It is best to remove this tissue with clean, but not necessarily sterile, instruments. Avoid areas with obvious bacterial contamination.

Important Issues to Address in Your Surgical Pathology Report on Placentas

- What procedure was performed (was the placenta removed via spontaneous delivery or manually), and what structures/organs are present?
- What is the trimester maturation of the villi (second or third trimester)?
- Are any abnormalities of the placental shape, membrane insertion, or cord insertion present?
- Are any anomalous vessels or vessels with thrombi present?
- Is a normal three-vessel cord present?
- Is there inflammation of the membranes, umbilical cord, or chorionic villi?
- Are the maternal cotyledons disrupted, or is there compression by hematomas?
- Does the parenchyma show any infarction? If so, what percentage is involved?
- Are any villous thrombi or neoplasms identified in the parenchyma?
- In twin gestations, is a dividing membrane present? If so, is it diamniotic–monochorionic or diamniotic–dichorionic?

IX The Urinary Tract and Male Genital System

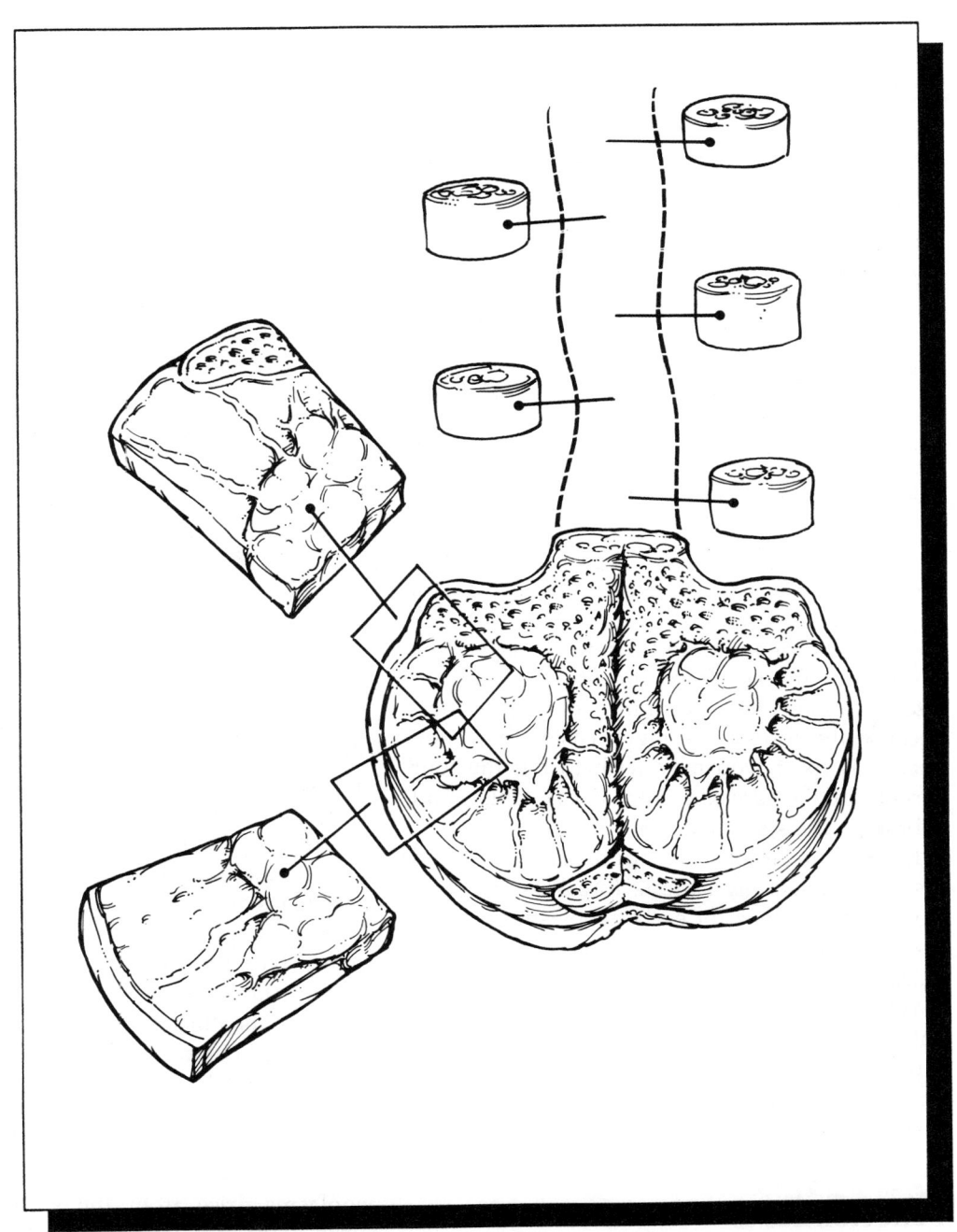

30 Penis

Foreskin

Foreskins removed from infants are usually not submitted to the surgical pathology laboratory for examination. If you do receive one of these specimens, measure it, describe its appearance, and submit a section for histologic evaluation. Foreskins removed from older patients are routinely submitted for evaluation, because they are more likely to harbor pathology. You need to sample these specimens more extensively and pay close attention to the margin of resection. Ink the epithelial margin, and carefully inspect the surfaces of the specimen. Record the number, size, location, and appearance of any lesions. Because the foreskin is much easier to section once it is fixed, you may wish to pin the four corners of the foreskin onto a wax tablet, and submerge the specimen in formalin.

Even if no lesions are appreciated on gross inspection, liberally sample foreskins removed from adults to look for early neoplastic changes. Use perpendicular sections so that the epithelial margin is included in the sections. When a neoplasm is suspected, each quadrant of the epithelial margin should be sampled. More extensive sampling may be necessary if a visible lesion is large or if the lesion approaches the margin at several sites.

Penectomies

The diverse findings encountered in penectomies range from the essentially normal penis removed from a patient undergoing a sex change operation to the penis grossly distorted by gangrene or infiltrating carcinoma. The best way to be prepared for virtually any penectomy specimen is to become familiar with the anatomy of the normal penis. This familiarity will allow you to answer those questions that should be foremost in mind when evaluating a penile lesion: Where on the penis does the lesion arise, into what anatomic compartments does the lesion extend, and how close is it to the resection margin?

Before beginning the dissection, identify the three basic structural components of the penis as illustrated. The *shaft*, as its name suggests, is the cylindrical rod-like portion of the penis. It is covered by a loosely attached layer of rugated skin, and it houses the three erectile bodies of the penis—the two corpora cavernosa (located dorsally and laterally) and the single corpus spongiosum (located ventrally, surrounding the urethra along the midline). The *glans* is the cone-shaped expansion of the distal corpus spongiosum. It sits like a bonnet on the end of the shaft. The edge of the glans at its base is referred to as the corona, and at the apex of the glans is the opening of the urethra (i.e., the urethral meatus). The *foreskin* is a retractable fold of skin that partially covers the glans. Its attachment to the skin of the shaft occurs just behind the corona. The foreskin will obviously not be present in penectomies from circumcised males.

Carefully examine the surfaces of the specimen, keeping in mind that the vast majority of penile neoplasms arise from the surface epithelium of the glans and from the undersurface of the foreskin. Neoplasms may be concealed by the foreskin, so be sure to retract this skin fold and look at the entire surface including the epithelium lining the deep recesses of the coronal sulcus. Other neoplasms—especially those that are not

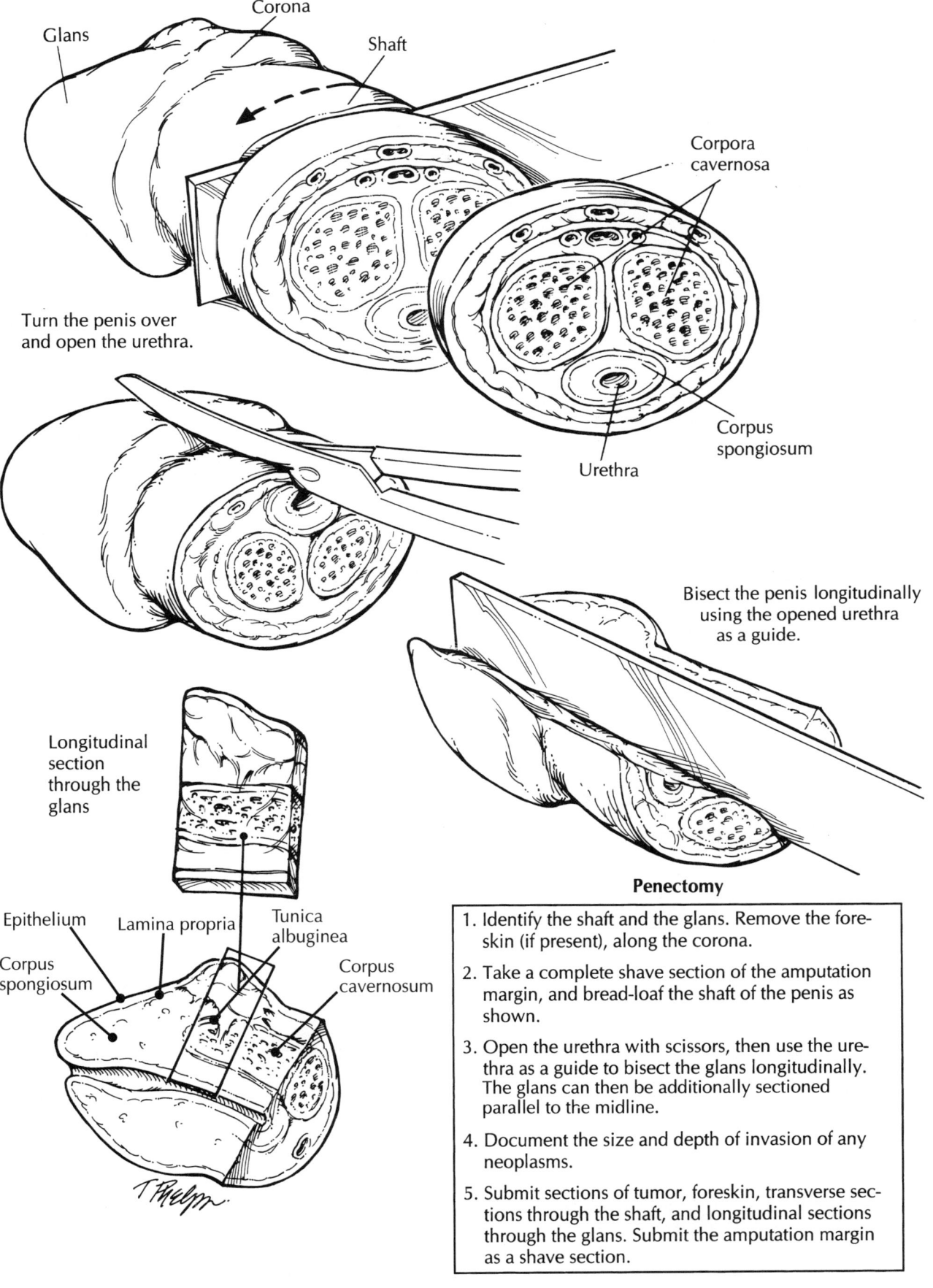

Penectomy

1. Identify the shaft and the glans. Remove the foreskin (if present), along the corona.

2. Take a complete shave section of the amputation margin, and bread-loaf the shaft of the penis as shown.

3. Open the urethra with scissors, then use the urethra as a guide to bisect the glans longitudinally. The glans can then be additionally sectioned parallel to the midline.

4. Document the size and depth of invasion of any neoplasms.

5. Submit sections of tumor, foreskin, transverse sections through the shaft, and longitudinal sections through the glans. Submit the amputation margin as a shave section.

deeply invasive—may be so subtle as to elude casual inspection; therefore, be sure to look carefully for discolored plaque-like irregularities that characterize superficial spreading carcinomas. Do not stop once one lesion has been found; keep looking for others. Squamous carcinomas of the penis tend to be multifocal, and these tumors will be overlooked if the entire epithelial surface is not examined.

In the gross description, record the dimensions of the entire specimen and the dimensions of each of its individual components (i.e., foreskin, glans, and shaft). Describe the surfaces of each component, and note the number, size, color, and distribution of any lesions found. Assess the tumor's macroscopic pattern of growth (e.g., nodular, ulcerative/infiltrative, verrucous, or flat).

Begin the dissection by taking a shave section from the penile shaft at the amputation site. This section represents the only margin. If it is carefully taken, this section will include margins of the skin, erectile bodies, and penile urethra. If all of these components cannot be included in a single section, submit each component individually. Remove the foreskin from the uncircumcised penectomy. This can be done with a circular cut leaving a 5-mm rim of foreskin attached to the corona. The foreskin should then be separately processed according to the guidelines given previously in the section on the foreskin. The deep structures of the penis are most easily visualized when the penis is sectioned in two different planes. Bread-loaf the shaft perpendicular to its long axis. Begin at the proximal end of the specimen, and stop 1 to 2 cm from the corona. Next, serially section the distal penis parallel to its long axis. The first of these parallel longitudinal sections should bisect the proximal penis into equal halves midline through the urethra. This is not a difficult section if you first use scissors to open the urethra at the 6-o'clock position (i.e., midventral plane), and then insert a knife into the opened urethra to complete the longitudinal section. Serially section the rest of the glans parallel to this initial midline cut in the sagittal plane.

Examine the cut surfaces of the specimen. Locate and describe the appearance of the penile urethra and the four anatomic levels of the glans. As described by Cubilla et al.,[15] they include: (1) the epithelium, the flat less than 1 mm layer of epithelium covering the surface of the glans; (2) the lamina propria, the approximately 2 mm thick layer of loose connective tissue beneath the epithelium; (3) the corpus spongiosum (grossly reddish, spongy tissue located between the lamina propria and the tunica albuginea) surrounding the distal urethra; and (4) the corpora cavernosa (spongy reddish brown tissue encased in a band of firm white tissue, the tunica albuginea). If a tumor is present, measure how deeply it infiltrates the penis, and try to determine which of the four anatomic structures the tumor involves. The standard sections that should be submitted for histologic evaluation include the following: (1) a shave section from the shaft margin (including the skin, erectile bodies, and urethra); (2) sections of foreskin; (3) transverse sections through the shaft at two or three different levels; and (4) longitudinal sections through the glans including a midline section with the urethra. When sampling the tumor, submit sections that demonstrate its relationships to the adjacent surface epithelium, to the urethra, and to the corpora spongiosum and cavernosum. For tumors that involve the urethra, determine the maximum tumor extension by submitting sections at regular intervals along the entire length of the penis.

Important Issues to Address in Your Surgical Pathology Report on Penectomies

- What procedure was performed, and what structures/organs are present?
- Is a neoplasm present?
- Where is the tumor located (e.g., foreskin, glans, shaft, and/or urethra)?
- Is the tumor *in situ* or infiltrating?
- What are the histologic type and grade of the tumor?
- What is the size of the tumor, and how deeply (in millimeters) does the tumor infiltrate the penis?
- Is vascular invasion identified?
- What deep structures does the tumor involve (e.g., lamina propria, corpus spongiosum, corpora cavernosa, urethra, prostate, adjacent structures)?
- Are the resection margins free of tumor?
- Does the non-neoplastic portion of the penis show any pathology?

31 Prostate

Biopsies

Needle biopsies of the prostate consist of delicate and thin cores of tan soft tissue. Measure each piece of tissue, and document the total number of pieces before carefully transferring them into a tissue cassette. As is true for any small biopsy, do not use forceps to pick up these biopsies, because forceps can squeeze and distort the tissue. Have the histology laboratory section these biopsies at multiple levels, then have them stain alternating levels for routine histology. If sections are later needed for additional studies (e.g., immunoperoxidase), the unstained slides will be readily available, and diagnostic material will not be lost during sectioning of the tissue block.

Transurethral Resections and Open Enucleations

Frequently, the central region of the prostate is removed—either by transurethral resection or by open enucleation—to relieve symptoms of urinary obstruction caused by nodules compressing the prostatic urethra. Although the majority of these nodules are entirely benign, a small, yet significant percentage (i.e., 10%) harbor a carcinoma.

Tissue fragments obtained from transurethral resections of the prostate—referred to as *prostate chips*—are generally tan, rubbery, and cylindrical. The total number of chips resected varies greatly from case to case. Measure the combined weight of the chips, and record their aggregate dimensions. For larger specimens, it is not practical to submit all of the chips for histologic evaluation. Although six to eight tissue cassettes are generally sufficient to detect the vast majority of incidental carcinomas, the sensitivity of sampling can be increased by selectively submitting those chips that appear yellow, indurated, or in any other way grossly suspicious for carcinoma. More extensive sampling is warranted in specimens from younger patients, since even a small focus of carcinoma in these men may require aggressive therapy. For patients under the age of 65, consider submitting the entire specimen for histologic evaluation. Similarly, if cancer is identified histologically in a specimen that was partially submitted, the entire specimen should be submitted so that the approximate volume of the cancer can be calculated.

Specimens obtained by open enucleation are either partially or totally intact nodules, but the anatomic orientation of these nodules is usually not practical or possible. After weighing and measuring the tissue, serially section the specimen at 2- to 3-mm intervals. Note the appearance of the cut surface. Again, extensively sample the specimen to detect incidental carcinomas. Submit up to six to eight cassettes of tissue. As was true for the prostate chips, remember to selectively sample areas that appear grossly suspicious for carcinoma.

Radical Prostatectomies

One of the challenges of the dissection of radical prostatectomies is to find a balance which will

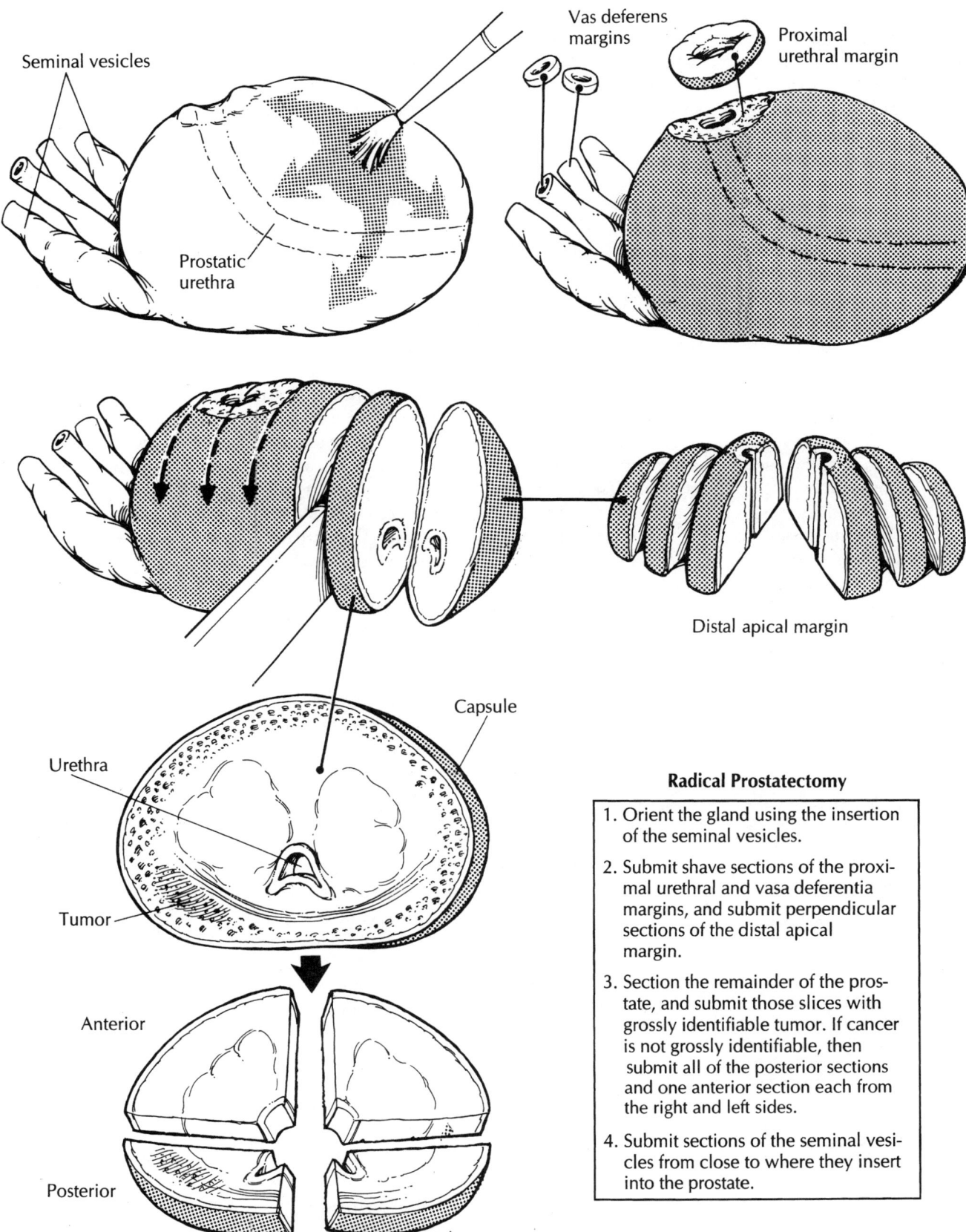

Radical Prostatectomy

1. Orient the gland using the insertion of the seminal vesicles.

2. Submit shave sections of the proximal urethral and vasa deferentia margins, and submit perpendicular sections of the distal apical margin.

3. Section the remainder of the prostate, and submit those slices with grossly identifiable tumor. If cancer is not grossly identifiable, then submit all of the posterior sections and one anterior section each from the right and left sides.

4. Submit sections of the seminal vesicles from close to where they insert into the prostate.

maximize prognostic information while minimizing the number of tissue cassettes submitted. Selective sampling of a carcinoma of the prostate can be difficult because subtle differences in the gross appearance of cancer and non-neo-plastic prostate tissue can be hard to recognize. This is why it is so important that you familiarize yourself with the subtleties of the gross appearance of prostate cancer. A number of the gross features of prostate cancer are outlined in Table 31-1 and can be helpful in distinguishing carcinoma from non-neoplastic tissue.

Orient the prostate by locating the seminal vesicles and vasa deferentia. These structures insert into the posterior aspect of the base (proximal end) of the gland and provide a landmark that is quick and easy to find. In contrast to the broad and flat base, the apex (distal end) of the prostate narrows and becomes cone shaped. The contour of the gland can be used to distinguish the anterior and posterior aspects of the prostate. The anterior surface of the prostate is rounded and convex, while the posterior surface is broad and flat. After orienting the specimen, weigh and measure it. Inspect the intact prostate for asymmetry, and palpate it for areas of induration. Paint the surfaces of the prostate with ink. Fixation of the prostate before sectioning permits thinner sectioning of the gland and better assessment of the margins. Relatively recent fixation protocols that utilize microwave fixation, such as that described by Ruijter and coworkers,[16] have significantly reduced fixation times. Indeed, radical prostatectomy specimens can now be fixed and sectioned on the same day as the surgery.

Following fixation, thinly shave the vasa deferentia and the proximal (bladder neck) margins. The distal (apical) margin can be submitted in one of two ways. One method is to submit this margin as a thinly shaved section. A second method is illustrated. Amputate the distal 1 cm of the apex, then section this apical cone at right angles to the cut edge in thin parallel slices. The latter technique allows for a more accurate assessment of exactly how close the cancer approaches the distal (apical) margin. If the proximal (bladder neck) and distal (apical) margins are taken as shave sections, these sections should be very thin (1 mm in thickness). A common misunderstanding among pathologists is that these sections are taken to assess the status of the prostatic urethral margins. They are not. These sections are taken to sample the bladder neck margin. Once transected during surgery, the urethra retracts into the gland. Thus there is no need to obtain urothelium on these margin sections, and you should avoid the tendency to submit thick doughnut-shaped sections with urothelium in the center. The seminal vesicles are evaluated by taking a section through the base of the seminal vesicle where it joins the prostate. It is not necessary to submit entire tips of the seminal vesicles.

After the margins have been taken, serially section the prostate at 2- to 3-mm intervals from apex to base. Do not use the urethra as a point of reference for these sections, because this structure follows a curved course through the prostate. Instead, section the prostate perpendicular to the broad flat posterior surface of the gland. The carefully sectioned prostate can be likened to a loaf of sliced bread. Each individual slice should be intact, uniformly thin, and surrounded by a "crust" of prostatic capsule and inked soft tissue. You will come to realize the importance of this crust when you later have to evaluate the histologic sections for extraprostatic extension of the tumor.

Lay the individual slices out sequentially from apex (distal) to base (proximal). Be careful to maintain the orientation (i.e., right vs. left, anterior vs. posterior) of each slice. Beginning at the apex and proceeding to the base, designate

---

TABLE 31-1. Gross appearance of prostate cancer.

Location: The cut surface of the normal prostate shows a fibromuscular band that divides the prostate into a peripheral zone and a transitional zone (i.e., periurethral area). Most carcinomas arise peripherally in the posterior and posterolateral portion of the gland. In contrast, hyperplastic nodules tend to be located centrally around the urethra.

Texture: Carcinomas tend to be solid and homogeneous, while non-neoplastic prostate tissue is often spongy and cystic.

Color: Carcinomas vary in color from gray to brown to yellow. Sometimes these colors contrast sharply with the uniform tan appearance of non-neoplastic prostate. Perhaps more commonly, the color of the cancer and non-neoplastic tissue overlap, and color cannot be used to distinguish the two.

Structural Alterations: Prostatic carcinomas often cause structural changes that are apparent on close inspection of the cut surface. Important clues to search for are asymmetry between the two sides of the gland and displacement of the fibromuscular band that normally divides the transitional and peripheral zones of the gland.

each slice (e.g., A, B, C). This will enable you to remember the location of each individual slice within the prostate.

Several key landmarks guide the examination of the individual slices. The prostatic urethra is located near the center of each slice. It has a roughly U-shaped appearance on cut section. The arms of the U point to the posterior surface of the gland, and its convexity points to the anterior surface. Find the fibromuscular band of tissue that separates the central/anterior portion of the gland from the horseshoe-shaped peripheral portion of the gland. Try to find the cancer using the guidelines outlined in Table 31-1. Describe the appearance of any lesions, carefully noting their location (left or right, anterior or posterior) and size. Because each slice has already been designated, you can precisely indicate in your gross description which of the slices appear involved.

The slices may have to be sectioned further to fit into standard tissue cassettes. A median section through the urethra will divide the slice into roughly equal right and left sides, and a coronal section through the urethra will, when necessary, further divide the slice into anterior and posterior quadrants. Although it is common practice in many academic centers to submit the entire prostate for histologic examination, such processing significantly increases the cost of handling specimens and can impose strains on a laboratory's resources. As a more efficient alternative, these specimens can be partially sampled using protocols that vary depending on the presence or absence of grossly apparent tumor. If you can confidently identify the cancer grossly, submit slices that contain the entire gross lesion. The question arises as to how thoroughly to sample the prostate when the tumor is not grossly visible. We recommend sampling the entire posterior aspect of the prostate along with one anterior section from the both the right and left sides of the middle of the gland. If one of these mid-gland sections shows significant tumor, go back to the specimen and submit the entire anterior portion of the gland on the side involved.

After the specimen has been appropriately sampled, retain the remaining tissue sections in their original order and orientation in case additional sections must be submitted. One simple method is to fasten the slices together with a safety pin or rubber band.

Pelvic Lymph Node Dissection

Radical prostatectomies are usually accompanied by a dissection of the pelvic lymph nodes. These dissections are generally submitted by the surgeon as separate specimens.

Pelvic lymph node dissections consist of variable numbers of lymph nodes embedded in fibrofatty connective tissue. Each lymph node should be submitted for histologic evaluation. Keep in mind that in a small but significant number of cases the metastatic implants are present in adipose tissues (not in the grossly recognized lymph nodes). Based on this finding, we submit all adipose tissue from pelvic lymphadenectomy specimens, at least for cases with biopsy Gleason scores of 7 or higher.

Important Issues to Address in Your Surgical Pathology Report on Radical Prostatectomies

- What procedure was performed, and what structures/organs are present?
- Where in the prostate is the bulk of the tumor located? Does it involve both sides of the gland?
- What are the histologic type and grade of the tumor?
- Does the tumor involve greater than 5% of the tissue resected?
- Does the tumor extend beyond the prostate (i.e., "extraprostatic extension").
- Is vascular or perineural invasion identified?
- Does the tumor infiltrate the seminal vesicles?
- Is the tumor present at any of the following margins: proximal (bladder neck) margin, distal (apical) margin, vasa deferentia margins, or soft tissue margins?
- Has the tumor metastasized to regional lymph nodes or pelvic adipose tissue? Record the number of metastases and the total number of lymph nodes examined.

32 Testis

Biopsies

The most important thing to remember when processing a testicular biopsy is to treat it gently. The delicate sponge-like consistency of the testicular parenchyma makes it particularly susceptible to desiccation and compression. Be sure that the tissue remains in fixative during transportation and processing. Bouin's solution is a better fixative for these biopsies than is formalin. Take care not to crush the tissue when transferring the specimen to the tissue cassette. Do not use forceps; instead, gently filter the specimen into tissue paper. The entire specimen should be embedded and sectioned at multiple levels.

Radical Orchiectomies

When the entire testis is resected, it is usually removed in continuity with the epididymis and a variable length of the spermatic cord. Orchiectomy specimens can be oriented with relative ease using the epididymis as a landmark. The epididymis is roughly a C-shaped structure that cups the testis along its posterior aspect. Between the posterior aspect of the testis and epididymis is the mediastinum testis, where ducts, nerves, and vessels enter and exit the testis. The rete testis is a network formed in the mediastinum testis by the seminiferous tubules. Always be aware of the location of the mediastinum during your dissection because neoplasms and infections may extend beyond or into the testis at this site.

After the specimen has been oriented and all the structures attached to the testis have been identified, weigh and measure the testis and epididymis, and record the dimensions of the spermatic cord. The tunica vaginalis is a thin membranous sac that covers the external surface of the testis. After noting the appearance of its outer surface, open the tunica vaginalis along the anterior surface of the testis. Record the volume and appearance of any fluid that may have accumulated within this space, and examine the inner surface of the tunica for thickening or exophytic growths. Due to the noncohesive nature of germ cell tumors, it is a good idea to obtain sections of the spermatic cord before incising the main tumor to avoid contamination. Shave the spermatic cord margin and also submit cross sections from each of the three levels of the spermatic cord (proximal, mid, and distal).

The tunica albuginea is the thick fibrous capsule of the testis. Keep in mind that this resilient covering makes for an effective barrier to the diffusion of formalin and an equally formidable barrier to a dull knife. The testis should therefore be sectioned with a sharp knife before it is placed in fixative. As illustrated, partially bisect the testis along its long axis. Begin the cut along the anterior surface (the side opposite the epididymis), and extend the section into the mediastinum testis. The testis can now be opened much like a book, with the epididymis serving as the bookbinding. This initial section will optimize your ability to assess the relationship between any focal lesions and the testicular parenchyma, the tunica albuginea, and the epididymis. Furthermore, this section will allow formalin to penetrate and fix the testicular parenchyma. After making the initial section, photograph the specimen and collect tissue for special studies as indicated. A frozen section or touch preparation from the surface of the lesion may be used to determine

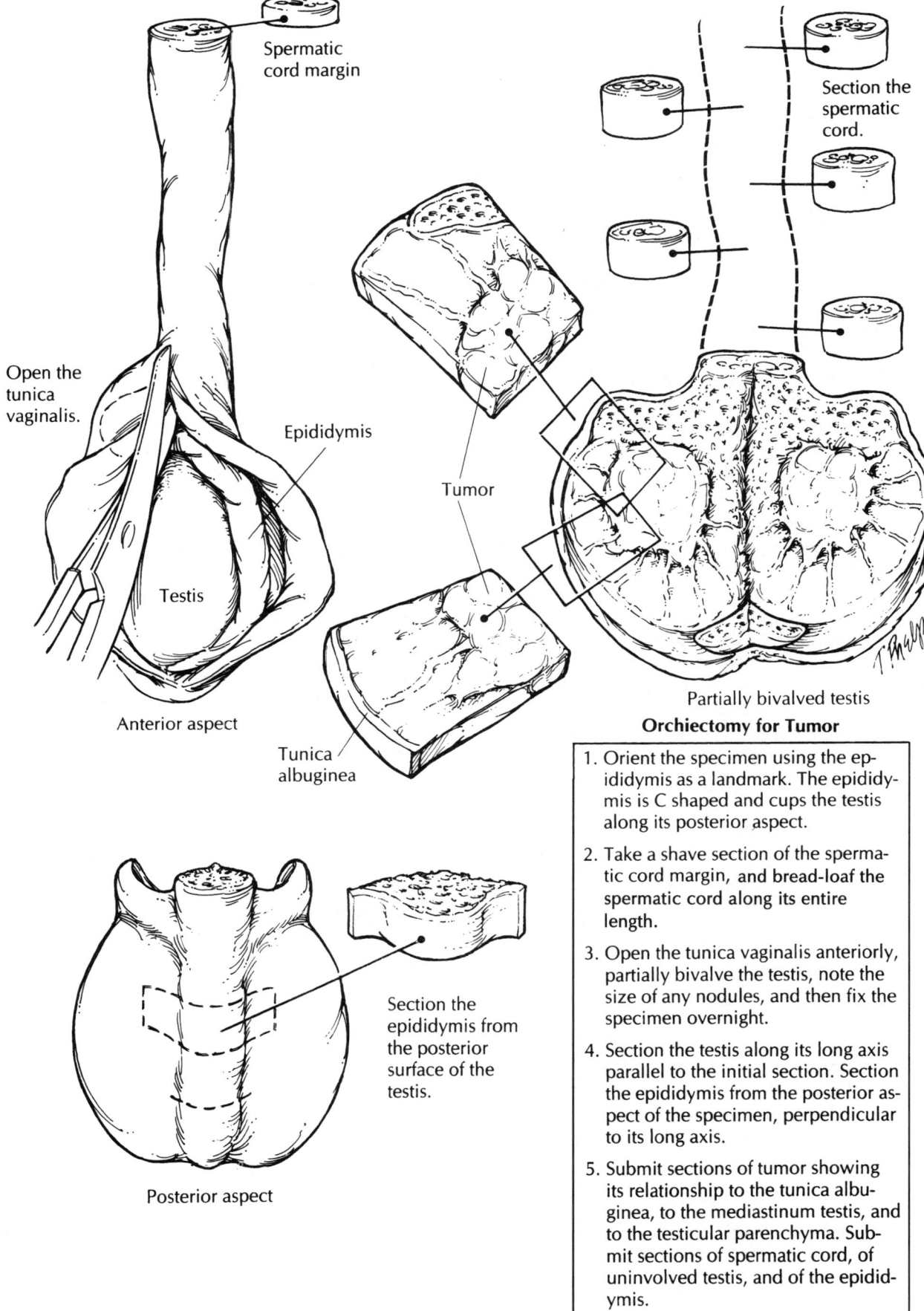

Orchiectomy for Tumor

1. Orient the specimen using the epididymis as a landmark. The epididymis is C shaped and cups the testis along its posterior aspect.

2. Take a shave section of the spermatic cord margin, and bread-loaf the spermatic cord along its entire length.

3. Open the tunica vaginalis anteriorly, partially bivalve the testis, note the size of any nodules, and then fix the specimen overnight.

4. Section the testis along its long axis parallel to the initial section. Section the epididymis from the posterior aspect of the specimen, perpendicular to its long axis.

5. Submit sections of tumor showing its relationship to the tunica albuginea, to the mediastinum testis, and to the testicular parenchyma. Submit sections of spermatic cord, of uninvolved testis, and of the epididymis.

if tissue needs to be sent for microbiologic studies, for a lymphoma workup, or for electron microscopy.

After the specimen is well fixed, it can be thinly sectioned at 3-mm intervals. Bread-loaf the testis along its long axis parallel to the initial section. The epididymis should be sectioned from its head to its tail at right angles to its long axis. As illustrated, this is best accomplished from the posterior aspect of the specimen. If you have not already done so, serially section the remaining cord at regular intervals along its entire length.

Carefully examine the cut surface of the testis and paratesticular tissues. Give a detailed description of the appearance of any lesions, and try to determine their location in the testis or paratestis (e.g., central, inferior pole, superior pole, testicular hilum, epididymis, paratesticular soft tissue, spermatic cord). When describing the appearance of a testicular mass, be sure to note its size and areas of hemorrhage and/or necrosis, even if these areas appear small and inconsequential. Try to determine if the tumor is confined to the testicular parenchyma, or if there is extratesticular extension, either beyond the tunica albuginea or into the epididymis. If a testicular neoplasm is clinically suspected, but one cannot be found on gross inspection, do not give up. Instead, scrupulously inspect the thin sections for any scars or areas of gritty calcification. These findings may represent regressive changes in a pre-existing neoplasm.

The standard sections to be submitted from any orchiectomy specimen include: (1) sections of tumor showing its relationship to the tunica albuginea and to the mediastinum testis; (2) sections of the testicular parenchyma; (3) sections of the epididymis; (4) sections of the spermatic cord margin; and (5) sections from three levels of the spermatic cord (i.e., proximal, mid, and distal). The number of sections that should be submitted is highly dependent on the clinical setting. Some of the more common reasons for which the testis is resected are cited below, along with some guidelines to keep in mind when sampling these specimens.

Sampling Testicular Neoplasms

Primary testicular neoplasms often exhibit more than one morphologic component (e.g., semioma and embryonal carcinoma). Because even the focal presence of an aggressive component may affect the treatment and prognosis, it is critical that all of the components present be demonstrated histologically. When submitting sections of primary testicular neoplasms, aim to be both thorough and selective. To be thorough, submit at least one section of tumor for every 1 cm of its greatest diameter. To be selective, sample the areas of the tumor that appear distinct on gross examination. For example, be sure to submit sections from areas of hemorrhage, necrosis, or mucinous change, even if these areas represent only a minor component of the tumor's gross appearance. These gross changes often correlate with important histologic features.

Sometimes a primary testicular tumor can regress, leaving only a small scar. When a tumor cannot be identified in a testis removed from a patient with a metastatic germ cell tumor, the testis should be entirely submitted for microscopic examination.

Undescended Testis

The undescended testis is vulnerable to torsion, infarction, and most importantly, the development of germ cell neoplasms. Thus, a testis that is maldescended is often resected even when a tumor is not clinically apparent. Your principal role in the processing of the undescended testis is to determine if a neoplasm is present. Because early neoplastic changes or regressed tumors may not be apparent on gross examination, sample generously all areas of the testis even when a focal lesion is not seen. Just as in the normally positioned testis, an undescended testis removed from a patient with a metastatic germ cell tumor should be entirely submitted if a testicular tumor is not grossly apparent.

Bilateral Orchiectomies for Prostate Cancer

The testes removed from patients with metastatic prostatic carcinoma are not necessarily abnormal. Instead, bilateral orchiectomies in these patients are usually done as a therapeutic procedure to remove a source of testosterone. Nonetheless, carefully examine the specimen for a metastasis or an unsuspected primary tumor. If none is found, submit one section of the testicular parenchyma from each testis.

Torsion, Infarction, and Infectious Disease

For infectious processes, infarcts, and torsion, be sure to submit sections from both the periphery and the center of any lesions. The duration of testicular torsion and the host response to an infectious agent are best evaluated in the viable tissue at the periphery of a lesion. Also, when dealing with inflammatory lesions of the testis, always remember to submit fresh tissue for microbiologic studies.

Anorchia and Intersex Syndromes

Sometimes the pathologist is called on to determine the presence and/or type of gonadal tissue in a surgical specimen. In these instances, it is of critical importance that the specimen be reviewed and oriented with the surgeon. Label all of the grossly identifiable structures, and photograph the specimen so that the histologic findings can be correlated with the structures identified grossly. Always submit a section for histologic evaluation of each structure identified grossly. When the testis cannot be grossly identified, submit the entire tissue so that it can be evaluated for histologic evidence of testicular regression.

Important Issues to Address in Your Surgical Pathology Report on Orchiectomies

- What procedure was performed, and what structures/organs are present?
- Is a neoplasm present?
- Where does the tumor originate (i.e., testis, epididymis, spermatic cord)?
- What is the size of the tumor?
- What are the histologic type and grade of the neoplasm? Is intratubular germ cell neoplasia present?
- Is the tumor limited to the testis? Does the tumor extend into any of the adjacent structures: rete testis, epididymis, spermatic cord, tunica albuginea, or scrotum?
- Can vascular invasion be identified histologically?
- If a neoplasm cannot be identified, is there histologic evidence of intratubular germ cell neoplasia, calcification, or scar formation?
- Does the tumor involve any of the margins?

33 Kidney

General Comments

The gross examination plays an important role in the evaluation of kidney specimens. Macroscopic features often provide important clues to the underlying pathologic process. For example, the accurate pathologic staging of renal neoplasms can usually be accomplished simply by noting relationships between the tumor and certain anatomic landmarks. As with other tissues, no kidney specimen should be dissected without prior knowledge of the patient's clinical history. This fundamental rule is especially important when handling kidney specimens in which the evaluation of glomerular disease relies on immunofluorescence and ultrastructural analysis. Thus, before processing even the smallest kidney biopsy, determine from the clinical history whether fresh tissue should be submitted for these special studies.

Biopsies

Electron microscopy and immunofluorescence studies are central to the diagnostic evaluation of kidney biopsies for non-neoplastic disease. Even small specimens must be properly oriented because glomeruli should be included in the tissue submitted for each of these tests. The goal of orienting kidney biopsies is to distinguish cortex from medulla. While this distinction is usually quite simple with the larger wedge biopsies, the identification of cortex and medulla in small-needle biopsies often requires the use of a magnifying lens or dissection microscope. Under magnification, the cortex can be recognized by its red sunburst pattern corresponding to the vascular tufts of the glomeruli. In contrast, the straight vessels of the medulla are seen as thin red streaks coursing through tan/white tissue. From the tips of the cortical end, freeze a 1-mm section for immunofluorescence, and submit an adjacent 1-mm section in glutaraldehyde for electron microscopy. If multiple cores are received, do the same for each core. If you cannot confidently identify an end with cortex, do not guess. Rather, submit 1-mm sections from both ends of the core. For larger wedge biopsies, freeze a full-thickness section of cortex for immunofluorescence, and submit 1-mm^3 cubes from the cortex in glutaraldehyde for electron microscopy. Submit the remainder of the tissue in fixative for routine histologic processing.

Nephrectomies for Neoplastic Disease

The purpose of evaluating kidneys resected for neoplasms is to determine the type of tumor, its extent, and the completeness of the resection. This can easily be achieved if you approach the nephrectomy as if it were made up of three individual compartments: the kidney, the renal hilum, and the perinephric fat. Describe each component of the kidney individually and systematically (Table 33-1).

First, weigh and measure the entire specimen. The renal capsule and the perinephric fat should not be stripped from the kidney until after their relationships to the tumor are established. Anatomically orient the specimen. The ureter will provide a useful landmark: the downward

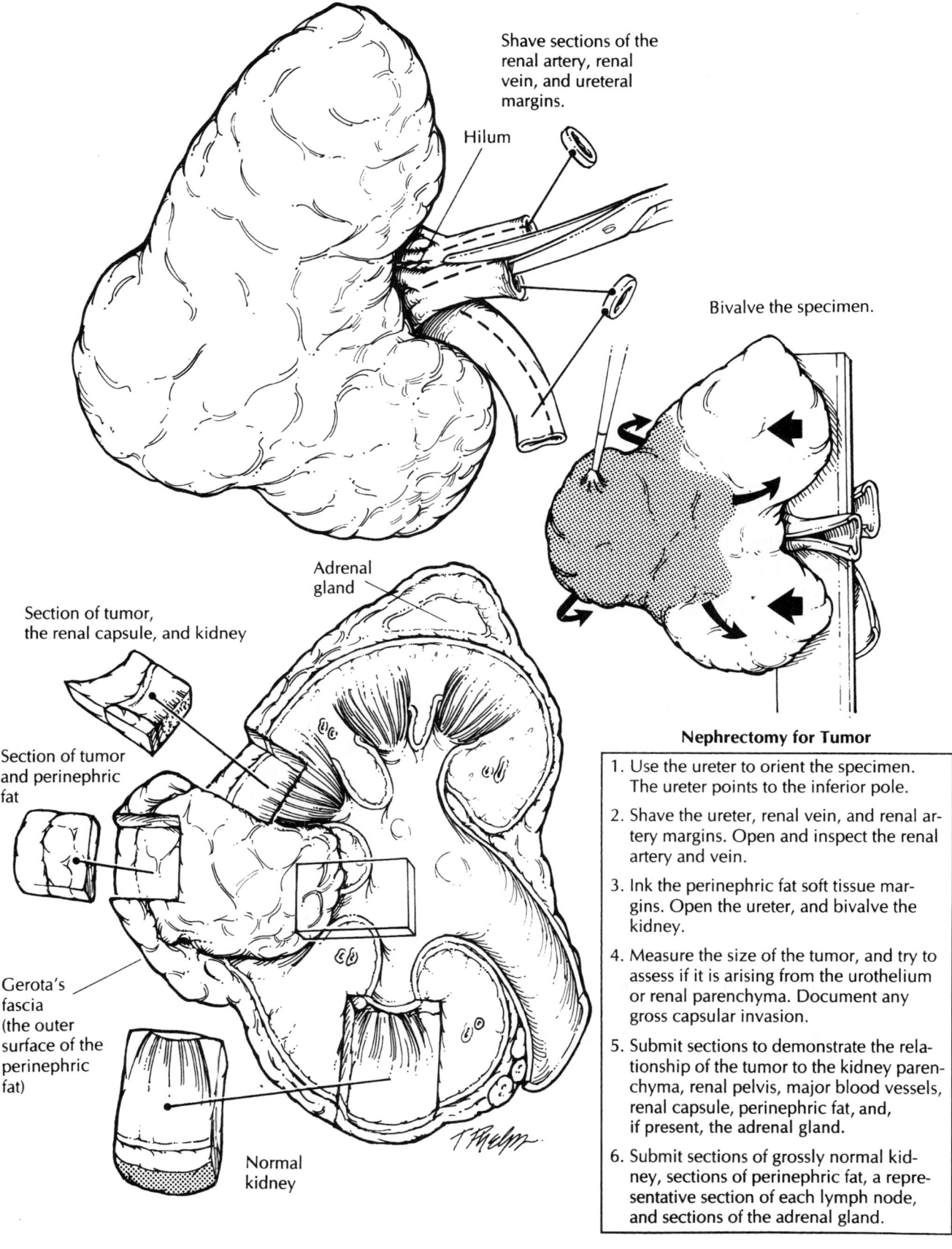

TABLE 33-1. Non-neoplastic components of nephrectomy specimen to be inspected and described.

Hilum		
	Vessels	• Patency (e.g., atherosclerotic plaque, thrombosis)
	Lymph nodes	• Number and size
	Ureter	• Size (e.g., stenosis or dilatation)
		• Appearance of mucosa (e.g., red, purulent)
Kidney		
	Capsular surface	• Contour (e.g., smooth, granular, coarsely scarred)
		• Character of capsule (e.g., strips with ease, scarred, adherent)
	Cortex	• Thickness and color
	Medulla	• Thickness and color
		• Shape of the pyramids
	Collecting system	• Configuration (e.g., distortion, dilatation, stenosis)
		• Contents (e.g., stones)
		• Appearance of mucosa (e.g., red, purulent)
Perinephric fat		• Appearance
Adrenal gland		• Size and appearance

course of the ureter points to the inferior pole of the kidney. By knowing whether the kidney is from the right or left side, you can easily identify its anterior and posterior surfaces.

Begin the dissection at the kidney hilum. Identify the ureter, renal artery, and renal vein. Shave the margin from each, and then open each with a small pair of scissors to the point at which they enter the kidney. Look for the presence of vascular invasion, atherosclerosis, and thrombosis. Carefully inspect the mucosa and wall of the ureter. Is the ureter dilated or strictured? Are any masses present? Occasionally, lymph nodes will be present in the soft tissues of the hilum, and these should be individually measured and sampled. Other lymph node groups are usually submitted separately by the surgeon.

Next, ink the soft tissue margins and direct your attention to the dissection of the kidney itself. The objective of the initial section is to bivalve the kidney so that the relationship of the tumor to the kidney can be easily visualized. The plane of this initial section may vary depending on the location of the tumor, but in general it will be a sagittal cut that begins at the hilum and exits laterally through the perinephric fat. It may be helpful to insert probes into the calyces of the upper and lower poles of the kidney to guide the knife through the renal pelvis. Once the tumor is exposed, obtain fresh tissue for special studies such as electron microscopy, immunofluorescence, and cytogenetics, as is indicated. Describe the size, shape, color, and consistency of the tumor. Does the tumor appear to be centered in the cortex, medulla, or pelvis? Measure the distance of the tumor to the nearest margin, and note its relationship to the perinephric fat, renal pelvis, renal vein, ureter, and adrenal gland. Photograph the bivalved specimen. At this point you may choose to complete the dissection of the kidney in its fresh state, or you may want to submerge the specimen in formalin until it is well fixed.

The outer surface of the fat represents Gerota's fascia. Ink this surface where it overlies the tumor, and submit perpendicular sections to show the relationship of the tumor to the soft tissue margin. Then carefully peel back the perinephric fat from the kidney, examine the capsular surface, and look for tumor extension through the renal capsule. Keep in mind that when renal tumors invade through the capsule, they tend to bulge from the surface of the kidney. Note any bulges, and document any disruption of the normal contour of the kidney surface by submitting sections that include the tumor, the adjacent non-neoplastic kidney, and the overlaying capsule. Make additional sections through the tumor and surrounding kidney. Look for any satellite tumors.

Submit at least four sections of tumor (or more if necessary) to demonstrate the relationship of the tumor to the kidney parenchyma, renal pelvis, major blood vessels, renal capsule, and perinephric fat. Because some renal neoplasms are multifocal, section through the remainder of the kidney, looking for smaller tumors. Do not forget to describe the cortex, medulla, and collecting system of the non-neoplastic kidney. Also, submit one or two sections of the non-neoplastic kidney for histology. Finally, dissect the fibrofatty tissue enveloping the kidney, and submit one or two sections of the fat to assess infiltration by tumor.

Nephrectomy specimens often will include the adrenal gland. Be sure to look for it in the superior perinephric fat; if it is present, weigh it, measure it, and submit a section. Keep in mind that the lymph nodes will be found in the soft tissues at the kidney hilum. A misdirected search for lymph nodes in the perinephric fat outside of the hilum will be a waste of your time.

Important Issues to Address in Your Surgical Pathology Report on Nephrectomies for Tumor

- What procedure was performed, and what structures/organs are present?
- Is a neoplasm present?
- Where is the tumor located?
- How large is the tumor?
- Does the tumor invade the renal capsule, Gerota's fascia, major veins, or the adrenal gland?
- What are the histologic type and grade of the neoplasm?
- What is the status of each of the margins (ureter, renal vein, soft tissue)?
- Are metastases identified? Record the number of nodes involved and the number examined.
- Does the non-neoplastic portion of the kidney show any pathology?

Partial Nephrectomies

Occasionally, you may receive a partial nephrectomy—that is, a tumor removed with only a small portion of surrounding renal parenchyma. Take the same approach as you would for a total nephrectomy, only remember to sample the renal parenchymal margins. Ink these margins, and submit perpendicular sections to demonstrate the distance of the tumor's edge to the margin. Given the much more limited extent of these resections, you will often not be able to assess the relationship of the tumor to the perinephric fat, renal vein, ureter, or other important structures.

Nephrectomies for Non-neoplastic Disease

Dissection of the nephrectomy specimen is essentially the same for neoplastic and non-neoplastic diseases. Before beginning the dissection, try to establish from the patient's clinical history whether fresh cortical tissue should be taken for immunofluorescence studies or electron microscopy. Evaluate the kidney, the hilum, and the perinephric fat as three separate compartments, using the guidelines of dissection given earlier. When the specimen shows some modification (e.g., the absence of a perinephric soft tissue compartment), simply alter the dissection accordingly. Some pathologists may prefer to evaluate the texture of the cortical surface by stripping the capsule from the fresh specimen, and this can be done before the kidney is sectioned and fixed.

If calculi are identified during the dissection, submit some for chemical analysis if indicated. Because the macroscopic findings often provide crucial clues to the pathologic process involving the kidney, describe each component of the kidney individually and systematically (see Table 33-1).

Cystic Kidneys

Sometimes kidneys are resected for congenital or acquired non-neoplastic cystic disease. Even for massively enlarged and distorted kidneys, the dissection should follow the same guidelines given above, only remember to pay particular attention to the following points: (1) Probe the ureters before opening them to check for patency. (2) Note the location of the cysts in terms of their relationship to the cortex and medulla. (3) Document the size and contents of the cysts. (4) Last, because cystic kidneys can harbor unsuspected neoplasms, thoroughly section and inspect the kidney. Submit sections of any suspicious areas, including solid foci, cysts with thickened walls, and cysts with a papillary lining.

34 Bladder

Biopsies

Biopsy specimens of the urinary bladder are generally removed through the cystoscope. They vary from single and minute to numerous, large, and papillary. Orientation of these specimens is generally impossible, even for the larger papillary fragments. Biopsies of neoplasms potentially hold important information regarding tumor type, tumor grade, and extent of tumor invasion into the various layers of the bladder wall. By following two simple rules, you can avoid missing this crucial information. First, be sure to submit all of the pieces of tissue for processing and multiple sectioning. Second, avoid the common mistake of overfilling specimen cassettes with tissue fragments. Keep in mind that portions of the specimen will not be sampled if they are "buried" within a crowded cassette. In addition, we strongly recommend that the urologist submit superficial and deep tumor biopsies as separate specimens to facilitate the detection of deep muscle invasion.

Total Cystectomies

The processing of resected urinary bladders can be accomplished in three steps: (1) orientation of the specimen and identification of relevant structures (e.g., ureters); (2) fixation of the specimen; and (3) dissection of the specimen. Given the almost spherical shape of the bladder, this first step, orientation, is not necessarily an easy one. The peritoneum covering the surface of the bladder can be used as a reliable, though subtle, anatomic landmark. As illustrated, the peritoneum descends further along the posterior wall of the bladder than it does along the anterior wall. If they are present, other pelvic organs can also be used to orient the specimen. For example, the seminal vesicles and uterus mark the posterior aspect of the bladder. Once the specimen is oriented, locate both ureters and, when present, the vasa deferentia. The best place to look for the ureters is in the lateral perivesicular fatty connective tissues. The ureters are much easier to locate and dissect in the fresh state than they are once the specimen is fixed. Tag the end of each ureter with a safety pin so that you can locate them later.

The next step is to fix the specimen. Some prefer to fix bladders in distention, either through the urethra via a catheter or through the bladder wall using a large-gauge needle. The method we prefer and describe below is to open the bladder and pin it out before submerging it in formalin. The advantage of this latter method is that by exposing the tumor before fixation samples can be collected for ancillary studies requiring fresh tissue. Begin by inking the surface of the perivesicular soft tissues, and then open the anterior bladder wall from the urethra to the bladder dome using scissors. Avoid disrupting the posterior wall, because the ureteral orifices are located in this region, and they will serve as important anatomic landmarks later in the dissection. Examine the mucosa for ulcerations, exophytic tumors, or more subtle mucosal alterations. Note the size, gross morphology (flat, papillary, or ulcerated), and location (e.g., dome, trigone, free walls) of any lesions in the bladder. Photograph the opened specimen. Collect fresh tissue for special studies if warranted. Pin the specimen to a wax block such that the bladder cavity is opened and the luminal surface is fully exposed, and submerge the entire specimen in formalin.

After the specimen is well fixed, resume the dissection by shaving the margins from each of the ureters and (when present) the vasa deferentia. These already should have been located and tagged in the fresh specimen. The urethral margin should also be taken as a thin shave section. When the specimen includes the prostate (see En Bloc Resections, next page), amputate the distal 1 cm of the prostate at its apex; then section this apical cone at right angles to the cut edge in thin, parallel sections. These sections will include the distal portion of the prostatic urethra, and will permit you to determine precisely the status of the distal margin at the prostatic apex. Next, using a small pair of scissors, open the ureters on both sides, beginning at their trigone orifices. Look for ureteral strictures and dilatations, and examine the mucosa for ulcerations or exophytic lesions. Document these findings in the gross dictation. Submit transverse sections of the ureters at regular intervals along their entire length.

If a tumor is identified in the bladder, try to determine its depth of invasion. To do this, make a full-thickness cut through the tumor and bladder wall. See whether the tumor appears to infiltrate the muscularis propria of the bladder and, if so, whether it extends into the surrounding soft tissues. Take sections of the tumor to demonstrate its relationship to the adjacent urothelium and, importantly, its maximal depth of invasion. Keep in mind that for large exophytic tumors sections will be more informative when they are taken from the base of the tumor than when they are taken from its surface.

Urothelial neoplasms often arise in a background of widespread epithelial alterations. Furthermore, many urothelial neoplasms are treated before surgical resection, and residual tumors may not be grossly apparent. For these reasons, it is important that bladders resected for urothelial neoplasia be extensively sampled for histology, even at sites that appear distant from the tumor. As a guide for sampling, treat the bladder as though it were a box with six walls including the floor (trigone), roof (dome), right and left lateral walls, anterior wall, and posterior wall. Submit two sections from each of these, as well as longitudinal sections through the ureteral orifices on both sides. Selectively sample areas where the mucosa appears abnormal. Carefully inspect the bladder mucosa because many *in situ* neoplasms of the bladder are flat and are characterized by a subtle red velvety appearance, in contrast to the tan, smooth appearance of normal mucosa.

Section through the perivesicular soft tissues, and look for tumor extension beyond the bladder wall. Submit perpendicular sections from the soft tissue margins. Be sure to search for lymph nodes, which are sometimes present in the perivesicular soft tissues. If any are found, measure them individually, and submit each for histologic evaluation.

Partial Cystectomies

Less frequently, only a portion of the bladder is removed as a sheet-like piece of tissue. In general, these partial cystectomies should be fixed and dissected according to the guidelines given for complete bladder specimens, keeping in mind that orientation of these specimens may not always be possible. Rather than a three-dimensional box, the partial cystectomy can be thought of as a rectangular sheet with four edges. These edges are important, because they represent the surgical margins of the bladder wall. Ink the edges and assess these margins for tumor involvement by taking perpendicular sections from all edges of the rectangle at regular intervals. Remember to include mucosa as well as the wall of the bladder in these sections. Sections should also be taken to demonstrate the maximum depth of invasion of the tumor.

A peculiar variation of the partial cystectomy is seen in resections of neoplasms arising from the urachal tract. These specimens consist of the dome of the bladder in continuity with the urachal tract up to and including the umbilicus. As illustrated, the bladder portion of the specimen should be routinely processed as you would any ordinary partial cystectomy. As for the urachal tract, first ink the surrounding soft tissue margins, and then serially section through the tract from the bladder to the umbilicus. These sections should be taken at right angles to the long axis of the urachal tract. Submit a number of these cross sections from the urachal tract for histology as well as the standard bladder sections. Remember to sample the two additional margins introduced by this resection: the soft tissue margin

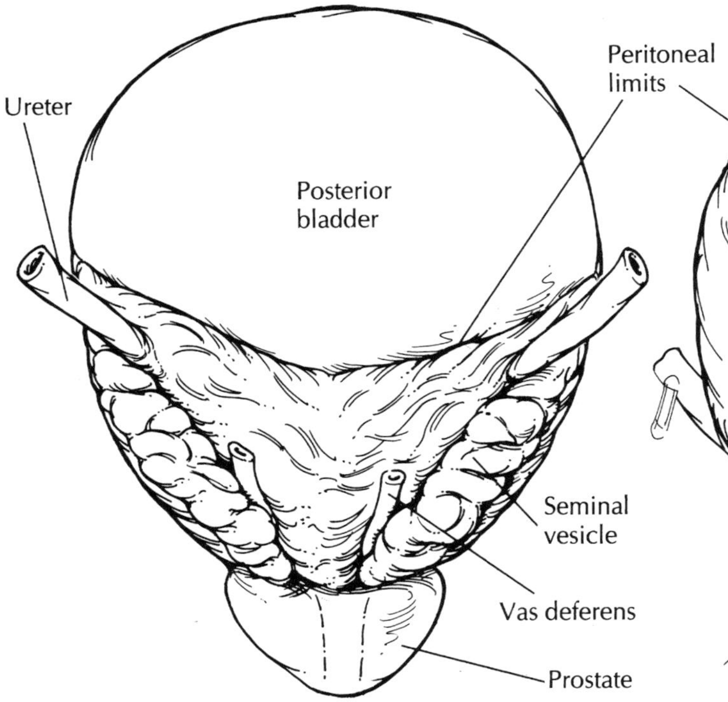

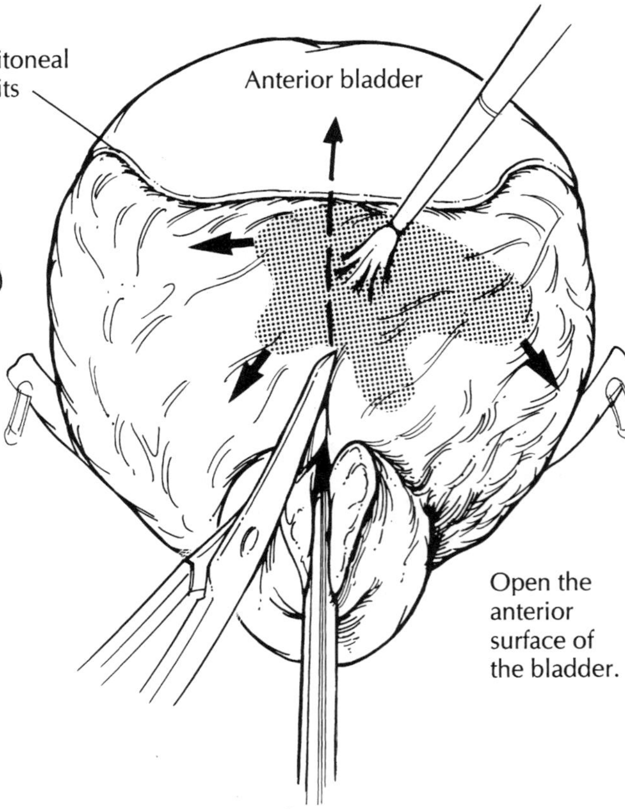

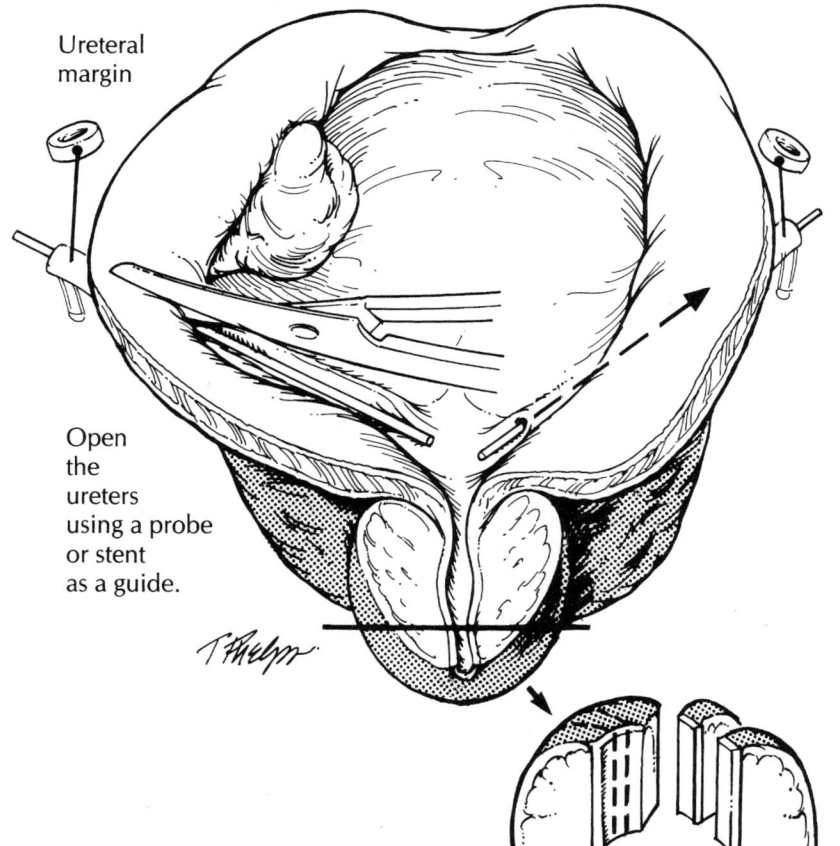

Cystoprostatectomy

1. Orient the bladder. The peritoneum extends further down the posterior wall than it does anteriorly.

2. Open the prostate and bladder along the anterior surface, beginning at the distal urethra.

3. Think of the bladder as a box with sides made up of the trigone, dome, anterior wall, posterior wall, left lateral wall, and the right lateral wall.

4. Submit shave sections of distal urethral and ureteral margins and perpendicular sections from the closest soft tissue margin.

5. Submit sections of the tumor to demonstrate its maximal depth of invasion and the relationship of the tumor to the bladder mucosa. Submit two sections of the trigone, dome, anterior wall, posterior wall, left lateral wall, and right lateral wall. Submit transverse sections of the ureters and a longitudinal section through the ureteral orifices. Include standard prostate sections. Submit sections of any lymph nodes.

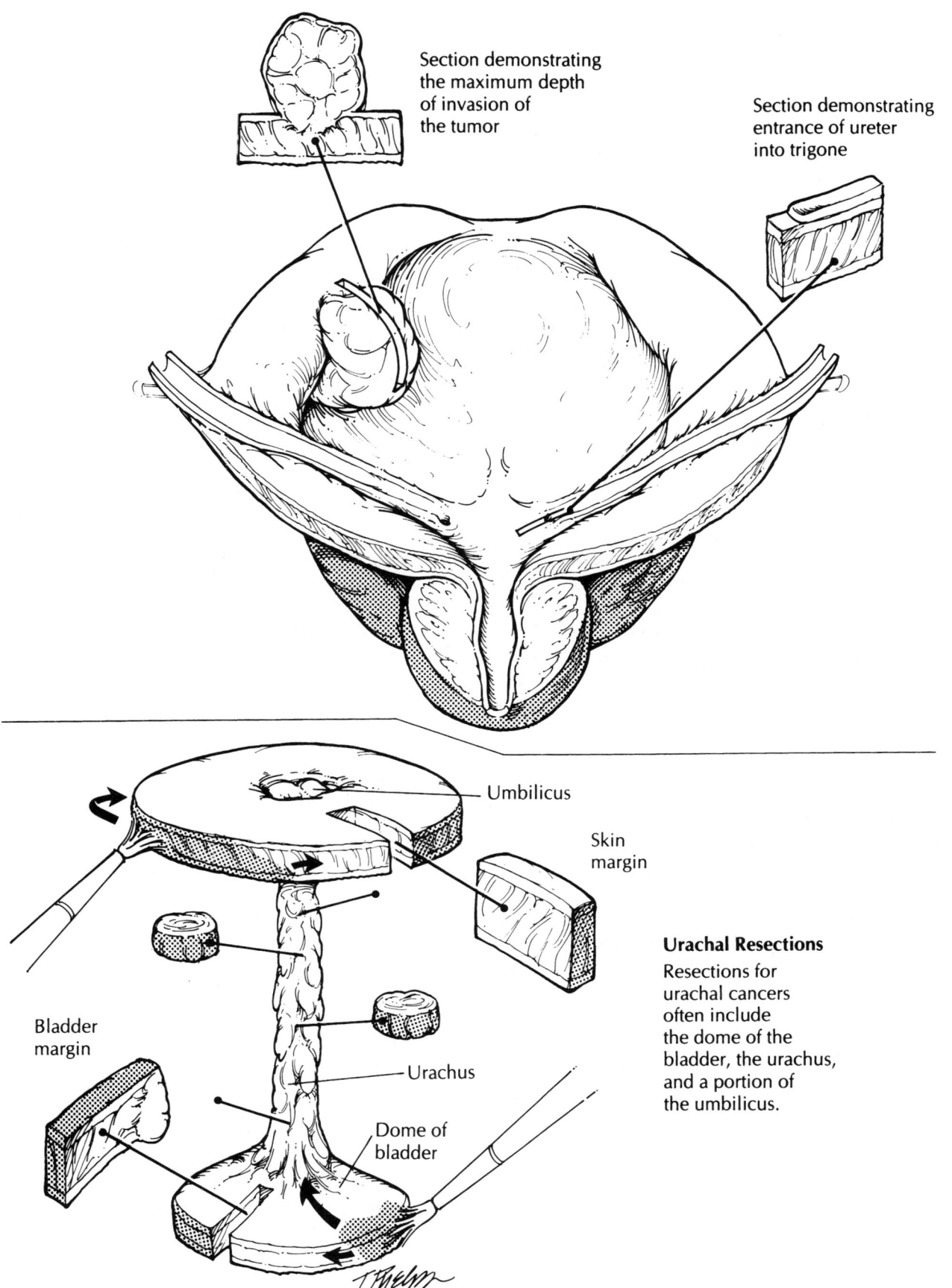

surrounding the urachus and the skin margin rimming the umbilicus.

En Bloc Resections

Commonly, the bladder is removed in continuity with the prostate, uterus, or other pelvic organs. The added complexity of these specimens introduces only minor alterations to the guidelines given above. For cystoprostatectomies, you will again need to open the specimen anteriorly before fixing it; only now begin the incision at the distal prostatic urethra. Using a pair of scissors, open the prostate anteriorly by cutting along the prostatic urethra, and continue the incision through the anterior bladder wall all the way to the dome. Try not to disrupt the posterior aspect of the prostate with this first longitudinal cut. After the specimen has been opened, carefully examine the urethral mucosa for evidence of extension of tumor into the prostatic urethra. Once the specimen is fixed, serially section the prostate from apex to base at 2- to 3-mm intervals. These sections should be transverse sections through the posterior surface of the gland. Examine the cut surface of the prostate. If a tumor is identified, try to determine if it is arising centrally from the prostatic urethra or if it is more peripherally located, as is common for cancer of the prostate. This observation is important, because the prostate should be processed differently (see Chapter 31) if a primary prostate carcinoma is present. If no peripheral tumors are noted, then a more limited sampling of the prostate is in order. These prostate sections should include (1) shaved margins from the distal vasa deferentia; (2) perpendicular sections from the distal (apical) margin of the prostate including the prostatic urethra; (3) a posterior transverse section from the apical, mid, and basilar regions of the gland; (4) two cross sections of the prostatic urethra; and (5) a section of each seminal vesicle.

Because the other pelvic organs commonly removed with the bladder (e.g., uterus and rectum) are situated posteriorly, use the same anterior approach to open the bladder without altering its relationship to these other organs. Section these additional structures, keeping four objectives in mind: (1) document the presence of these structures; (2) demonstrate the relationship between the tumor and each of these structures; (3) evaluate the resection margins for each organ; and (4) examine the attached pelvic organs for other diseases. For example, when a portion of rectum accompanies the bladder specimen, sections should be submitted (1) to document the presence of rectum and any incidental rectal pathologic findings; (2) to demonstrate the relationship between the rectum and the tumor; and (3) to assess the status of the proximal and distal rectal margins.

Important Issues to Address in Your Surgical Pathology Report on Cystectomies

- What procedure was performed, and what structures/organs are present?
- Is a neoplasm present?
- Where in the bladder is the tumor located (trigone, anterior wall, posterior wall, left lateral wall, right lateral wall, dome)?
- How large is the tumor?
- What is its pattern of growth? Is it papillary, flat, or ulcerated?
- Is the neoplasm *in situ* or infiltrating?
- What are the size, histologic type, and grade of the neoplasm?
- What is the maximal depth of invasion of the neoplasm? Does it extend into the lamina propria, the inner half of the muscularis propria, or the outer half of the muscularis propria?
- Does the tumor extend beyond the bladder into the perivesicular fat, prostate, uterus, vagina, pelvic wall, or abdominal wall?
- For bladder carcinomas involving the prostate, specify the nature of prostatic involvement. Specifically, does the carcinoma directly invade the prostate at the bladder neck? Does the carcinoma involve the prostatic urethra? Is there involvement of prostatic ducts with or without stromal invasion?
- What is the status of each of the margins (the ureters, urethra, soft tissue, etc.)?
- Is the tumor multifocal or unifocal?
- Does the tumor involve blood vessels, nerves, or regional lymph nodes? How many lymph nodes were examined, and how many harbor a metastasis?

X   The Ocular System

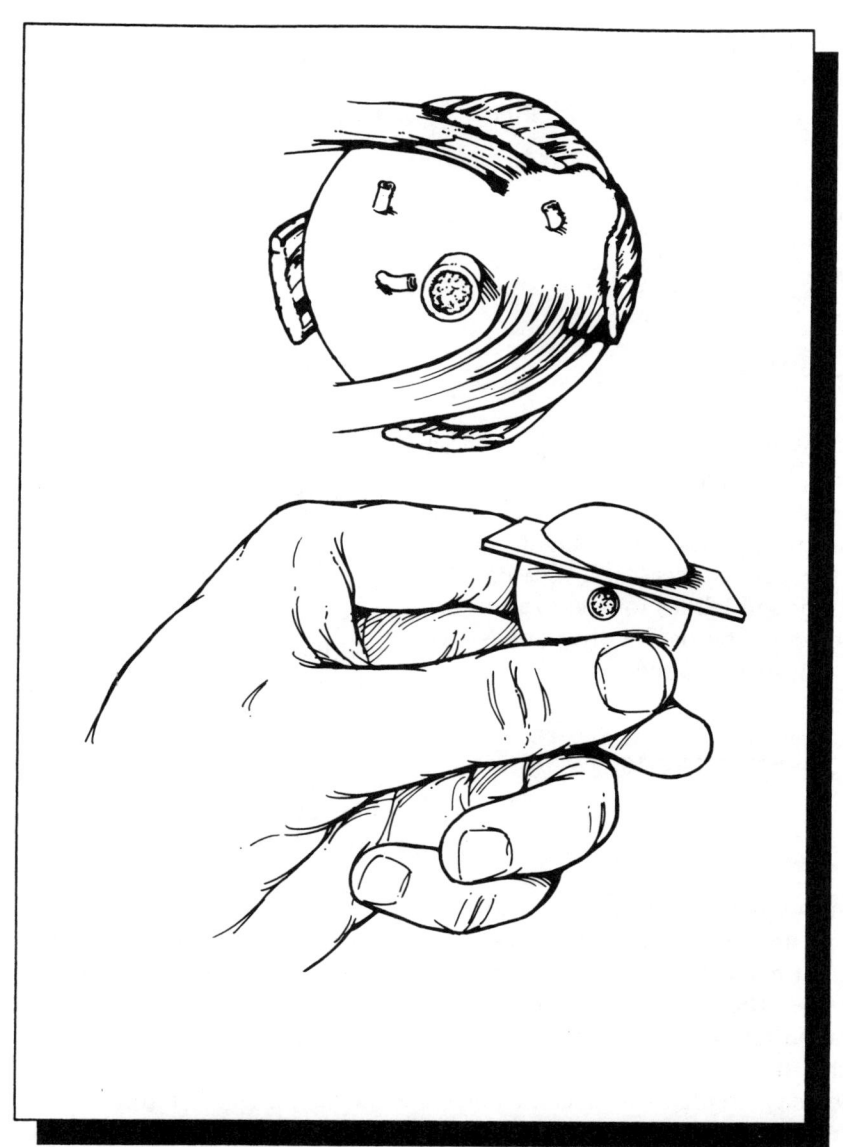

35 Eye

Robert H. Rosa, Jr., M.D., and W. Richard Green, M.D.

General Comments

The eye is a unique neurosensory organ. Much information can be gathered from the gross and microscopic examination of enucleated globes regarding the pathogenesis and manifestations of ocular and systemic diseases. In this chapter, we provide basic guidelines for the fixation and sectioning of ocular tissues, with emphasis on grossing the enucleated globe.

Enucleation Specimens

Fixation

The most commonly used fixative for ocular tissues is 10% neutral buffered formalin (4% formaldehyde), but even this standard fixative has its disadvantages. The relatively high osmolarity of 10% neutral buffered formalin may cause contraction of the anterior chamber and vitreous cavity, which may result in artifactual detachment of the retina. Moreover, formalin tends to dissolve water-soluble substances such as glycogen, resulting in shrinkage of fixed tissue. Thus, it is even a less suitable fixative when electron microscopy studies are required. The amount of 10% neutral buffered formalin required for adequate fixation varies with the size of the ocular specimen. For example, a small specimen such as a cornea or lid biopsy may require only 5 to 10 ml of formalin; an enucleated globe, 150 to 300 ml of formalin; and an orbital exenteration, 500 ml of formalin.

One alternative to formalin is glutaraldehyde 4%. This solution provides adequate fixation for both light and electron microscopy, while causing much less tissue shrinkage because of its lower osmolarity. For specimens less than 2 mm in diameter, glutaraldehyde 2.0% to 2.5% may be the preferred primary fixative for electron microscopy. Glutaraldehyde, however, causes tissues to become hard and brittle and may adversely affect the staining of tissues. For example, ocular tissues fixed in glutaraldehyde 4% stain less vividly with alcian blue and colloidal iron techniques, and they stain diffusely and nonspecifically with the periodic acid-Schiff (PAS) reaction. Yet another alternative is to combine fixatives to achieve optimal preservation for both light and electron microscopy. For example, a solution that combines 4% formaldehyde and 1% glutaraldehyde in phosphate buffer 0.1 mol/L can be used.

Fixation of ocular tissues requires patience. Practices that are designed to speed up the process (e.g., opening the globe, cutting windows into the sclera, or injecting fixative directly into the vitreous) are strongly discouraged because they are likely to induce artifactual disruption of the ocular tissues. The fixation of an enucleated globe in formalin generally requires 24 to 48 hours. After fixation, gently rinse the globe in running water for 16 hours, then place it in ethyl alcohol 60% for grossing.

Eyes that contain excessive calcium deposits or even bone formation may require special decalcifying agents in addition to routine fixatives. In these cases, first fix the globe and then decalcify it in a solution of sodium citrate and formic acid for 24 to 72 hours. When the specimen is soft enough to section, wash it overnight in running tap water to remove all traces of acid, and then place the specimen in ethyl alcohol 60% before further processing. Because decalcification obscures histologic detail and interferes with staining, check the specimen daily while it is in solution to avoid excessive decalcification.

External Examination

Proper orientation of the eye is essential to document the location of a lesion within the eye. Although the eye is roughly spherical, careful attention to external landmarks allows one to orient this structure with respect to the horizontal median and nasal aspect. One such landmark is the cornea. The cornea occupies the anterior one sixth of the globe, measuring about 11 mm in its vertical plane and 11.5 mm in its horizontal plane. Thus, the longer axis of the cornea indicates the horizontal meridian. Other external landmarks are even more helpful in orienting the eye. The posterior ciliary arteries, for example, can be used to determine both the horizontal plane and the nasal aspect of the specimen. These vessels enter the sclera in the region of the optic nerve and then extend horizontally. Importantly, the nasal vessel is usually more prominent and therefore can be used to identify the nasal aspect of the eye. The nasal aspect can also be identified by measuring the distance between the limbus (the periphery of the cornea where it joins the sclera) and the optic nerve. This distance is shortest along the nasal aspect.

Perhaps the most reliable landmarks for orienting the eye are the insertions of the extraocular muscles. The use of these landmarks, however, requires a good understanding of ocular anatomy (Fig. 35-1). The tendon of the superior oblique muscle extends temporally from the trochlea in the nasal orbital wall to insert into the sclera superotemporally posterior and just temporal to the superior rectus insertion and superior to the optic nerve. The inferior oblique muscle extends temporally from the inferonasal orbital wall to insert into the sclera (as a muscular rather than as a tendinous insertion) just temporal to the optic nerve and posterior ciliary vessel. The insertion of the inferior oblique muscle overlies an area of the sclera corresponding to the macula inside the eye.

Once the eye has been properly oriented, measure its anteroposterior, horizontal, and vertical dimensions. Record all measurements in millimeters. Also record the dimensions of the cornea and the length of the optic nerve stump. Describe any abnormal external features such as corneal opacities and lacerations or wounds of the cornea and/or sclera. A careful external examination will often disclose important information regarding a history of eye pathology. Scars located at the superior limbus suggest prior surgery for cataracts or glaucoma, and the presence of a silicone band or sponge suggests prior surgery for retinal detachment. If these silicone bands and sponges are encountered, they need not be dislodged, because they will dissolve during processing. On the other hand, metal clips should be meticulously removed from any area submitted for histologic evaluation.

For cases of suspected melanoma, carefully examine the outer surface of the specimen for tumor spread. Specifically, examine the vortex veins for engorgement by tumor, check the episcleral soft tissues for pigment deposition, and look for gross extrabulbar extension by the tumor. In cases of suspected retinoblastoma, carefully examine the optic nerve grossly, and take the surgical margin of the optic nerve for microscopic examination. A dissecting microscope is extremely helpful in identifying minute lesions, and it should be employed during the external and intraocular examinations.

Photography plays an integral part of the gross examination of ocular tissues. As discussed in Chapter 4, photographs are useful for documenting any abnormal features of the external globe and are very helpful in correlating these gross features with the clinical findings. Likewise, photographs should be taken of intraocular lesions after the eye has been opened. The best photographs are obtained with the specimen submerged in alcohol (60%) and with even illumination.

Transillumination of the globe plays an important role in the localization of intraocular tumors that cannot be directly visualized on external examination. To transilluminate the specimen, place the eye in front of a small intense light against a dark background. One method is to use a substage microscope lamp in a dark room. Rotate the globe over the light source, and look for areas of increased or decreased transmission of light. Increased transmission of light may be seen in defects of the iris as occur in pigmentary dispersion syndrome and following peripheral iridectomy or cataract surgery. Decreased transmission of light may be due to intraocular hemorrhage or intraocular tumors. Mark these transillumination

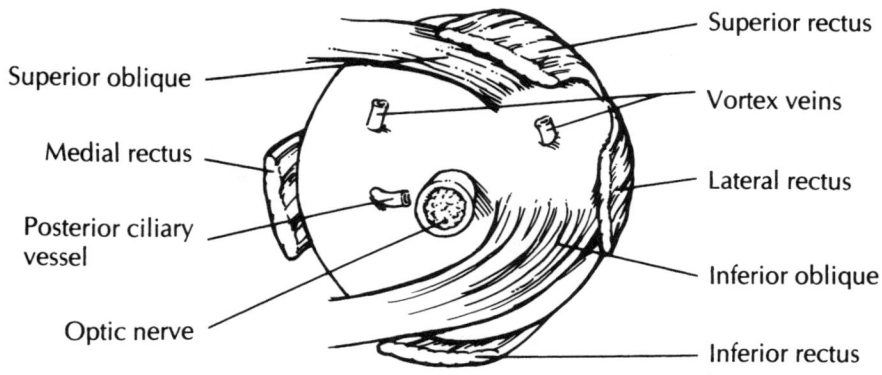

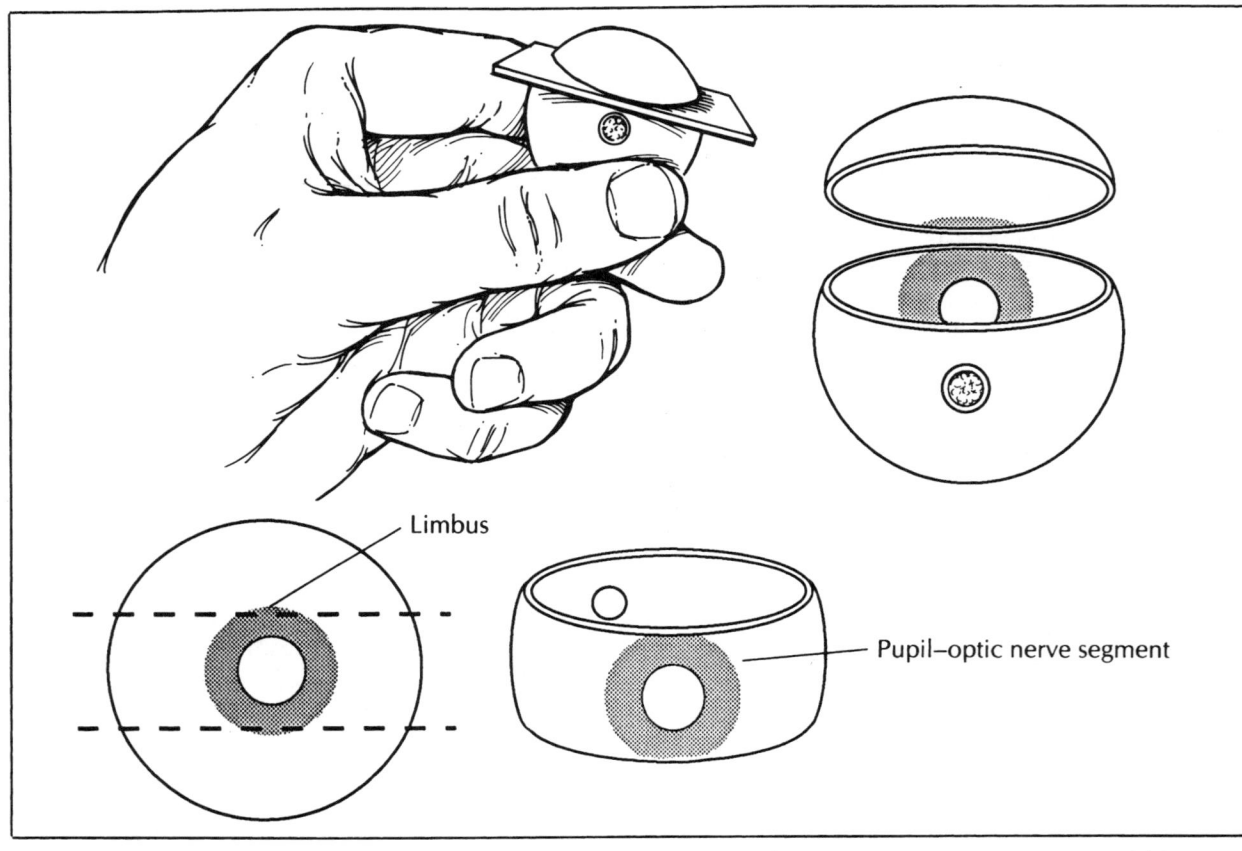

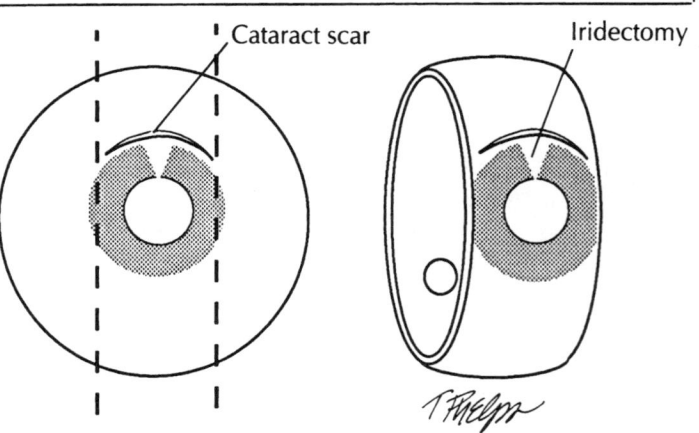

Figure 35-1 (Top). The posterior external aspect of a normal right globe.

Figure 35-2 (Middle). Routine sectioning of the globe with horizontal cuts. The pupil, optic nerve, and macula are all in the same plane (see anterior and posterior views).

Figure 35-3 (Bottom). Sectioning of the globe with vertical cuts to incorporate the cataract scar into the pupil–optic nerve segment.

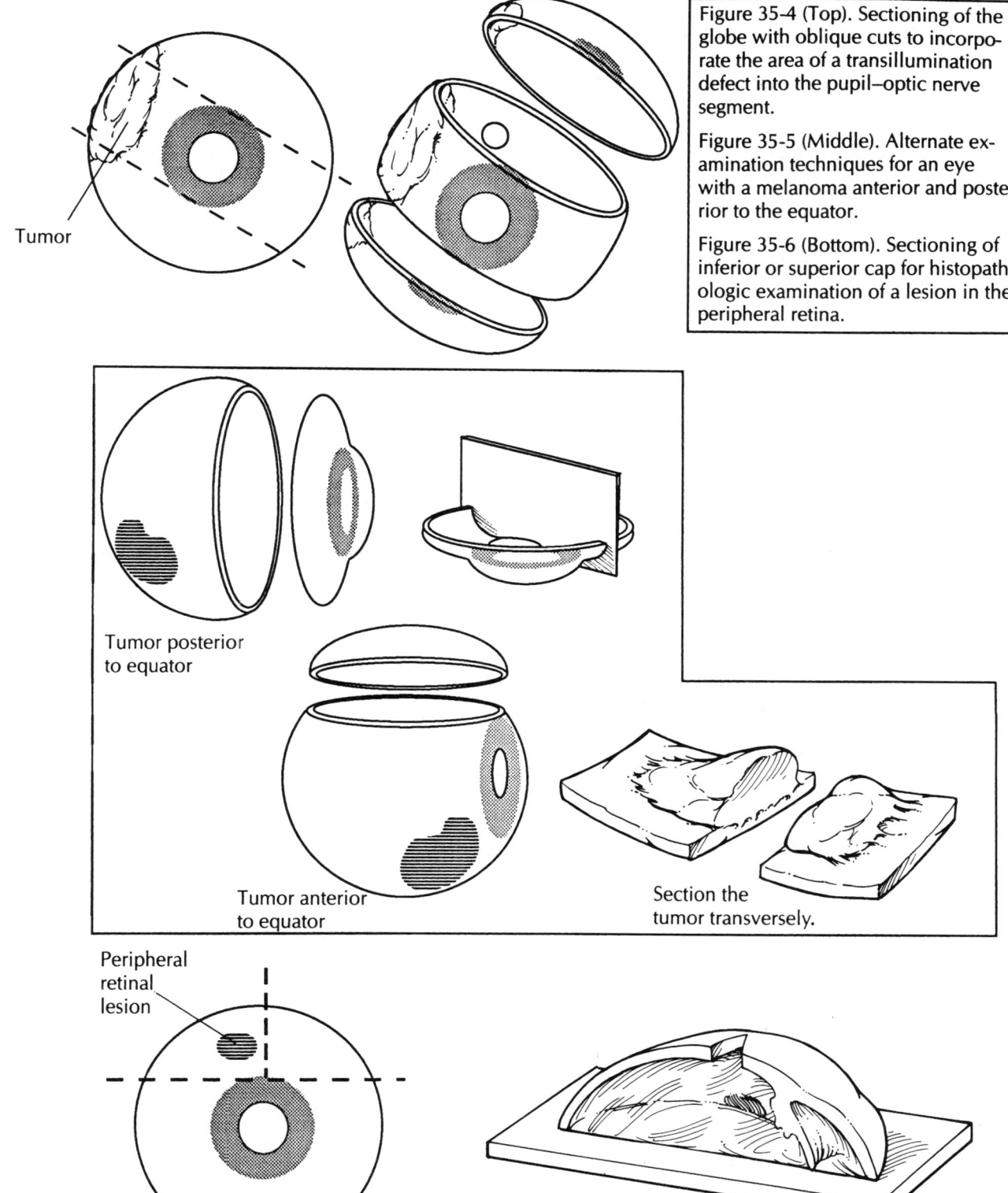

Figure 35-4 (Top). Sectioning of the globe with oblique cuts to incorporate the area of a transillumination defect into the pupil–optic nerve segment.

Figure 35-5 (Middle). Alternate examination techniques for an eye with a melanoma anterior and posterior to the equator.

Figure 35-6 (Bottom). Sectioning of inferior or superior cap for histopathologic examination of a lesion in the peripheral retina.

defects on the corresponding sclera with a pencil. The location of these transillumination defects will determine how the eye should be sectioned.

Sectioning

The planes of section through the globe depend on the presence and location of a lesion. Begin by cutting off the distal 3-mm portion of the optic nerve, and submit this portion on end for histologic examination. If no focal lesions are apparent after external examination, transillumination, and review of the clinical and surgical findings, open the eye in a horizontal plane parallel to the center of the optic nerve and macula. The ultimate aim is to provide a median section along the pupil and optic nerve axis—the pupil–optic nerve (P-O) section—which includes the pupil, optic nerve head, and macula in the same section. Approaching the eye from its posterior aspect, place a razor blade 5 mm superior to the center of the optic nerve. Do not aim the blade toward the center of the pupil, as the lens is a hard structure that is easily dislodged if you try to cut through it. Instead, avoid the lens by aiming 0.5 mm central to the limbus. Once the razor blade is engaged, turn the eye, and view it from the side to help maintain the proper plane of sectioning. Using a sawing motion, continue the section all the way through the limbus (Fig. 35-2).

Before sectioning further, stop to examine the intraocular components. This examination should be performed with a dissecting microscope. Systematically evaluate the lens, iris, ciliary body, vitreous, choroid, retina, and optic nerve head. Note the size and location of any lesions. If an intraocular tumor is present, document its location using the ora serrata, optic disk, and macula as points of reference. Record its size in all dimensions. Try to determine which ocular structures are involved. Specifically note the relationship of the tumor to the optic nerve.

Once the intraocular examination is complete, finish sectioning the eye. Place the cut surface of the globe on a flat surface, and then cut the eye in a plane parallel to the initial section. Again, the razor blade should enter the posterior aspect of the eye 5 mm from the center of the optic nerve, and it should exit the anterior surface of the eye through the periphery of the cornea (i.e., 0.5 mm central to the limbus). The completion of this second cut will result in two caps (or callottes) and the P-O segment.

For eyes with focal lesions, the eye can be sectioned vertically or obliquely to include the lesion in the P-O plane. A few common examples are worthy of specific description. If evidence of prior cataract surgery is present, cut the globe vertically in a plane perpendicular to the wound (Fig. 35-3). If a corneal laceration is present, cut the globe perpendicular to the long axis of the lesion. If a transillumination defect (e.g., melanoma) is present, cut the globe so that the center of the tumor is in the plane of the P-O segment (Fig. 35-4).

An alternative technique for sectioning an eye with melanoma has been designed to permit direct visualization of the tumor from the perspective of the clinician and thus enhance clinicopathologic correlations.[17] For melanomas located posterior to the equator, the anterior segment (cornea, iris, lens, and pars plicata) is removed en bloc by a coronal cut through the pars plana just anterior to the ora serrata. For melanomas that extend anterior to the equator, a cap is removed by a cut along the P-O plane. Either of these cuts permits the examiner to look into the globe and directly visualize the apex of the tumor (Fig. 35-5).

Tissue Sampling

In most cases, only the P-O segment is submitted for histologic evaluation. Important exceptions are when a cap contains the macula (as when the P-O segment is taken in the vertical plane) or a lesion. If a lesion is present in the cap, then the cap may be further sectioned into superonasal, superotemporal, inferonasal, and/or inferotemporal segments, as necessary, and submitted for processing. A mark on the tissue section and a note to the histotechnologist may help guide proper orientation of the tissue during embedding. For example, a small V may be cut into the segment opposite the margin of interest with instructions provided to "embed V up" (Fig. 35-6). The pathologist may wish to supervise the embedding of the tissue to ensure proper orientation. Store any remaining tissue in formalin, taking care to designate the tissue properly.

Cataract Specimens

The handling of cataract specimens varies from institution to institution. In general, cataracts are difficult to evaluate by light microscopy. Hence, the histopathologic examination of cataract specimens is performed only for special indications (such as with congenital cataracts and pseudoexfoliation syndrome). If the submission of cataract specimens is required, document the color, diameter, and thickness of the lens nucleus.

Intracapsular cataract extraction (ICCE) is a surgical technique that allows for the best evaluation of the lens, as the lens is removed in its entirety (capsule, cortex, and nucleus). ICCE was the procedure of choice for cataract extraction for many years; however, this technique is used today only in rare circumstances (such as in conditions with zonular weakness).

Phacoemulsification is a type of small-incision extracapsular cataract extraction (ECCE) that was initially introduced in 1967. Recently, this technique has gained popularity over the more traditional technique of ECCE. With phacoemulsification, there is a smaller incision, less induced astigmatism, and perhaps a faster recovery of vision. The lens nucleus is emulsified ultrasonically; therefore, no cataract specimen is submitted.

Eyelid Excisions

Basal cell carcinoma accounts for 85% to 95% of all malignant epithelial tumors of the eyelids. Most excised specimens with basal cell carcinoma are elliptical. If the long axis of the specimen is less than 10 mm, the specimen should be bisected perpendicular to its long axis through the center of the tumor. This technique allows for the evaluation of three surgical margins (two skin margins and the deep margin). If the ellipse is larger than 10 mm, the specimen can be cut in a cruciate configuration, resulting in a 3- to 4-mm central portion and two end portions. The two end portions are bisected in a plane perpendicular to the central portion. Separately label and submit the central portion and end sections. With this technique, all five surgical margins (e.g., deep, lateral, medial, superior, and inferior) are evaluated.

Special Techniques

Given the easy accessibility of the eye, small tissue samples for diagnostic purposes are readily obtained using a variety of methods. Although these specimens do not require complex dissections, they do require careful handling to preserve cellular detail. Scrapings of the cornea and conjunctiva can be processed as wet-fixed smears. This technique is useful in cases of conjunctival intraepithelial neoplasia. Rapid fixation of the slides in 95% ethyl alcohol is essential in this technique. Do not allow the specimen to air dry. After fixation, the slides may be stained with a modified Papanicolaou technique. Air-dried smears are often useful to look for infectious agents in cases of suspected exogenous or endogenous endophthalmitis. Drops of the specimen are placed on the center of three or more slides and allowed to air dry. The slides can then be fixed in 100% methanol for 5 minutes. Microorganisms can then be detected using Gram, Giemsa, periodic acid-Schiff (PAS), and Papanicolaou stains.

The Millipore filter preparation technique can be used to examine ocular fluid specimens in cases of vitreous hemorrhage, proliferative vitreoretinopathy, and suspected intraocular tumors. This procedure provides for excellent cytologic preservation. The specimen may be received in a plastic syringe or a vitrectomy cassette and must be fresh and unfixed before filtration. After filtration, the cells are fixed with 95% ethyl alcohol. Do not allow the filter to air dry at any time during the procedure. If a specimen is very cellular, divide it among several filters. During filtration, direct the washings along the sides of the funnel to avoid disturbing the cells on the filter. Fix the filters for a minimum of 15 minutes in a Petri dish with 95% ethyl alcohol. A modified Papanicolaou technique, Gomori's stain for iron, and the PAS stain are routinely used to stain the Millipore filter. Absolute propylalcohol rather than absolute ethyl alcohol should be used during staining to avoid dissolution of the filter. The stained Millipore filters are then mounted on glass slides for microscopic examination.

The celloidin bag technique is useful for the retrieval of tissue fragments and cellular material suspended in a fluid. Place 10% neutral buffered formalin and the specimen into a centrifuge-tube lined by a celloidin bag. Centrifuge for 10 minutes. Decant the supernatant, remove the celloidin bag, and tie the bag with a string just above the pellet. Fix the specimen again in formalin for at least 30 minutes. The specimen may now be submitted for routine paraffin processing and sectioning.

Important Issues to Address in Your Surgical Pathology Report on the Eye

- What procedure was performed?
- Is the specimen a right or left eye? What is the size of the eye? (What are the anteroposterior, horizontal, and vertical dimensions? What is the length of the optic nerve? What are the horizontal and vertical dimensions of the cornea?)
- What is the status of the anterior segment (surgical incisions, corneal opacification, iris or lens abnormalities)?
- Are any transillumination defects present? What are the measurements of these defects, and where are they in relation to external landmarks?
- Note the condition of the iris, ciliary body, and lens. Is an intraocular lens present? If so, is it in the anterior or posterior chamber? If in the posterior chamber, is it in the capsular bag or in the sulcus (between the ciliary body and the root of the iris)?
- Is there a posterior vitreous or retinal detachment? Is any hemorrhage present in the vitreous or retina? Is the choroid thickened? Is the optic nerve head cupped or swollen?
- Is an intraocular tumor present? Describe its type, location, size, color, margins, and consistency. Is any associated hemorrhage or necrosis present? What ocular structures are involved? Does the tumor extend into the optic nerve? Is the tumor present grossly at the cranial or surgical margin of the optic nerve?

XI The Endocrine System

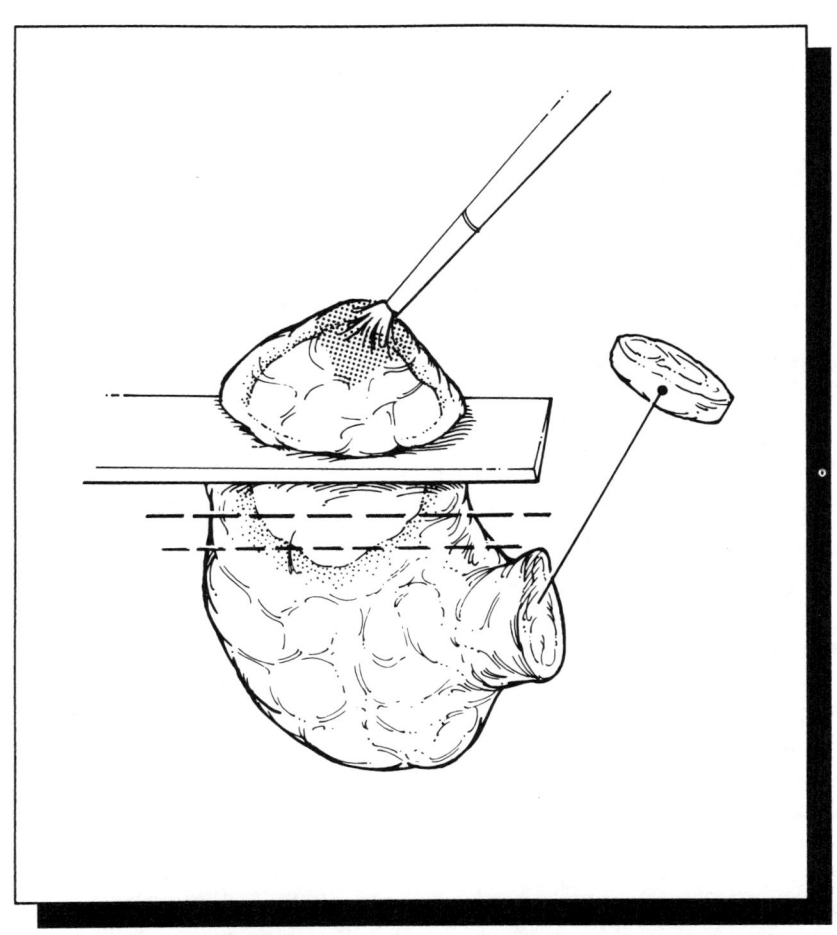

36 Thyroid

Thyroidectomies

One major task of the surgical pathologist evaluating a thyroid specimen is to identify the infrequent thyroid neoplasm from among the vast majority of harmless thyroid nodules—an effort that is shared with the cytopathologist, endocrinologist, and surgeon. Thorough inspection and appropriate sampling of the thyroid is central to the diagnosis and subsequent treatment of thyroid lesions.

The thyroid gland has a relatively simple anatomy. As illustrated, its shape resembles that of a butterfly with open wings: two expanded lateral lobes are bridged at the midline by the isthmus. In some specimens, a small triangular midline lobe (i.e., the pyramidal lobe) is also present. When present, the pyramidal lobe extends superiorly from the isthmus. The two most common resections of the thyroid are total thyroidectomy, in which the entire gland is removed intact, and hemithyroidectomy, in which a single lobe is removed by an incision through the isthmus. Orientation of these specimens is seldom problematic. The isthmus can be used to identify the inferior and medial aspects of the gland, and the posterior surfaces of the lateral lobes have a concave shape caused by the trachea.

Once the specimen has been oriented, it should be weighed and measured. Describe its shape, contours, and symmetry. Be sure to note the presence and appearance of any extrathyroidal tissues. In particular, inspect the posterior aspect of the specimen for parathyroid glands and lymph nodes, and inspect the anterior aspect for fragments of adherent skeletal muscle. Palpate the specimen to assess the consistency of the thyroid and to localize any focal lesions before cutting the specimen.

Paint the outer surfaces of the thyroid with ink; and in the case of hemithyroidectomy, remove the isthmic margin as a thin shave section. Although the specimen can be serially sectioned in either the coronal, sagittal, or transverse plane, the relationship of a focal lesion to the thyroid capsule is often best demonstrated by cutting perpendicular to the long axis of each individual lobe. Once the thyroid is sectioned, sequentially lay out the individual slices in such a way as to maintain the proper orientation of the specimen.

Carefully inspect the cut surfaces of the specimen. Assess whether the thyroid is diffusely or focally abnormal. For diffuse lesions, ask yourself the following questions: Is the gland symmetrically or asymmetrically involved? Is the lesion confined to the thyroid, or does it extend beyond the capsule of the thyroid into the surrounding soft tissues? Is the lesion cystic or solid, soft or hard, well demarcated or poorly defined? If an isolated lesion is identified, record its size and location, and determine if it is surrounded by a capsule. Keep in mind that the presence of a discrete nodule does not exclude the presence of additional lesions. Always look for multifocal lesions. Gentle palpation of each slice will sometimes reveal small but firm carcinomas that are not apparent simply by looking at the cut surface.

Imprints of the tumor allow quick and easy evaluation of its cytologic features and will nicely supplement the histologic findings of a frozen section. Simply touch the surface of a glass slide to the cut surface of the tumor, or smear a small piece of the tumor between two slides, and immediately fix the slides in 95% alcohol. These

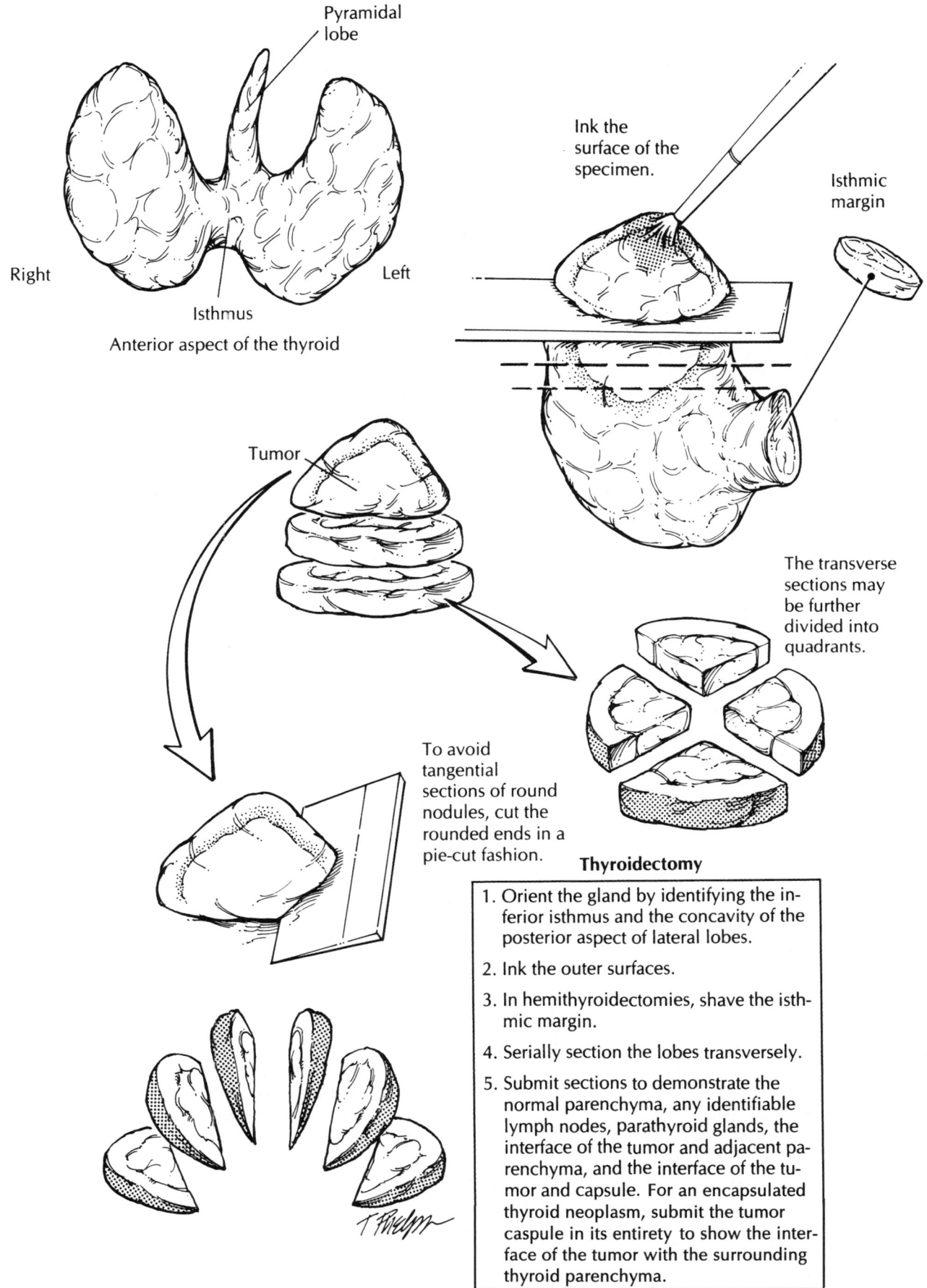

Thyroidectomy

1. Orient the gland by identifying the inferior isthmus and the concavity of the posterior aspect of lateral lobes.
2. Ink the outer surfaces.
3. In hemithyroidectomies, shave the isthmic margin.
4. Serially section the lobes transversely.
5. Submit sections to demonstrate the normal parenchyma, any identifiable lymph nodes, parathyroid glands, the interface of the tumor and adjacent parenchyma, and the interface of the tumor and capsule. For an encapsulated thyroid neoplasm, submit the tumor caspule in its entirety to show the interface of the tumor with the surrounding thyroid parenchyma.

slides can be used for Diff-Quik or hematoxylin and eosin staining.

Sections for histology should be taken to demonstrate the following: (1) all components of a lesion (e.g., solid areas and cystic areas); (2) the interface of the tumor (and its surrounding capsule) with the adjacent non-neoplastic thyroid parenchyma; (3) the relationship of the tumor to the thyroid capsule and extrathyroidal soft tissues; and (4) the presence of parathyroids, lymph nodes, and normal-appearing thyroid parenchyma (one or two sections from each lobe). Since the histologic evaluation will be hampered if the tissue blocks are thick and bulky, you may want to consider fixing the slices in formalin until they are firm enough to section thinly. Although these general guidelines should direct the sampling of any thyroid lesions, two frequently asked questions deserve special consideration:

1. *How many sections do I need to submit to avoid sampling error?* This question often arises in cases of multinodular goiters and encapsulated nodules. In multinodular goiters, the thyroid is often massively enlarged, and its cut surface may show numerous nodules, hemorrhage, calcification, scarring, and even necrosis. In these instances, try to avoid the common error of submitting too many sections. Instead, document the finding with a photograph and a detailed gross description. Sampling a multinodular goiter should be limited to one or two sections selectively taken from the periphery of each nodule (up to five nodules per lobe). Conversely, the more common error when sampling encapsulated nodules is to submit too few sections. Your primary task in sampling these lesions is to make sure that areas of transcapsular or vascular invasion are not missed. Since these areas usually cannot be seen by the naked eye, they can easily be missed unless the peripheral portion of the nodule is extensively sampled. The more capsule sampled, the greater chance of finding invasive foci. Therefore, the tumor–capsule–thyroid interface of any encapsulated nodule should be submitted in its entirety for histologic evaluation.

Similarly, thyroids removed from patients with one of the multiple endocrine neoplasia (MEN) syndromes should be extensively sampled for histology. Many pathology laboratories are beginning to receive thyroids prophylactically removed from young patients with germline mutations of the *ret* proto-oncogene. Even though these glands may appear grossly normal, each lobe should be blocked and submitted in its entirety in an effort to detect C-cell hyperplasia and small medullary carcinomas. In your gross report, note those sections taken from the middle third of each lobe, as this area is where C-cell hyperplasia and small medullary carcinomas are most likely to be detected.

2. *How can I avoid tangential sections of a round nodule?* Tangential sections through a round nodule may give the artifactual microscopic impression that the tumor infiltrates the capsule. Whereas tangential sectioning is usually not a problem at the equator of a nodule where the knife easily passes perpendicular to the tumor capsule, it becomes increasingly difficult to avoid as one approaches the rounded ends of the nodule while bread-loafing the specimen. One method to minimize tangential sectioning is to cut these rounded ends like a pie rather than a loaf of bread.[18] Decapitate the rounded ends from the tumor nodule, place the flat surface of each end on the cutting board, and then, as illustrated, direct each cut perpendicular to the tumor capsule as though you were dividing a pie into equal pieces.

Regional neck lymph nodes are usually removed separately by the surgeon and submitted as separate specimens. These should be anatomically oriented, and each level should be carefully dissected (see Chapter 10). Each lymph node identified should be submitted for histologic evaluation.

Important Issues to Address in Your Surgical Pathology Report on Thyroidectomies

- What procedure was performed, and what structures/organs are present?
- What is the size of the lesion, and where is it located? Is the tumor multifocal? If so, record the number of tumors and the size of each.
- What are the histologic type and grade of the tumor (e.g., follicular, papillary, medullary, anaplastic)?
- For encapsulated neoplasms, does the tumor infiltrate its surrounding capsule?
- Is vascular invasion present?
- Is the lesion confined to the thyroid, or does it extend beyond the thyroid capsule into the extrathyroidal soft tissues?

- Are any abnormalities present in the non-neoplastic thyroid tissue (e.g., nodular hyperplasia, thyroiditis, C-cell hyperplasia)?
- Is evidence of metastatic disease present? Record the number of lymph nodes with metastases and the total number of lymph nodes examined. If present, note the presence of tumor extension into the extranodal fat.
- If identified, note the presence and number of parathyroid glands. Whenever possible, the location of the gland(s) should be specified.

37 Parathyroid Glands

Parathyroidectomies

Parathyroid glands are usually removed from patients with hypercalcemia. During the removal of these glands, the surgeon often needs help identifying parathyroid tissue, determining whether the parathyroid tissue is proliferative, and distinguishing between hyperplasia involving multiple glands and a neoplasm confined to a single gland. For the surgical pathologist, these issues translate into two simple questions that can be promptly addressed: (1) Is parathyroid tissue present? (2) How large is the parathyroid gland?

1. *Is it parathyroid tissue*? Parathyroid glands are oval, encapsulated nodules that have a homogeneous red-brown cut surface. This gross appearance of the parathyroid is not specific and may resemble a lymph node or a thyroid nodule. Fortunately, this distinction can be made with speed and relative ease by resorting to frozen section evaluation and/or with a touch imprint from the surface of the encapsulated nodule.
2. *How big is it*? Perhaps the biggest oversight when evaluating parathyroid tissue is forgetting to weigh the tissue. While histologic examination is important in confirming the presence of a parathyroid gland, the histologic findings may not reliably distinguish between normal and proliferative parathyroid tissue. Instead, this distinction is best made by weighing the gland. Therefore, it is critical that every specimen potentially representing parathyroid tissue be accurately weighed. Once an enlarged parathyroid gland is removed, remain alert. Remember to weigh additional specimens, since their size may be critical in distinguishing between an isolated adenoma and diffuse hyperplasia.

With these two questions in mind, the dissection of parathyroid tissue is simple. Measure and weigh the specimen, and note its gross appearance including its shape and color. Use a scale that is accurate to the nearest milligram. If a portion of the gland has been harvested by the surgeon for the purpose of autotransplantation, ask the surgeon to estimate the weight of the gland that was harvested and record this value in the gross report. Sometimes, instead of a grossly apparent parathyroid gland, you may receive a portion of thyroid or thymus. Because the parathyroids may lie hidden deep in the parenchyma of these organs, they should be rapidly yet thoroughly dissected and inspected. In these cases, weigh the entire specimen before dissecting it, and then weigh the potential parathyroid gland alone once any associated tissues have been delicately removed. Bisect the parathyroid, and note the appearance of its cut surface.

Although the intraoperative parathyroid hormone assay is being increasingly used intraoperatively to guide the surgical management of primary hyperparathyroidism, in many practices surgeons still request frozen sections to confirm the removal of parathyroid tissue. Touch imprints of the cut surface of the specimen (immediately fixed in 95% alcohol and stained with hematoxylin and eosin) can be used to differentiate parathyroid from thyroid and lymphoid tissue, and they often serve as a valuable adjunct to the frozen section.

In addition to the parathyroid gland, remember to sample other tissues that may be part of the specimen (e.g., thyroid gland, thymus, and associated soft tissues). Indeed, when these structures are removed in a search for an occult parathyroid gland, the entire specimen should be submitted for histologic evaluation if the parathyroid gland is not grossly apparent. In the rare case of a parathyroid carcinoma, sections should be submitted in an attempt to document local invasion by the tumor. These sections should demonstrate the relationship of the tumor to its capsule and to any adjacent structures (e.g., thyroid gland).

Important Issues to Address in Your Surgical Pathology Report on the Parathyroid

- What procedure was performed, and what structures/organs are present?
- Is parathyroid tissue present? How many glands were removed?
- What is the weight of each parathyroid gland (to the nearest milligram)?
- Based on the comparative weights and histologic features, is the tissue most consistent with normal parathyroid tissue, multiglandular hyperplasia, or an adenoma? Keep in mind that the distinction between multiglandular hyperplasia and an adenoma requires correlation with the clinical and surgical findings.
- For parathyroid carcinomas: What is the size of the carcinoma? Does the carcinoma extend beyond the tumor capsule? Is angiolymphatic invasion present? Does the carcinoma infiltrate into adjacent soft tissues and/or the thyroid? Are the margins involved by tumor?

38 Adrenal Glands

Adrenalectomies

Extrinsic hormonal influences and intrinsic pathologic processes have profound and predictable effects on the size, color, and shape of the adrenal gland. For example, the pathogenesis of hypercortisolism is frequently suggested by the size and color of the adrenal cortex, and the distinction between benign and potentially malignant cortical neoplasms is often based on the dimensions and weight of the tumor. Therefore, careful examination of the gross specimen plays an important role in recognizing and interpreting pathologic processes involving the adrenal gland.

A thorough evaluation of the specimen requires a certain familiarity with the anatomy and weight of the normal adrenal gland. As illustrated, the right adrenal gland has the shape of a pyramid and the left adrenal gland the shape of a crescent. The average weight of each is approximately 4 g in the adult. Weights of 6 g or more are abnormal. Specimen orientation is easily achieved by locating the concave surface of the specimen. This concavity is the point at which the adrenal abuts the ipsilateral kidney, and thus it represents the inferolateral aspect of the specimen. The adrenal gland is considered a tripartite structure composed of a head, body, and tail. The head is the thickest and broadest portion of the adrenal and is situated most medially. The middle third represents the body. The thinnest and most lateral third represents the tail. Unlike the kidney, blood does not enter the adrenal at a single vascular pedicle. Instead, numerous small arteries pierce the cortex at multiple sites. Most of these vessels are too small to appreciate grossly. In contrast, the adrenal is drained by a single vein. This vein exits the adrenal at the junction of the body and the head of the gland and is usually visible to the naked eye, especially when filled and distended by tumor.

Examine the contours of the adrenal gland. Be sure to ink the soft tissues overlying any areas where tumor bulges from the surface of the adrenal, since these areas represent soft tissue margins. Look for and sample the adrenal vein. The entire specimen should then be measured and weighed. Distinguishing between a benign and malignant adrenal neoplasm is often done by weight. It is therefore critical that you accurately weigh the intact fresh specimen before it is fixed and before tissue is procured for additional studies. For tumors between 50 and 100 g we recommend that you carefully remove any extraneous soft tissue not near margins closely approached by the tumor before weighing. If the gland appears enlarged, determine and document whether this enlargement is due to a solitary mass, multiple nodules, or diffuse hyperplasia. Extended resections of primary adrenal tumors may also include portions of adjacent kidney, liver, and/or abdominal wall. The presence and appearance of these structures should be noted, and their relationships to the adrenal tumor should be described.

Unless otherwise indicated, the adrenal should always be sectioned in the transverse plane. This plane of sectioning optimizes evaluation of the relative sizes of the cortical and medullary compartments. Serially section the adrenal gland at 2- to 3-mm intervals perpendicular to the long axis of the specimen. Keep in mind that although the adrenal gland is removed as a single structure, it is both structurally and functionally compartmentalized into a steroid-secreting

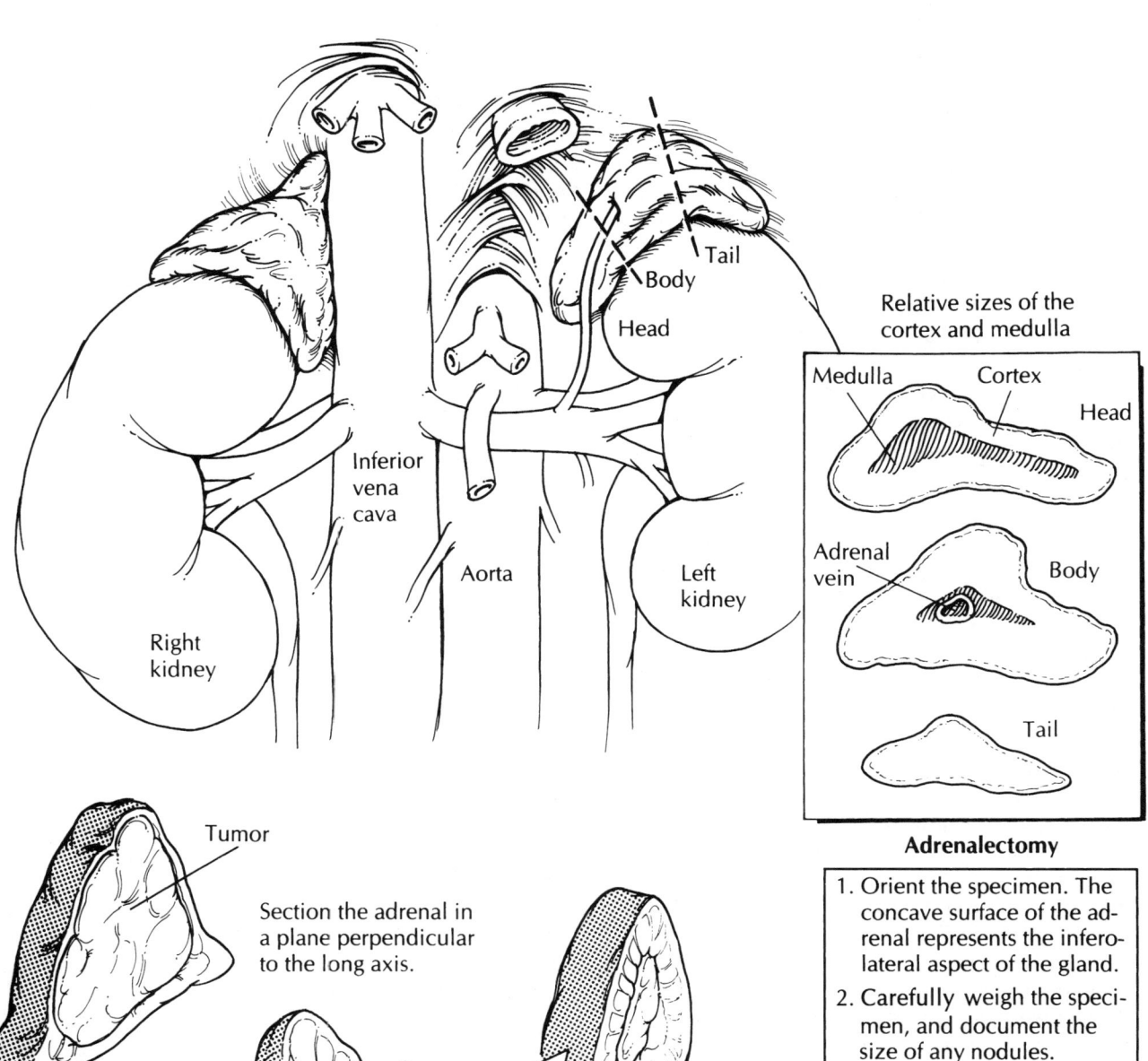

Relative sizes of the cortex and medulla

Adrenalectomy

1. Orient the specimen. The concave surface of the adrenal represents the inferolateral aspect of the gland.
2. Carefully weigh the specimen, and document the size of any nodules.
3. Ink the specimen. If a tumor is present, dissect away any extraneous soft tissues not near a closely approached margin and document the weight of the tumor. Section it perpendicular to the long axis of the gland.
4. Measure the thickness of the cortex and medulla in the head, body, and tail.
5. Submit sections of the tumor to show its relationship to the capsule and to the adjacent adrenal tissue.
6. Submit sections of grossly uninvolved adrenal tissue.

cortex and a chromaffin-positive medulla. This compartmentalization will become most apparent when the adrenal is sectioned. The medulla is seen as an inner gray or white band confined mostly to the head of the adrenal. This central band is sharply demarcated from the outer yellow-brown cortex. The inner zone of the cortex is typically brown, while the outer zone of the cortex is often yellow. The inner zone corresponds to the lipofuscin-laden zona reticularis and the outer zone to the lipid-laden zona glomerulosa and zona fasciculata. Measure and record the thickness of these compartments at three levels—the head, body, and tail. Remember to document the exact dimensions of any tumors and to record the appearance of the tumor's cut surface: What is its color? Is it necrotic and/or hemorrhagic? Is it encapsulated? Does it extend beyond the adrenal and into adjacent tissues?

Before the specimen is fixed in formalin, ask yourself if fresh tissue should be specially processed. For example, adrenal cortical neoplasms are sometimes evaluated for steroid content. Viable fresh tissue from these tumors can be snap frozen in liquid nitrogen and stored in a −70°C freezer for easy retrieval if tissue is later needed for biochemical analysis. Fresh tissues from adrenal medullary neoplasms have historically been processed in dichromate fixatives (e.g., Zenker's solution) to preserve cytoplasmic chromaffin granules. Today, this practice has limited value because these same catecholamines can be more precisely characterized and quantified from the patient's serum. Perhaps the strongest indication for special tissue processing is if the tumor was resected from a young patient. For adrenal tumors from pediatric patients—where a primitive neuroblastic tumor is often suspected—fresh tissue should be set aside for cytogenetic, molecular (e.g., N-myc amplification), and ultrastructural analysis (see Chapter 39).

Sections from a tumor should be taken to demonstrate the relationship of the tumor to the adrenal, to the tumor capsule, and to any associated soft tissues and visceral organs. Do not forget to take sections from the surgical margins, including an appropriate margin from all structures represented in the extended resection (e.g., abdominal wall, kidney) and from the periadrenal fat overlying a bulging tumor. Large adrenal tumors should be sampled to include all components contributing to its often variegated appearance on cut section. For the uninvolved adrenal gland and for specimens that do not have a discrete lesion, submit a representative section from the head, body, and tail. To best demonstrate the cortex and medulla, these sections should be taken perpendicular to the long axis of the gland.

Regional lymph nodes will generally not be found in the specimen but may be separately submitted by the surgeon. Any lymph nodes that are present should, of course, be sampled for histologic evaluation.

Important Issues to Address in Your Surgical Pathology Report on Adrenalectomies

- What procedure was performed, and what structures/organs are present?
- What are the dimensions and weight of the adrenal gland?
- For focal tumors: From which compartment (cortex or medulla) does the tumor appear to arise? What are the dimensions and weight of the tumor? Is the tumor benign, malignant, or of uncertain malignant potential? Does the tumor infiltrate vessels, the tumor capsule, and/or the surrounding tissues? What is the status of the surgical margins? Has the tumor metastasized to regional lymph nodes? If so, how many lymph nodes were removed, and how many are involved by tumor?
- For diffuse processes: Which compartment (cortex or medulla) is expanded? Is the compartment uniformly enlarged, or is the enlargement due to multiple nodules?

XII Pediatric Tumors

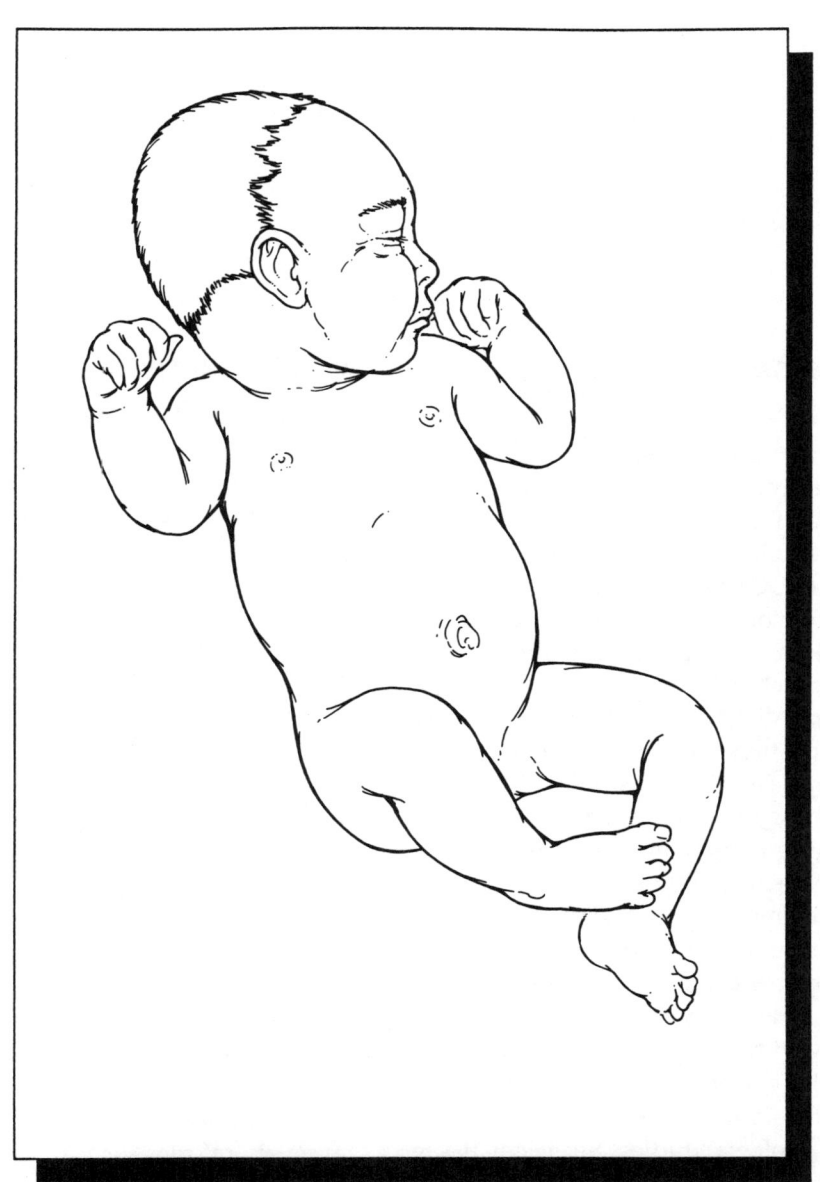

39 Pediatric Tumors

Elizabeth J. Perlman, M.D.

General Comments

A number of tumors are unique to children. These tumors frequently require special processing to ensure that the diagnosis can be established and appropriate treatment given. The Children's Oncology Group (COG) creates, monitors, and evaluates therapeutic protocols for pediatric tumors. In the United States, COG frequently requires that pathologic material be sent to review pathologists to verify the diagnosis and to further classify the tumor. Additional fresh and frozen tissue is often required for biologic studies, which are performed at specialized reference laboratories. If this tissue is not collected at the time of surgery, the patient may not be eligible for the appropriate treatment protocol. Furthermore, as knowledge is accumulated and protocols change, tissue requirements change. Therefore, pathologists who are processing pediatric tumors need to work closely with their pediatric oncologists to be aware of the current protocol requirements. Conversely, the entire specimen cannot be submitted for biologic studies. Sufficient tissue must be available to establish a histologic diagnosis. It is vital that the pathologist be responsible for the appropriate triage of this tissue. In many cases, tissue also needs to be submitted for ancillary diagnostic studies (such as electron microscopy and cytogenetic analysis). Despite these demands, pediatric tumors can be processed easily if a series of steps is routinely performed at the time of initial processing. Establishing a routine is particularly important because many biopsies are performed during off-hours.

Overall Guidelines

1. Ensure that *all* pediatric tumors are promptly received in the fresh state. This may entail processing during off-hours by on-call personnel.
2. Decide how much of the specimen is needed for routine histology. This will depend on the tumor type suspected and the size of the biopsy.
3. Submit tissue for electron microscopy if appropriate. It is good practice to put a small piece of every pediatric tumor in glutaraldehyde. This can then be embedded, and the decision of whether to section and process can be made at a later time.
4. Place ½ to 1 cc of minced tumor in Roswell Park Memorial Institute medium (RPMI) or equivalent tissue culture medium and refrigerate. This material can be submitted for cytogenetic analysis, flow cytometry, or mailed to a reference laboratory for special studies (such as ploidy, gene amplification studies, or fluorescence in situ hybridization).
5. Freeze a minimum of 1 cc of tumor tissue in liquid nitrogen. This can be submitted to reference laboratories for protocol studies or held locally in a tumor bank if available. Normal tissue should also be frozen. If you have limited tissue, remember that the frozen section control is often inadequate for permanent histology, yet if it is kept frozen it can be used for these studies.

Small Blue Cell Tumors of Childhood

Pediatric tumors are often embryonal neoplasms showing little or no differentiation by routine histology. In particular, at the time of frozen section, these tumors appear to be primitive, small, round blue cell tumors. Their diagnosis often depends on ancillary studies such as immunohistochemistry, electron microscopy, and cytogenetics or molecular genetic analysis. If all pediatric specimens are processed as delineated in the first section, all necessary information should be available in a timely fashion. Table 39-1 lists the most common small blue tumors of childhood and their pertinent diagnostic features.

Pediatric Renal Neoplasms

Pediatric renal tumors are often primarily resected and must be carefully processed to ensure accurate staging.[19] Since these tumors are often bulky and friable and are therefore easily distorted, processing must be undertaken with care. (Refer also to Chapter 33.)

1. Photograph the nephrectomy specimen before bivalving. Carefully examine the contour of the kidney and the tumor, and identify potential sites of capsular penetration.
2. Ink the surface (do not strip the capsule).
3. Submit shave sections of the vascular and ureteral margins. The renal vein margin is particularly important.
4. Bivalve the specimen. The kidney should always be bivalved by the pathologist *after* steps 1–3 are performed, not by the surgeon and not in the operating room. Choose your plane of incision carefully, as the placement of the original incision determines your ability to document the relationship between the tumor and kidney, the tumor and the renal sinus, etc. The incision should be at or near the vertical midplane of the kidney. This cut should avoid sites of capsular penetration if possible.
5. Obtain fresh tissues needed for special studies (cytogenetics, frozen, etc.), as outlined previously. Photograph the bivalved specimen.
6. Make cuts parallel to the initial bivalving incision at 2- to 3-cm intervals. Submerge the specimen in a large container of formalin. If the formalin can be refrigerated, color preservation will be enhanced and autolysis slowed.
7. After a few hours or overnight fixation, the remaining sections may be obtained. Two slides should be prepared from all tissue blocks to expedite the mailing of slides to the external review pathologist. The majority of the routine tumor sections should be taken from the periphery of the lesion, showing the following:
   a. Nature of the tumor–kidney junction.

TABLE 39-1. Common small blue cell tumors of childhood and diagnostic parameters.

Tumor type	Immunohistochemistry				EM	Common cytogenetic changes
	NSE	Actin	CD99	CLA		
Neuroblastoma	+++	−	−	−	Neurosecretory granules, processes containing neurofilaments or neurotubules	1p del n-myc amplification
Peripheral neuroectodermal tumor	+	−	++	−	Scant neurosecretory granules, rare processes	t(11;22) and variants
Ewing's sarcoma	±	−	++	−	Glycogen lakes	t(11;22) and variants
Rhabdomyo sarcoma						
Alveolar	±	++	±	−	Myofilaments	t(2;13), t(1;13)
Embryonal	±	++	±	−	Myofilaments	11p15 abnormalities
Lymphoblastic lymphoma	−	−	++	+	−	Variable
Burkitt's lymphoma	−	−	−	++	−	t(8;14)
Synovial sarcoma	−	−	±	−		t(X;18)
Desmoplastic small round cell tumor	±	±	±	−		t(11;22) (p13; q24)

CLA, common leukocyte antigen; EM, electron microscopy; MIC2, antibody to the protein coded for by the *MIC2* gene; NSE, neuron-specific enolase.

b. Relationship of the tumor to the renal capsule, particularly in areas of concern for capsular penetration.
c. Relationship of the tumor to the renal sinus.
d. Areas of the tumor that appear different (e.g., necrosis, hemorrhage). Always indicate the exact site from which each section is taken. This is most easily done by taking Polaroid or digital photographs (see Chapter 4). Drawings are often insufficient.
8. Carefully section and inspect the normal kidney, particularly adjacent to the tumor. These areas may show microscopic foci of persistent embryonal tissue known as nephrogenic rests, the potential precursor lesion of nephroblastomas.
9. Carefully dissect the hilar and perinephric tissues for lymph nodes. Failure to submit regional lymph nodes may render patients ineligible for some low-stage protocols.

Using the above guidelines for submission of blocks, histologic evaluation should then provide the specific tumor diagnosis as well as the stage. The staging currently used for pediatric tumors is provided in Table 39-2. The diagnosis of stage II neoplasms depends on the identification of either renal capsular penetration or invasion of vessels of the "renal sinus." The renal sinus is the principal portal of exit for tumor cells from the kidney and therefore deserves careful study. The renal sinus is the concave portion of the kidney that contains much of the pelvicalyceal system and the principal arteries, veins, lymphatics, and nerves that pass through this sinus. It is largely filled with vascularized adipose tissue. The renal sinus can be recognized histologically by the fact that the renal cortex lining the sinus lacks a capsule. A thick capsule surrounds the pelvicalyceal structures and continues to cover the medullary pyramids. The distinction between stage I and stage II tumors includes either penetration of the renal capsule or infiltration of vessels of the sinus. Some stage I tumors can distort the renal sinus and protrude with a smoothly encapsulated surface without invading the soft tissue of the renal sinus. Such tumors do not meet the criteria for upstaging, unless they show renal capsular penetration.

TABLE 39-2. Staging of pediatric renal neoplasms (From National Wilms' Tumor Study).

Stage I: Tumor confined to kidney, completely excised.
  Intact renal capsule
  Infiltrated but not penetrated renal capsule
  Renal sinus vessels not infiltrated
  Renal vein contains no tumor (intrarenal vessels may be involved)
  Lymph nodes contain no tumor
  No distant metastases
Stage II: Tumor extends out of the kidney but is completely excised, and there is no evidence of nodal or distant metastases.
  Tumor penetrates renal capsule into perirenal fat
  Tumor capsule biopsied, without diffuse peritoneal spillage
  Tumor infiltrates renal sinus vessels
  Tumor in renal vein, removed without cutting across tumor
  Tumor infiltrates adjacent organs or vena cava, but is completely resected
Stage III: Tumor is incompletely excised.
  Tumor incompletely excised
  Surgical margins involved by tumor
  Tumor in lymph nodes
  Tumor thrombus transected
  Peritoneal implants present
  Tumor removed in more than one part

Important Issues to Address in Your Report on Pediatric Renal Neoplasms

- What procedure was performed, and what structures/organs are present?
- What type of neoplasm is present? The most common diagnoses in children are Wilms tumor, clear cell sarcoma of kidney, rhabdoid tumor, congenital mesoblastic nephroma, and renal cell carcinoma. If Wilms tumor, state whether the histology is *favorable* or *unfavorable*. Unfavorable histology is based on the presence of cells with nuclei four times the size of surrounding blastemal cells and the presence of aberrant, multipolar mitotic figures. If unfavorable histology (also called *anaplasia*) is present, comment on its extent (focal or diffuse).
- What is the size of the tumor (weight and greatest dimension)?
- Are any margins involved?
- Is the renal vein involved by tumor?
- Is renal capsular penetration present?
- Is renal sinus invasion present?
- Has the tumor metastasized to regional lymph nodes? Record the number of metastases and the total number of lymph nodes examined.

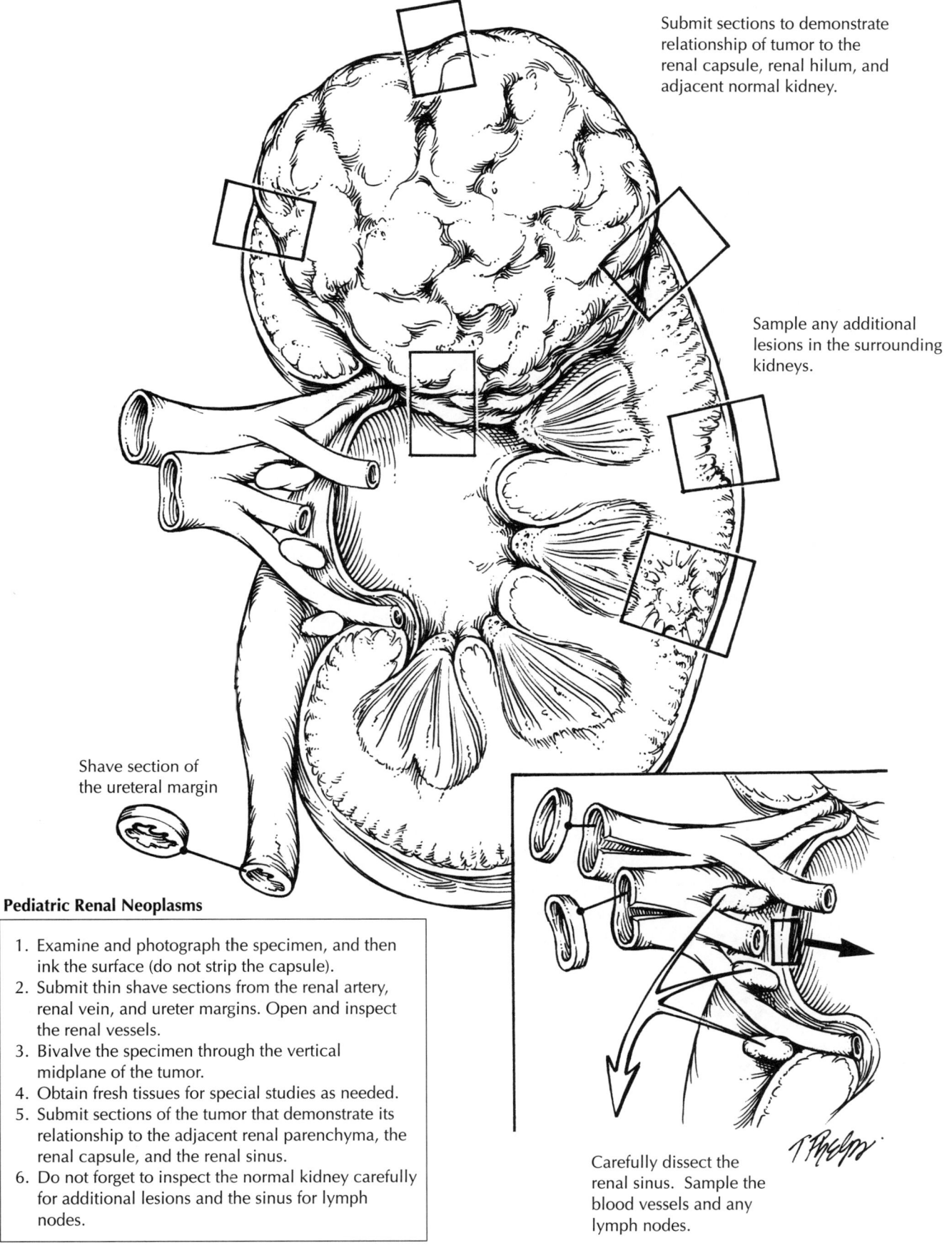

Submit sections to demonstrate relationship of tumor to the renal capsule, renal hilum, and adjacent normal kidney.

Sample any additional lesions in the surrounding kidneys.

Shave section of the ureteral margin

Carefully dissect the renal sinus. Sample the blood vessels and any lymph nodes.

Pediatric Renal Neoplasms

1. Examine and photograph the specimen, and then ink the surface (do not strip the capsule).
2. Submit thin shave sections from the renal artery, renal vein, and ureter margins. Open and inspect the renal vessels.
3. Bivalve the specimen through the vertical midplane of the tumor.
4. Obtain fresh tissues for special studies as needed.
5. Submit sections of the tumor that demonstrate its relationship to the adjacent renal parenchyma, the renal capsule, and the renal sinus.
6. Do not forget to inspect the normal kidney carefully for additional lesions and the sinus for lymph nodes.

ing

XIII   The Central Nervous System

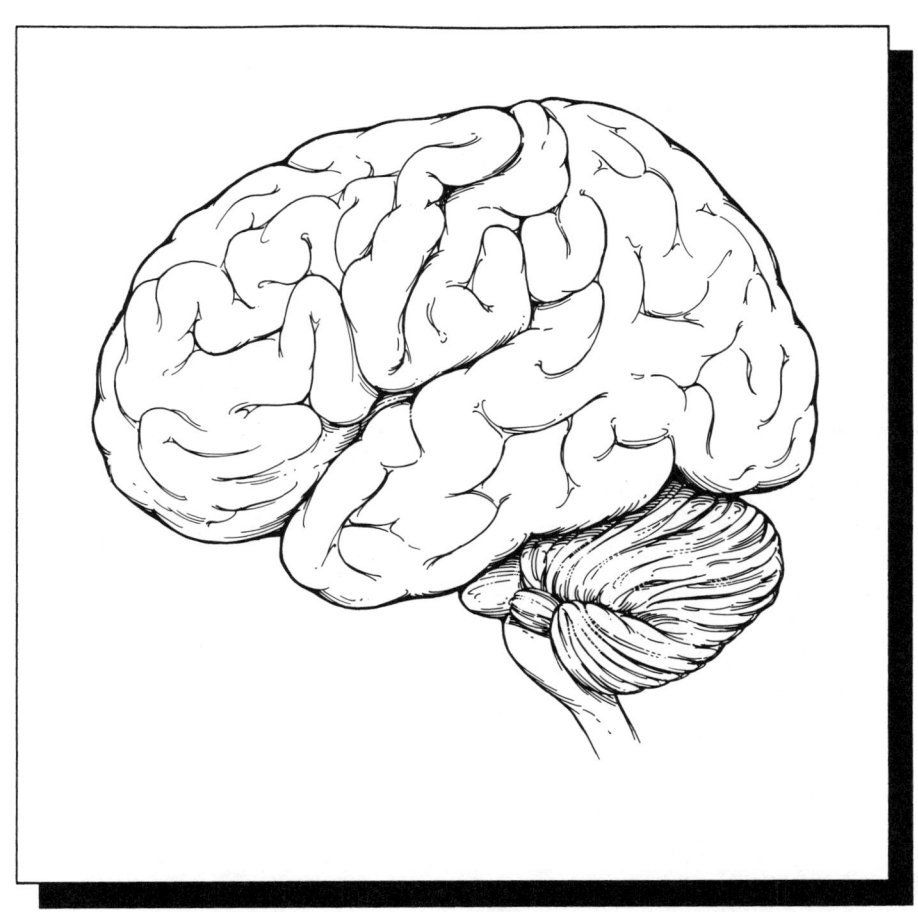

40 Brain and Spinal Cord

Peter C. Burger, M.D.

General Comments

In some respects, pathologic evaluation of specimens from the central nervous system (CNS) is less complicated than evaluation of other organs, because requests for margins and the need for extensive specimen dissections are unusual. On the other hand, CNS specimens are usually small, and care must be taken to preserve the tissue. Do not use all of the tissue by freezing the entire specimen. This is especially true for specimens of the spinal cord. These can be minute, yet major therapeutic decisions often depend on the results of the pathology studies. In all cases, it is essential to keep the clinical and radiologic findings in mind when processing specimens from the CNS.

Ultrasonic aspirations are widely used for tumor resections. As a consequence, much of the specimen may be lost unless it is recovered from the instrument's bag receptacle. The fragments may be difficult to interpret histologically but can be invaluable. They are entirely suitable for molecular or cytogenetic studies.

Cytologic Preparations

Cytologic preparations are essential in the frozen section and permanent section evaluation of all surgically excised brain lesions. These should be prepared in every case for which a frozen section is requested. As illustrated, the preferred procedure is as follows: A minute portion of the fresh specimen is placed on a glass slide and, with considerable pressure, smeared between an opposing slide. The slides are separated and immersed *immediately* in 95% alcohol. Following fixation for 45 to 60 seconds, the preparation is stained and coverslipped. I prefer routine staining with hematoxylin and eosin.

Needle Biopsy Specimens

Needle biopsy specimens need to be interpreted and handled with special care. The evaluation should begin with cognizance of the clinical and radiographic findings. The chance of making an error is vastly increased when these specimens are studied in a vacuum devoid of clinical or radiographic information.

Begin your examination with the cytologic preparation as described above. One of the remaining fragments of tissue can then be used for a frozen section if desired. If an abnormality is established by the smear, a frozen section may not be necessary. Unless you are assured of additional tissue, it is generally wise to freeze only one or two cores at the time of initial examination, holding others in reserve. Throughout the process, review these slides in reference to the radiographic images to ensure that abnormal tissue is obtained and that the findings are consistent with the images. Close contact with the surgeon is extremely important. As is true for biopsies from other body sites, small specimens can be colored with eosin to facilitate identification at the time of embedding and sectioning.

Frozen Sections/Permanent Sections

Freezing must be accomplished as rapidly as possible to minimize the formation of ice crystals.

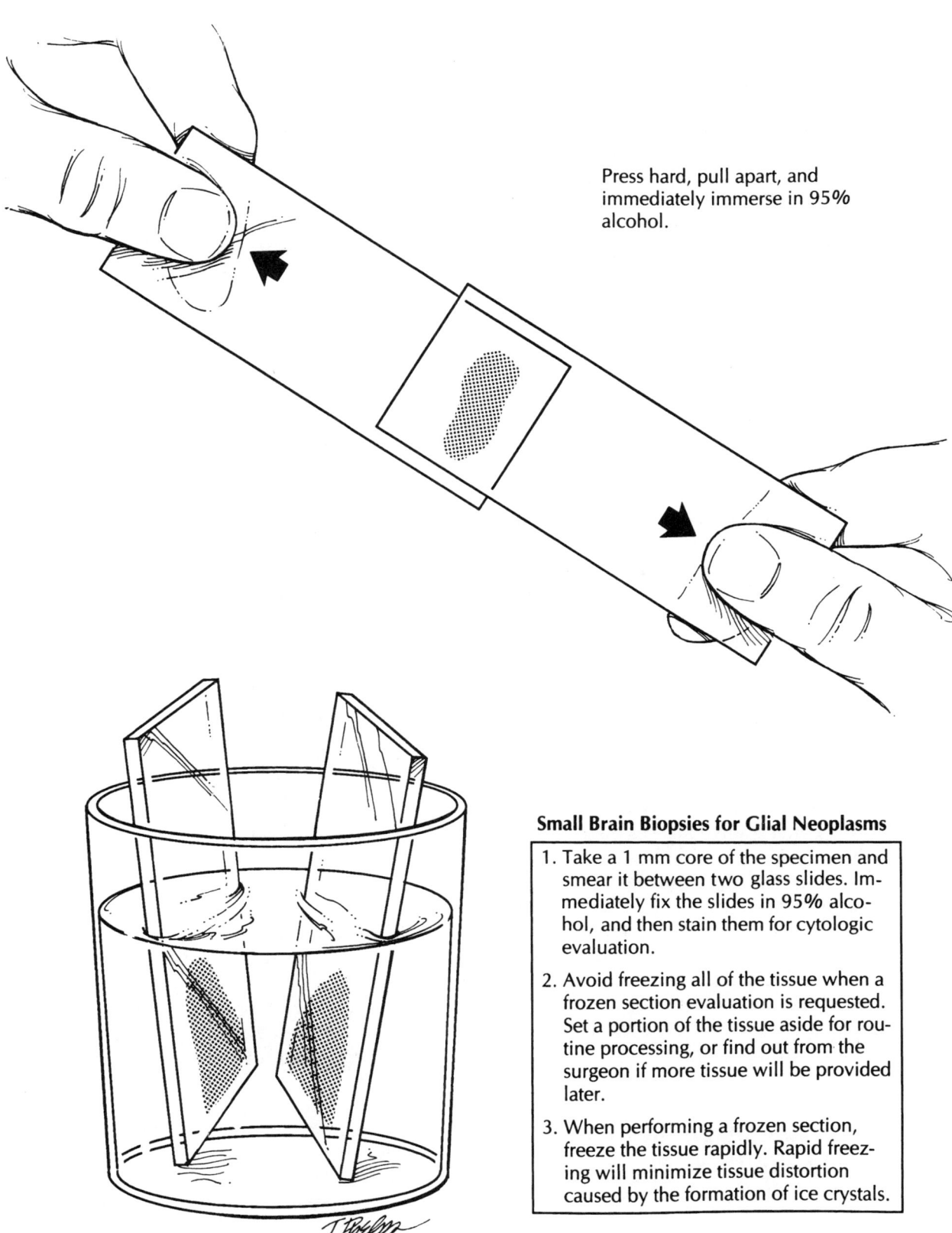

Press hard, pull apart, and immediately immerse in 95% alcohol.

Small Brain Biopsies for Glial Neoplasms

1. Take a 1 mm core of the specimen and smear it between two glass slides. Immediately fix the slides in 95% alcohol, and then stain them for cytologic evaluation.

2. Avoid freezing all of the tissue when a frozen section evaluation is requested. Set a portion of the tissue aside for routine processing, or find out from the surgeon if more tissue will be provided later.

3. When performing a frozen section, freeze the tissue rapidly. Rapid freezing will minimize tissue distortion caused by the formation of ice crystals.

Ice crystals are generally avoidable in certain neoplasms, such as meningiomas, but frequently not in infiltrating gliomas from edema-rich white matter. The recommended procedure is to establish a base of semifrozen mounting medium on a cold chuck. The medium should not be completely frozen, because solidly frozen medium will slowly freeze the tissue and encourage the formation of ice crystals by gradually drawing heat from the small specimen. Therefore, place the specimen on the partially frozen base, and immediately immerse it in liquid nitrogen. After freezing, the specimen can then be covered with additional mounting medium and refrozen. Cut and stain sections by standard methods.

In the case of gliomas, especially the well-differentiated variety (e.g., astrocytoma and oligodendroglioma), it is extremely important that blocks be available from tissue that is *not* subject to prior frozen section. Prior freezing produces nuclear angulation and hyperchromatism, which can make it difficult to distinguish between gliomas and to distinguish reactive or normal brain from an infiltrating glioma. Unless you are assured of more tissue by the surgeon, use only a portion of the specimen for a frozen section.

Electron Microscopy

To a large extent, immunohistochemistry has replaced electron microscopy as a diagnostic tool; however, in certain instances the latter technique is invaluable. Accordingly, it is appropriate to hold some tissue in reserve in glutaraldehyde (embedding later if necessary) for neoplasms for which classification may be difficult after review of the frozen section. Tissue may also be embedded from encephalitic lesions if viruses are suspected, because no immunohistochemical agents are commercially available for many classes of potential viral pathogens.

Processing of Tissues From Specific Entities

Meningiomas are frequently submitted with a dural attachment and arrive as either a complete en bloc excision or, more often, as a series of small fragments. Prognostically significant information relates to histologic features of the lesion as well as the interface of the tumor with surrounding tissues, that is, the brain and the skull. The surface of the mass adjacent to the brain should be sectioned, if identified, particularly if portions of the brain adhere to the surface. At least one section through the base of the tumor on the dura should also be taken. Decalcified sections of bone are appropriate to evaluate skull invasion.

Gliomas are an exceedingly heterogeneous group in terms of their macroscopic and microscopic characteristics. Generally, margins are not an issue and do not, unless specifically stated by the surgeon, affect the treatment of the patient. Fragments of ependymomas, oligodendrogliomas, and astrocytomas, in which little normal brain is recognized, do not need to be sampled in regard to the extent of the disease, although it is prudent to attempt such a localization. In larger en bloc specimens of gliomas, however, a series of marked and recorded sections passing from the tumor into the macroscopically normal brain is appropriate. In the case of malignant gliomas with central necrosis, the most diagnostic tissue is usually found in the cellular rim immediately surrounding the necrotic area. Sections from this area are therefore appropriate. In the case of well-differentiated gliomas (e.g., astrocytoma and oligodendroglioma), the tissue may not appear markedly abnormal, and multiple sections are necessary, particularly from areas in which the white matter is discolored.

Malignant gliomas after radiotherapy may have extensive therapy-related changes, such as coagulation necrosis. In this setting, multiple tissue sections should be submitted so as not to miss potential foci of active recurrent tumor.

Oligodendrogliomas are increasingly diagnosed by molecular techniques. The molecular laboratory can be consulted in regard to specific tissue preparation (e.g., fresh frozen, etc...).

Lymphomas are generally recognized during the frozen section process and, in the sporadic form in the nonimmunocompromised patient, they are often suspected on the basis of the neuroimaging features. In this setting, tissue can be reserved frozen for special marker studies (see Chapter 41), although most of the relevant markers for the simple purpose of establishing a clinical diagnosis can be performed on paraffin-embedded sections. A clinical history of prebiopsy steroid treatment is significant, as CNS lymphomas in this setting may be little more than a mass of macrophages and few if any residual neoplastic cells.

Pituitary adenomas are often approached via the transsphenoidal route, and the specimens are often small. Care must be taken not to freeze all of the specimens, as the resultant artifact complicates interpretation of permanent sections. Close communication with the surgeon is essential.

Creutzfeldt-Jakob disease is a rare disorder that is occasionally diagnosed in a cortical biopsy specimen. Although there appears to be only a very small likelihood that pathology personnel will contract Creutzfeldt-Jakob disease from these specimens, caution is appropriate considering the devastating consequences of this disease. Details of this issue are discussed by Brown.[20] Basically, the tissues are fixed in a standard formalin solution for at least 48 hours. The tissues are then placed in a cassette and decontaminated by immersion with periodic agitation in a 95% formic acid solution. The tissue will turn clear. After this, the tissue is placed in formalin again for 1 to 2 days. The tissues can then be treated as any other routine specimen, although some laboratories prefer to hand process them separately. Generally, frozen sections are not recommended on tissues from demented patients.

Specimens taken to control seizures are usually from the temporal lobe. Often they consist of "lateral" and "medial" temporal lobe specimens. The latter contains the hippocampus, which must be examined carefully for the presence or absence of "mesial" or "hippocampal" sclerosis (i.e., neuronal loss and gliosis).

Important Issues to Address in Your Surgical Pathology Report on Brain and Spinal Cord Biopsies

- What procedure was performed?
- What are the type and grade of the neoplasm? (For glial neoplasms, be sure to document the grading system employed.)
- What is the size of the neoplasm?

XIV The Hematopoietic and Lymphatic System

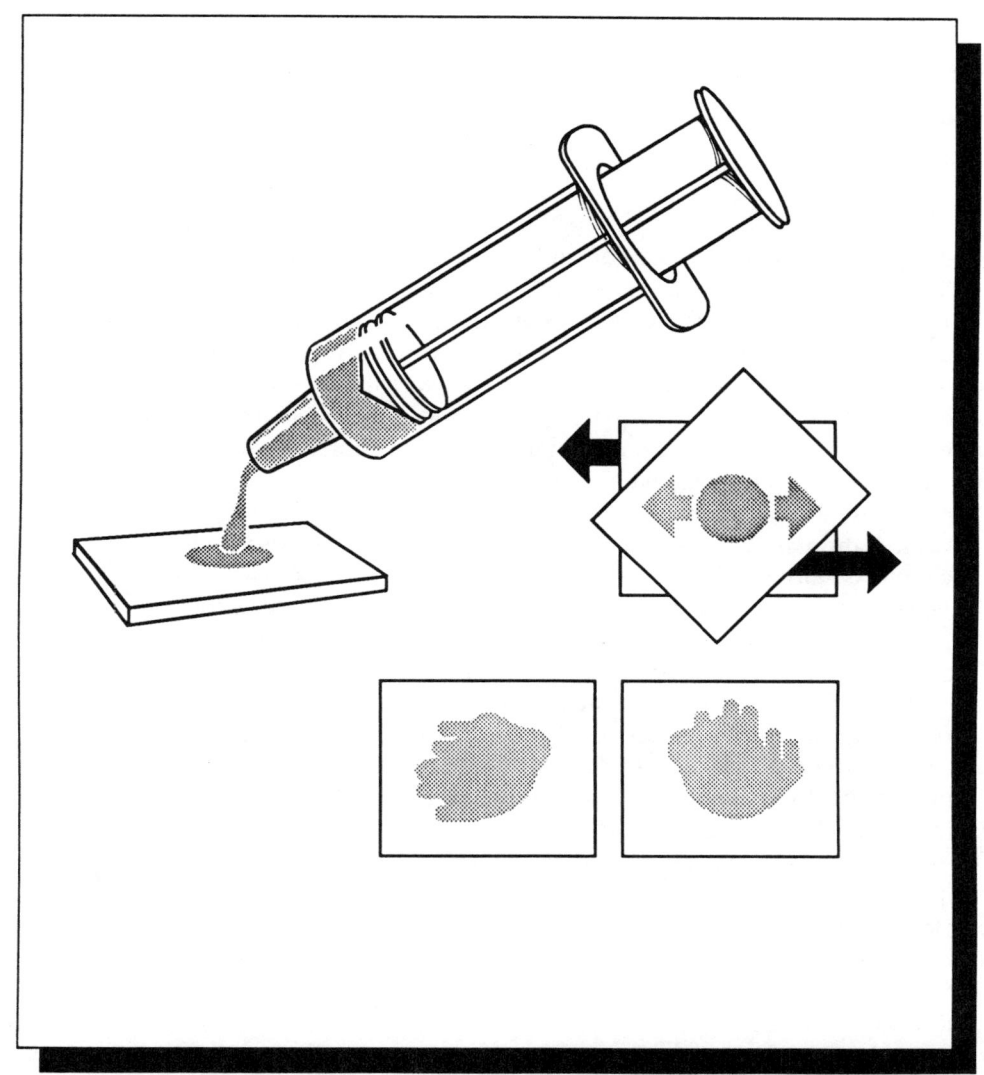

41 Lymph Nodes

High-quality sections for routine light microscopy are necessary, but not always sufficient, for the interpretation of lymph node biopsies. Immunophenotypic and genetic studies are often required for the diagnosis and classification of a hematopoietic neoplasm. Adequate fixation and timely and appropriate technical handling of lymph nodes are, therefore, even more important than with other specimens.

When lymph nodes are placed in an empty specimen container or in dry gauze, the edges of the specimen dry out, producing a prominent desiccation artifact at the edge of the node. Severe edge artifacts can be introduced into a lymph node even before the specimen reaches the surgical pathology laboratory. Surgeons should therefore be instructed to place resected lymph nodes immediately into a balanced physiologic solution such as Roswell Park Memorial Institute medium (RPMI) 640 or isotonic saline, and to transport lymph nodes immediately to the surgical pathology laboratory. Remember that lymph nodes can also dry out on the cutting table, so proceed quickly and efficiently after removing the specimen from the transport media.

Once the specimen is received, document its size, weight, and shape, and then slice it into uniformly thin 2- to 3-mm sections. Examine the cut surfaces of the node, and ask the following questions: Is the nodal architecture preserved? If the architecture is ablated, is the node grossly nodular, or is the process diffuse? Are any focal lesions present? Is the capsule intact? What is the appearance of the perinodal tissues?

Next, prepare touch imprints by placing the surface of a glass slide against the cut surface of the lymph node. At least five air-dried slides should be prepared, especially in cases of suspected Burkitt's lymphoma, lymphoblastic lymphoma, and myelogenous leukemia. These can be used later for Giemsa stains, oil red O stains, acid phosphatase stains, chloracetate esterase stains, and immunofluorescence for nuclear terminal transferase. Two additional imprints immediately fixed in 95% alcohol should be prepared for possible hematoxylin and eosin (H&E) staining.

Next, tissue should be submitted for light microscopy and, if sufficient tissue is available, for immunohistochemical and genetic studies. Sections for light microscopy should include not only the substance of the node, but also the capsule and perinodal soft tissues. Submit at least one section for fixation in neutral buffered formalin and at least one section in B-5 or an equivalent fixative. The B-5 fixative contains mercuric chloride as well as formaldehyde, and it provides crisp nuclear detail. If a section is submitted in a mercury-based fixative, remember to notify your tissue processing laboratory personnel because these sections require special processing.

When submitting fresh tissue for special studies, collect the sample from solid "fleshy" areas of the tumor. Avoid areas that appear necrotic or sclerotic as these areas may not contain a sufficient quantity of viable tumor cells. The best techniques for submitting fresh tissue for immunophenotyping will depend on your individual laboratory, but in general a representative section of the node should be snap-frozen in optimal controlled temperature embedding medium for frozen tissue specimens (OCT) for immunohistochemical studies, and a separate 0.5- to 0.7-cm cube should be submitted fresh for flow cytometry. Again, the rapid handling of tissue for these studies is crucial, because delays can

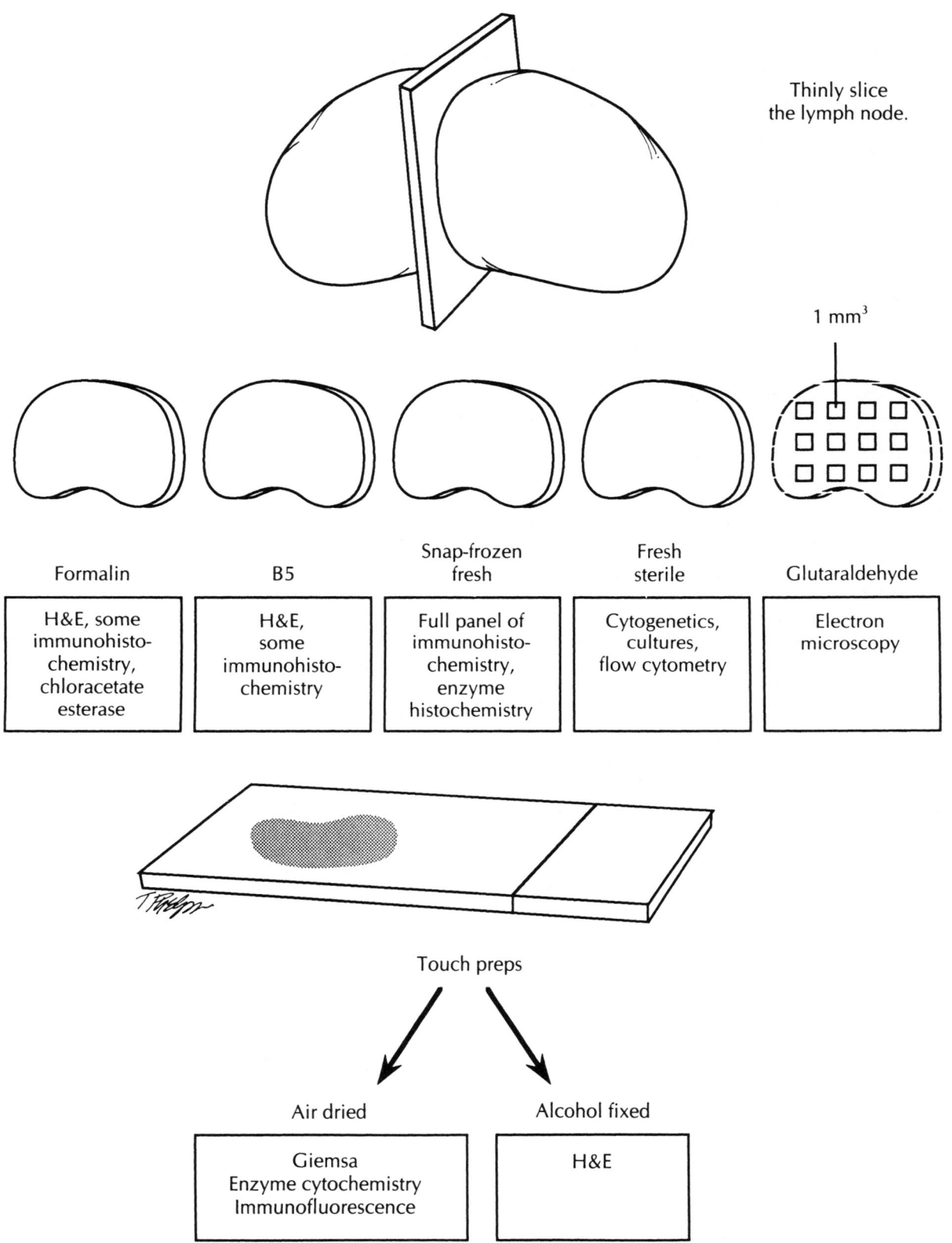

result in diffusion artifacts during immunostaining. If tissue will be sent off-site for these analyses, it should not be frozen, but instead it should be kept cool on ice and rapidly transported.

If adequate tissue is available, and it usually is, fresh tissue should also be sent for genetic studies such as gene rearrangements and karyotyping. Submitting this tissue is important because antigen receptor gene rearrangement analysis may be required in those rare cases for which morphology and immunohistochemistry alone cannot establish the diagnosis. Obtain instructions on how to submit these specimens properly from your genetics laboratory.

Finally, if an infection is suspected or granulomas are encountered on a preliminary frozen section evaluation, fresh sterile tissue should be submitted for microbiologic studies. If a solid tumor is in the differential diagnosis, then consider placing a small piece of tissue into glutaraldehyde for electron microscopy.

Clearly, the take-home message here is that "a stitch in time saves nine." Even the most challenging hematopoietic neoplasm can be diagnosed if well-fixed tissue for light microscopy and rapidly submitted fresh tissue for special studies are available. Table 41-1 summarizes the type of tissues to be submitted for specific staining methods and other analyses.

Important Issues to Address in Your Surgical Pathology Report on Lymph Nodes

- What procedure was performed, and what structures/organs are present?
- Anatomically, from where were the lymph nodes removed?
- What are the type and grade of the neoplasm?
- What are the number and size of the lymph nodes involved by tumor?
- What special studies were performed, and what were the results of these studies?

Extranodal Specimens

The lymphatic system is not limited to lymph nodes but encompasses diverse tissues and organs including the spleen, thymus, bone marrow, Waldeyer's ring, vermiform appendix, and mucosa-associated lymphoid tissue of the intestines and lung. Lymphomas can arise anywhere in this rather extensive lymphatic system. Moreover, they can arise in extranodal sites that are not part of the lymphatic system (e.g., thyroid, stomach). Although this chapter has focused on

TABLE 41-1. Tissues to submit.*

Tissue	Purpose
Air-dried touch imprints	Giemsa Enzyme cytochemistry—acid phosphatase, etc. Immunofluorescence for terminal transferase
Alcohol-fixed touch imprints	Hematoxylin and eosin
Formalin fixed, paraffin embedded	Hematoxylin and eosin Basic immunohistochemistry
B-5 fixed	Hematoxylin and eosin Basic immunohistochemistry
Snap-frozen fresh tissue	Detailed immunohistochemistry Enzyme histochemistry

Fresh sterile tissue	Cytogenetics
	   Gene rearrangements
	   Karyotyping
	Microbial cultures
	Flow cytometry

Glutaraldehyde	Electron microscopy

*Modified from Jaffee ES. *Surgical Pathology of the Lymph Nodes and Related Organs*. 2nd ed. Philadelphia, Pa: Saunders; 1995.

lymph nodes, it is important to recognize that a lymphoma can be encountered in almost any specimen.

If the nature of a tumor is unknown at the time of specimen processing, a touch prep or frozen section of the tumor is a fast, simple way to determine if you are dealing with lymphoid proliferation. This is important information to have as you begin the dissection because extranodal lymphoid proliferations, like their nodal counterparts, need to be submitted for special studies as appropriate. Once tissue has been obtained for special studies, the specimens can then be routinely processed in an organ-specific manner. There is no need to modify your approach in any significant way. Similar to dealing with some epithelial neoplasm, remember to document the dimensions of the tumor, determine the degree of involvement of adjacent structures, assess the status of the surgical margins, and evaluate the regional lymph nodes. The uninvolved tissues should also be sampled, and any additional pathologic processes (e.g., *Helicobacter pylori* infections in stomach resections, thyroiditis in thyroid resections) should be included in the final pathology report.

42 Spleen

Three elements are essential for the thorough dissection of the spleen: (1) Be familiar with the patient's clinical history. The dissection of a spleen removed for trauma is very different from the dissection of a spleen removed for a hematopoietic malignancy. (2) Remember that fresh tissue for immunophenotypic and genetic studies may be necessary to classify hematopoietic neoplasms involving the spleen. (3) Sections of the spleen for histology need to be very thinly sliced and well fixed.

Once resected, the spleen should immediately be brought fresh to the surgical pathology laboratory. The spleen should then be weighed and measured. Next, examine the appearance of the splenic capsule. This step is particularly important in cases of trauma. In particular, document whether the capsule is intact or lacerated, and if it is tense or wrinkled. Next, examine splenic hilum for lymph nodes. If any are found, they should be removed and a representative section of each submitted for histology.

Section the spleen in whichever plane you want, just make sure to section it thinly. Use a long sharp blade to cut the spleen into 2- to 3-mm slices. Examine both sides of each slice for any lesions. Carefully document both the white and red pulp. Expansion of the white pulp gives the cut surface the appearance of white nodules on a red background, while expansion of the red pulp gives the cut surface of the spleen a diffuse red appearance. This step is important because some diseases, such as non-Hodgkin's lymphoma, preferentially involve the white pulp, while others, such as Gaucher's disease, myeloproliferative disorders, and hairy cell leukemia, preferentially involve the red pulp. If nodules are present, count the number of discrete nodules. If the spleen was removed for trauma and if no nodules are found, submit two to four sections of the splenic parenchyma, including a section to demonstrate any parenchymal hemorrhage.

If nodules are present, or if the spleen was removed for a hematopoietic malignancy, then the rest of the approach to the spleen should now follow the approach taken for lymph nodes with suspected hematopoietic malignancies (see Chapter 41). First, prepare touch imprints. Take touch imprints from any discrete nodules. Before preparing these imprints, remove excess blood by blotting the surface of the spleen with a towel. Prepare at least five air-dried and two 95% alcohol-fixed slides.

Next, submit fresh tissue for immunophenotyping. Although the exact techniques vary among laboratories, in general, a representative section should be snap-frozen in optimal controlled temperature embedding medium for frozen tissue specimens (OCT) for immunohistochemical studies, and a separate 0.5- to 0.7-cm cube should be submitted fresh for flow cytometry. Fresh tissue should also be sent for genetic studies such as gene rearrangements and karyotyping; and if clinically indicated, fresh sterile tissue should be submitted for microbiologic studies. If multiple dramatically distinct nodules are present, each type should be separately submitted for these ancillary studies.

Next, tissue should be submitted for light microscopy. Submit thin sections so that they can fix well, and submit at least one section representing each type of lesion seen and one section that includes the splenic capsule. It is not necessary, and in fact not desired, for sections to fill the tissue cassette completely. If multiple small nodules are present, submit two to four representative sections. If both large and small nodules are seen, each must be represented in sampling. If the spleen is enlarged but no lesions are noted, three to four sections are sufficient. As was true for lymph nodes, at least one section should be fixed in B-5 or an equivalent fixative. (If you do submit a section in B-5, remember to notify your tissue processing laboratory because these sections require special processing.) If a storage disease is suspected, tissue should also be fixed in glutaraldehyde for possible electron microscopy.

Important Issues to Address in Your Surgical Pathology Report on Splenectomies

- What procedure was performed, and what structures/organs are present?
- What is the weight of the spleen?
- Is the white pulp architecture normal, more prominent than usual, or obscured (as by a diffuse red pulp infiltrate)?
- In the case of splenic trauma, is the capsule torn, and how much intraparenchymal hemorrhage is present?
- In the case of hematopoietic neoplasm, what type and grade of neoplasm is present, and how many discrete neoplastic nodules are present? Does the neoplasm involve the lymph nodes in the splenic hilum?

43 Thymus

The thymus, along with the lower pair of parathyroid glands, is derived from the third and fourth pharyngeal pouches. The right and left halves of the gland fuse to form a pyramid-shaped organ enclosed by a thin fibrous capsule. The thymus has a vital location adjacent to the important organs of the mediastinum. The gland usually sits in the anterosuperior portion of the mediastinum, with the base of the thymus sitting on the pericardium and the upper poles of each lobe extending superiorly into the neck.

Your dissection should start with what is perhaps the most important step in examining the thymus—a careful examination of the surface of the specimen. Is the organ well encapsulated, or is there evidence of a tumor with invasion into adjacent structures? Are pieces of lung, pericardium, or blood vessels present? Document the degree of encapsulation. Next, weigh the specimen, measure it in all three dimensions, and ink the surfaces of the gland. The gland can then be sectioned at 2- to 3-mm intervals. In infants, the cut surface of the thymus is pink, but by adulthood much of the parenchyma has been replaced by yellow fat. Describe the cut surface of the gland. Is it uniform and lobated, cystic or solid? Is there evidence of necrosis or fibrosis? Any grossly identifiable lesions should be measured, and sections should be submitted from each lesion to demonstrate the relationship of the tumor to adjacent structures, to the inked margins, and to any attached tissues. Because invasion into adjacent organs is a critical feature used to identify malignant thymomas, sampling should be directed to areas suspicious for capsular invasion. Moreover, because thymomas can be histologically heterogeneous, it has been suggested by Moran and Suster[21] that a minimum of five sections should be submitted from all thymomas. If no grossly identifiable lesions are noted, submit four representative sections for histology. Save the specimen because you may have to go back to it, depending on the patient's clinical history.

Important Issues to Address in Your Surgical Pathology Report on Thymectomies

- What procedure was performed, and what structures/organs are present?
- What are the size and weight of the thymus?
- Is the thymus partially or totally encapsulated?
- What are the type and grade of any neoplasms identified?
- If a tumor is present, does it extend to a margin or into adjacent structures?

44 Bone Marrow

The evaluation of the bone marrow typically includes both a trephine core biopsy and fluid aspiration. The details of the preparation of these specimens are beyond the scope of this manual; however, you should be familiar with some basics.

Trephine core biopsies are usually 1.0 to 3.0 cm in length and 0.1 to 0.2 cm in diameter. Because of their small size, they generally do not have to be sectioned for further processing. After documenting the size of the biopsy, while it is still fresh prepare imprints from the biopsy by gently touching the bony fragments to glass slides. These smears should be air dried for later Wright's staining or other special studies such as cytochemical and immunohistochemical analyses. Next, submit the entire core biopsy for processing. The choice of fixatives will depend on your individual institution, but most laboratories like to fix bone marrow biopsies in either Zenker's fixative (for at least 4 hours), buffered formalin (for at least 18 to 24 hours), B-5 (for 4 hours), Bouin's (for 4 to 12 hours), or a mixture of buffered formalin and ethylenediaminetetraacetic acid (EDTA). Once fixed, the specimen can be embedded in either paraffin or plastic. Although paraffin embedding is certainly easier, plastic embedding has the advantage of minimizing artifacts produced by inadequate decalcification.

Usually, approximately 1 cc of liquid is obtained from a bone marrow aspirate. Nine to ten smears should be made *immediately*, before the fluid clots. These smears can be prepared much the same way as peripheral blood smears are made. To make smears on a coverslip, place a drop on the edge of one coverslip, cover it with another coverslip placed at a 45-degree angle, and as the drop spreads pull the two coverslips apart rapidly and smoothly. Alternatively, one drop of the aspirate can be placed at one end of a glass slide and then gently smeared using a pusher coverslip, as illustrated. These smears should be air dried. The remaining aspirate should be placed in an anticoagulant such as EDTA and taken to the hematology laboratory for further processing, which might include iron staining, the preparation of additional smears, and possible electron microscopy. Generally, additional aspirates should be obtained for ancillary studies such as cytogenetics and flow cytometry.

Finally, excess aspirate fluid that has been allowed to clot can be submitted to the laboratory for histologic processing after it has been fixed in formalin.

Important Issues to Address in Your Surgical Pathology Report on the Bone Marrow

- Describe the cellularity, the relative numbers of myeloid and erythroid elements, and their degree of maturation. The marrow biopsy can be used to assess quantitative aspects of maturation, but subtle qualitative aspects are best appreciated on the aspirate.
- Describe the number of megakaryocytes, their arrangement, and any cytologic abnormalities.
- Note the degree and pattern of marrow fibrosis.
- Are there any increases in lymphocytes or plasma cells (include the pattern of infiltration and their cytology)?
- Is an extrinsic tumor present?
- Is the bone itself normal or abnormal?

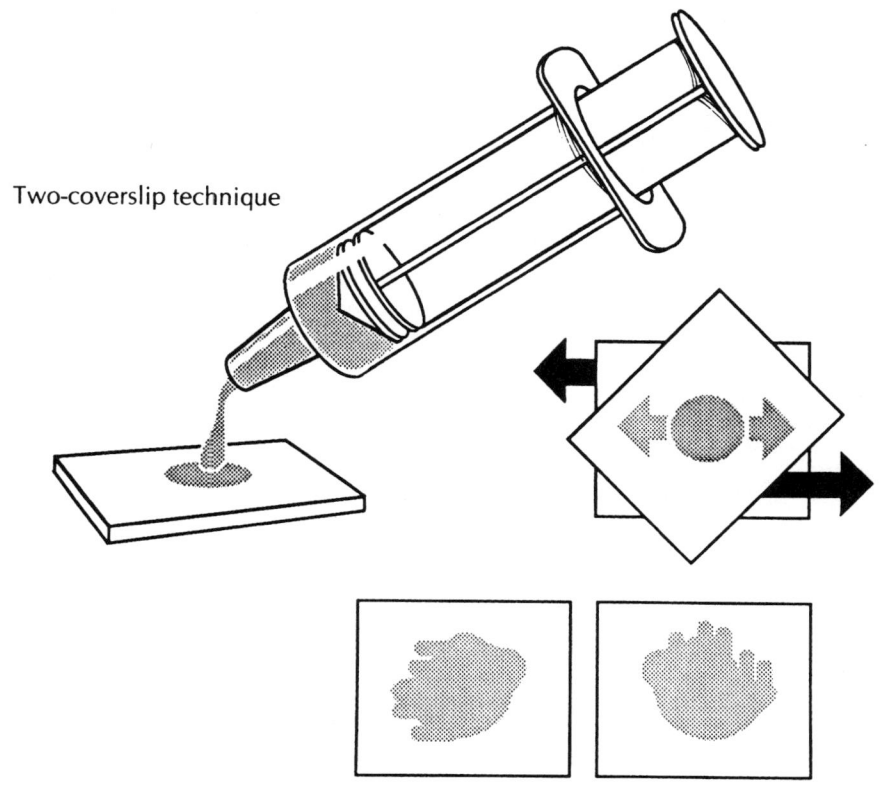

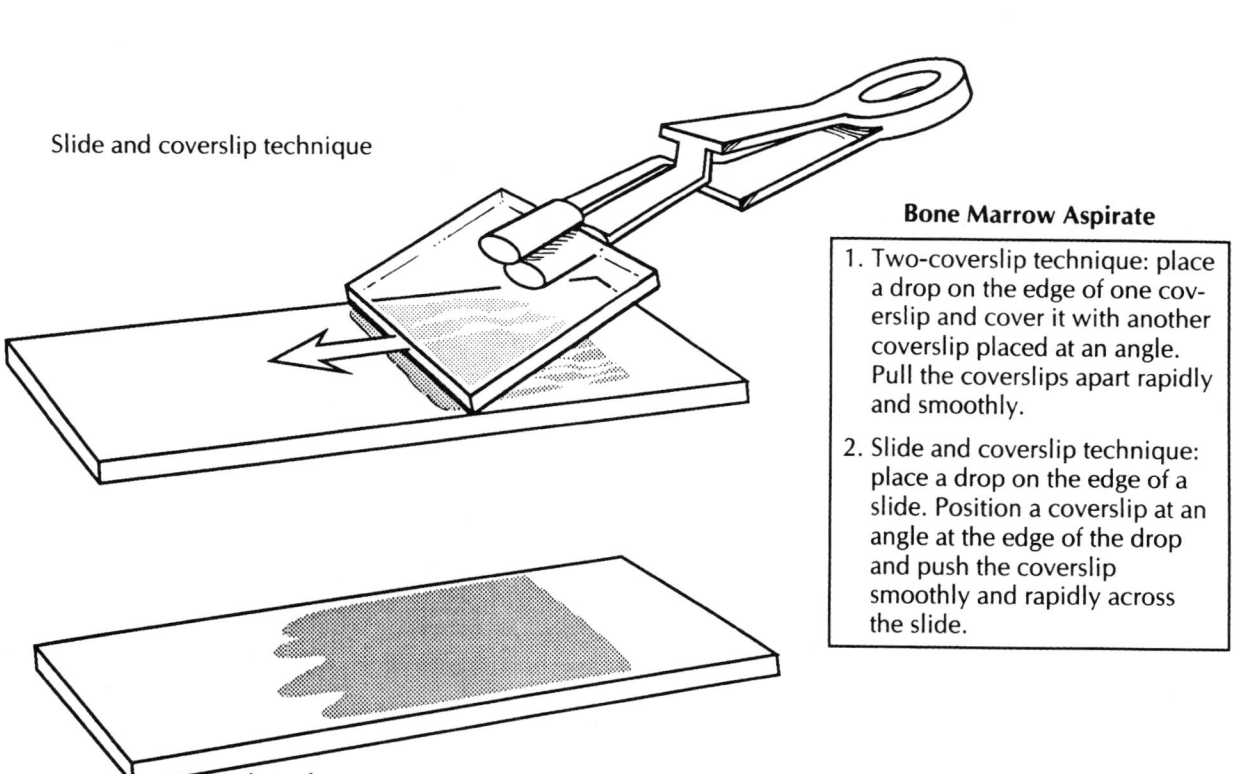

Bone Marrow Aspirate

1. Two-coverslip technique: place a drop on the edge of one coverslip and cover it with another coverslip placed at an angle. Pull the coverslips apart rapidly and smoothly.

2. Slide and coverslip technique: place a drop on the edge of a slide. Position a coverslip at an angle at the edge of the drop and push the coverslip smoothly and rapidly across the slide.

Each of these features should be commented on in the surgical pathology report, although a very brief description can suffice for features that are normal. Where possible, information from the biopsy, aspirate, and other ancillary studies should be combined to make a definitive diagnosis. In cases for which only a biopsy is available, sometimes only a descriptive diagnosis is given. This practice varies from institution to institution.

XV Odds and Ends

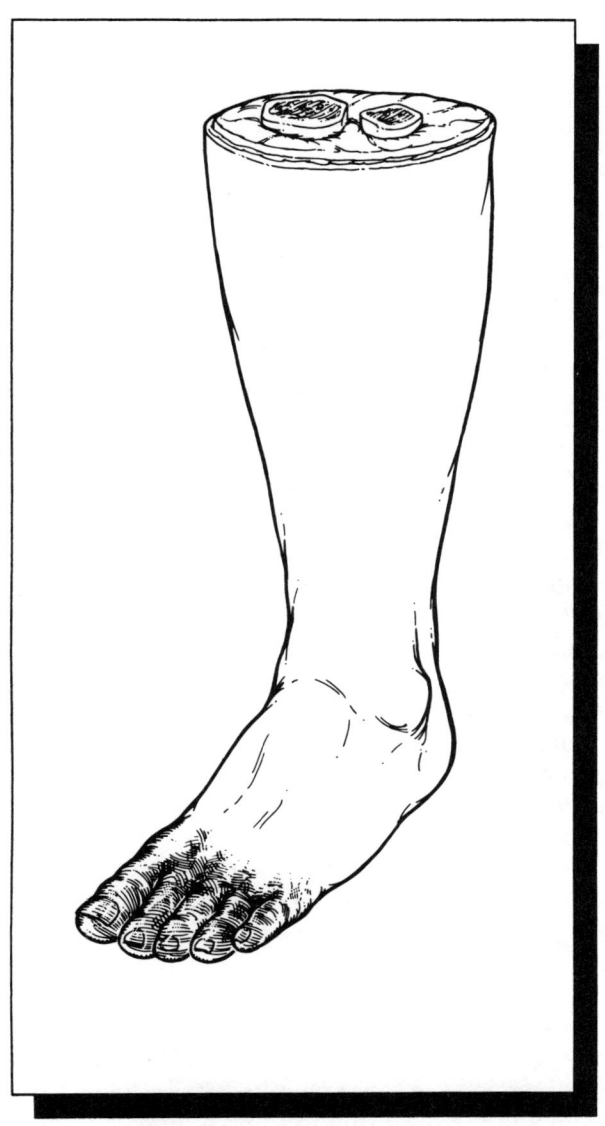

45 Common Uncomplicated Specimens

The dissection of tonsils, adenoids, hernia sacs, intervertebral discs, and amputations for gangrene are fairly straightforward, yet a brief discussion of the appropriate handling of these specimens is important for two reasons. First, because these specimens are so frequently encountered, even small mistakes in technique can be magnified over the course of handling numerous specimens. By getting it right the first time, you can avoid developing bad habits that are perpetuated with subsequent dissections. Second, mundane specimens are particularly susceptible to cursory and inattentive examinations. As is true for novel and complex specimens, the prosector should carefully examine the specimen and tailor a dissection that is attuned to the clinical context.

Tonsils and Adenoids

The term *tonsils* usually refers to the palatine tonsils. These are located laterally on each side of the oral cavity as it communicates with the oropharynx. The term *adenoids* refers to the pharyngeal tonsils. These are located along the roof of the nasal cavity as it communicates with the nasopharynx. Even when these two structures are received together in the same specimen container, they can easily be distinguished by their gross appearance. The palatine tonsils are oval-shaped nodules of tissue. They are longer vertically than they are horizontally. Their attached (i.e., lateral) surface is covered by a thick fibrous capsule with adherent soft tissues, while their free (i.e., medial) surface is covered by a tan, glistening mucosa and is somewhat cerebriform, which is due to a longitudinal cleft and stellate crypt openings. The adenoids, on the other hand, tend to be flat and are frequently fragmented when removed. Their free (mucosal) surfaces are disrupted by deep longitudinal clefts that extend into the underlying lymphoid tissue.

The palatine tonsils are usually removed from both sides of the oropharynx. Subtle changes in the size, shape, and consistency of the tonsils can be appreciated by comparing the two tonsils. For example, enlargement that is due to an infiltrative process may best be appreciated when the enlarged tonsil is compared to the normal tonsil from the opposite side. After the tonsils and adenoids are identified, they should be separately measured and described. Look for exophytic masses, ulcerations, bulky enlargement, and any other gross abnormalities. Bivalve the tonsils and adenoids along the long axis of each, and carefully inspect the cut surface for masses, abscess formation, or other lesions.

Tonsils and adenoids do not always need to be submitted for histologic evaluation. The decision to sample these specimens depends on the patient's clinical history and the gross findings. From our own experience, we have found that these specimens *should* be sampled for histologic evaluation if they meet any of the criteria listed below:

1. The age of the patient is greater than 10 or less than 3 years.
2. The tonsils or adenoids are grossly abnormal.
3. The tonsils or adenoids are greater than 3 cm.
4. There is a size disparity between the two tonsils.

5. Histologic evaluation is requested by the clinician or is indicated by the patient's clinical history.

If any one of the above criteria is met, the tonsils and adenoids should be appropriately sampled for histologic evaluation. One or two representative sections of the tonsils and adenoids are generally sufficient, but certain conditions may require special processing or more extensive sectioning. For example, diffusely enlarged tonsils or adenoids with architectural effacement may suggest involvement by a lymphoproliferative disorder, and these should be processed like a lymph node involved by a lymphoma (see Chapter 41). Sometimes the tonsils are removed in an attempt to find an "occult" primary neoplasm in a patient presenting with metastatic carcinoma to cervical lymph nodes. In this situation, the tonsils should be serially sectioned and submitted in their entirety for histologic evaluation. If the tonsils or adenoids do not meet any of the above criteria, they do not need to be sampled for histologic evaluation. After completing your gross description, place the specimen in formalin and store it for at least 2 weeks.

Hernia Sacs

Hernia sacs are pouches of peritoneum enclosing a hernia. Grossly and microscopically, these are unimpressive specimens. They consist of variable amounts of fat, fibroconnective tissue, and a mesothelium-lined peritoneum. Nonetheless, even hernia sacs attest to the dictum that unexpected but important pathologic findings can be discovered in the most mundane of specimens. Indeed, a wide range of pathologic findings have been documented in routinely resected hernia sacs, ranging from endometriosis to malignant mesothelioma.

Measure and describe the sac, taking note of any areas that appear hemorrhagic or discolored. Palpate the specimen, and document the contents of the hernia sac and whether any nodules are present. Small specimens do not require additional sectioning. Larger tissue fragments should be serially sectioned. Document the gross appearance of the cut sections. Standards for submitting grossly normal hernia sacs for histologic examination vary from institution to institution. In the current era of cost containment, some centers have eliminated the routine histologic examination of grossly normal pediatric hernia sacs. Nonetheless, all grossly abnormal hernia sacs, all hernia sacs excised from adults, and all hernia sacs from patients whose clinical history indicates a possible histology-based diagnosis should be submitted for histologic evaluation. Most hernia sacs can be entirely submitted in a single tissue cassette for histologic evaluation. For larger specimens, a single cassette with sections representing all components of the specimen is generally sufficient. More extensive sampling may be necessary when focal lesions are identified or when indicated by the patient's clinical history.

Intervertebral Disk Material

Intervertebral disks typically consist of multiple irregular fragments of fibrous tissue, cartilage, and bone in variable proportions. These fragments are small and generally do not require sectioning. Nonetheless, the prosector's role in handling these is not inconsequential. The appropriate sampling and processing of these specimens largely depends on the prosector's skill at recognizing the various components that are present.

Begin by measuring the specimen. This can be done most efficiently by measuring the aggregate dimensions of the specimen (not the dimensions of each individual piece). Describe the type and appearance of the tissue received. Separate the bone from the soft tissue fragments, and decalcify the pieces of bone so that they can be sectioned by the histology laboratory (see Chapter 2). Keep in mind that these small bone fragments do not require nearly as much time to decalcify as sections from large bone resections. As is true for tonsils, adenoids, and hernia sacs, some centers have eliminated histologic examination of disk tissue specimens after routine cervical and lumbar decompression. Nonetheless, routine disk tissue is submitted for histologic examination at most centers, and the tissues must be submitted when clinically indicated. After the bone has been separated, submit the soft tissues for histologic evaluation. Again, if all of the tissue does not easily fit into a single tissue cassette, submit fragments that are representative of the specimen as a whole. Sometimes the patient's clinical history may indicate more extensive sampling, as when metastatic carcinoma is suspected clinically.

Amputations for Gangrene

Admittedly, most amputation specimens are neither small nor anatomically simple. On the other hand, the dissection of amputations for gangrene is straightforward and need not entail an inordinate amount of time and effort. The dissection of these specimens, whether a resection of a digit or an entire limb, should focus on two key questions: What are the nature and extent of the lesion (e.g., ulceration and gangrene)? What is the underlying pathologic process (e.g., vascular occlusion)? As for all specimens, the patient's clinical history should be clarified before the dissection of an amputation specimen is begun. Clinical and radiographic findings may direct the dissection to the most relevant areas of the specimen.

First, measure the overall dimensions of the specimen. Make liberal use of anatomic landmarks (e.g., tibial tubercle, lateral tibial malleolus) when measuring the specimen and describing the location of any lesions. Next, examine the four components of the specimen—the skin, soft tissues, bone, and vasculature. Begin with the skin. Look for loss of hair, skin discoloration, and frank ulceration. Note the location of these findings. Next, evaluate the soft tissues. Section through any ulcers to determine the depth of the ulcer. Do the surrounding soft tissues appear necrotic? Also note whether the soft tissues at the surgical margin appear viable. The bone underlying areas of ulceration and necrosis is most likely to reveal pertinent pathology. Specifically, section through the deepest area of any ulcer, and determine if the underlying bone is grossly involved by the inflammatory process. Finally, evaluate the vasculature. For amputations of the lower limbs, occlusive vascular disease can usually be documented by performing a limited dissection of the anterior and posterior tibial arteries. These can be located by sectioning deeply into the anterior and posterior compartments of the calf. A deep transverse incision at midcalf can usually accomplish this. When a complete dissection of a particular vascular tree is indicated, an anatomy text outlining the distribution of the blood supply should be consulted.

Sections should be taken to demonstrate ischemic changes in the skin, necrosis of the soft tissue, inflammation in the underlying bone, occlusive disease of the vascular tree, and viability of the soft tissues at the surgical margin. When sampling the ulcer, include the adjacent epidermis and the underlying subcutaneous tissues. If the zone of ulceration and necrosis appears to extend to the bone, submit a section of the bone immediately underlying the ulcer. Submit cross sections of the major arteries, selectively sampling those regions where the lumen is most stenotic. Finally, submit a transverse section of the neurovascular bundle at the resection margin, along with some skin and soft tissue from this region.

Closing Comments

But if we are to be in the front lines, then we must make sure that we are better protected in all respects. I am living proof that it can happen to any of us. And no other health care worker should have to go through what I have endured.

Dr. Hacib Aoun
(from "When a House Officer Gets AIDS")[22]

It is our hope that this "hands-on" guide has provided the reader with a logical and concise approach to surgical pathology dissection. Although details of dissection vary from specimen to specimen, we have tried to emphasize some general principles: (1) understand the patient's clinical history before beginning the dissection; (2) approach each dissection in a systematic and orderly fashion; (3) document important findings with complete gross descriptions and specimen photography; (4) be thorough but selective in sampling tissues for histology; (5) remember ancillary studies, such as flow cytometry, cytogenetics, hormone receptor analyses and molecular studies, which may require specially processed tissue; and (6) communicate relevant findings in a complete yet concise manner.

While the routine application of these principles is certainly useful, a purely mechanical approach to surgical pathology is no substitute for compassion and caution. Remember that every specimen comes from a living patient who is anxiously awaiting your diagnosis. Try to imagine that the specimen you are handling came from a close relative. A timely and accurate diagnosis can have a significant positive impact on the patient's mental and physical well-being.

Likewise, a purely mechanical approach to specimen dissection can foster carelessness. Great physicians have lost their lives because they have contracted an infectious disease from a needle stick or knife cut.[22] Once the stick or cut has occurred, you cannot go back and reverse events. *Prevention is the key to your safety*. Wear protective clothing, a mask, and eye covers; do not rush; and pay attention to what you are doing! These simple steps may save your life.

References

1. Florell SR, Coffin CM, Holden JA, et al. Preservation of RNA for functional genomic studies: a multidisciplinary tumor bank protocol. *Mod Pathol.* 2001;14:116–128.
2. Robbins KT, Medina JE, Wolfe GT, Levine PA, Sessions RB, Pruet CW. Standardizing neck dissection terminology. *Arch Otolaryngol Head Neck Surg.* 1991;117:601–605.
3. Hutchins GM. Special studies on the heart and lungs. In: Hutchins GM, ed. *Autopsy: Performance & Reporting.* Northfield: College of American Pathologists, 1990;108–114.
4. Billingham ME, Cary NIR, Hammond ME, et al. A working formulation for the standardization of nomenclature in the diagnosis of heart and lung rejection: Heart Rejection Study Group; The International Society for Heart Transplantation. *J Heart Transplant.* 1990; 9:587–593.
5. Morse D, Steiner RM. Cardiac valve identification atlas and guide. In: Morse D, Steiner RM, Fernandez J, eds. *Guide to Prosthetic Cardiac Valves.* New York: Springer-Verlag, 1985;257.
6. Solez K, Axelsen IRA, Benediktsson H, et al. International standardization of criteria for the histologic diagnosis of renal allograft rejection: the Banff working classification of kidney transplant pathology. *Kidney Int.* 1993; 44:411–422.
7. Racusen LC, Solez K, Colvin RB, et al. The Banff 97 working classification of renal allograft pathology. *Kidney Int.* 1999;55:713–723.
8. Yousem SA, Berry GJ, Cagle PT, et al. Revision of the 1990 working formulation for the classification of pulmonary allograft rejection: Lung Rejection Study Group. *J Heart Lung Transplant.* 1996;15:1–15.
9. Banff schema for grading liver allograft rejection: an international consensus document. *Hepatology.* 1997;25:658–663.
10. Owings DV, Hann L, Schnitt SJ. How thoroughly should needle localization biopsies be sampled for microscopic examination? A retrospective mammographic/pathologic correlative study. *Am J Surg Pathol.* 1990;14: 578–583.
11. Schnitt SJ, Connolly JL. Processing and evaluation of breast excision specimens: a clinically oriented approach. *Am J Clin Pathol.* 1992; 98: 125–137.
12. Schnitt SJ, Wang HH. Histologic sampling of grossly benign breast biopsies: how much is enough? *Am J Surg Pathol.* 1989;13:505–512.
13. Association of Directors of Anatomic and Surgical Pathology: recommendations for the reporting of breast carcinoma. *Hum Pathol.* 1996;27:220–224.
14. Wigglesworth JS, Singer DB, eds. *Textbook of Fetal and Perinatal Pathology.* Boston: Blackwell Science, 1998.
15. Cubilla AL, Pirus A, Pfaanl R, Rodriguez I, Augero F, Young RH. Anatomic levels: important landmarks in penectomy specimens: a detailed anatomic and histologic study based on examination of 44 cases. *Am J Surg Pathol* 2001;25:1091–1094.
16. Ruijter ET, Miller GJ, Aalders TW, et al. Rapid microwave-stimulated fixation of entire prostatectomy specimens. Biomed-IIMPC Study Group. *J Pathol.* 1997;183:369–375.
17. Folberg R, Verdick R, Weingeist TA, Montague PR. The gross examination of eyes removed for choroidal and cilary body melanomas. *Ophthalmology.* 1986;93:1643–1647.
18. Yamashina M. Follicular neoplasms of the thyroid: total circumferential evaluation of the fibrous capsule. *Am J Surg Pathol.* 1992;16: 392–400.
19. Beckwith JB. Renal neoplasms of childhood. In Stemberg, ed. *Diagnostic Surgical Pathology,*

2nd edition. New York: Raven Press, 1994; 1741–1766.
20. Brown P. Guidelines for high risk autopsy cases: special precautions for Creutzfeldt-Jakob disease. In: Hutchins GM, ed. *Autopsy Performance and Reporting.* Northfield, IL: College of American Pathologists, 1990;68–74.
21. Moran CA, Suster S. On the histologic heterogeneity of thymic epithelial neoplasms. Impact of sampling in subtyping and classification of thymomas. *Am J Clin Pathol.* 2000;114:760–766.
22. Aoun H. When a house officer gets AIDS. *N Engl J Med.* 1989;321:693–696.

Suggested Web Sites

Association of Directors of Anatomic and Surgical Pathology: www.panix.com/~adasp/
The University of Pittsburgh Transplant Web Site: http://tpis.upmc.edu/

Suggested Readings

General Approach to Surgical Pathology Specimens

Association of Directors of Anatomic and Surgical Pathology. Standardization of the surgical pathology report. *Am J Surg Pathol.* 1992;16:84–86.

Bell JE, Ironside JW. How to tackle a possible Creutzfeldt-Jakob disease necropsy. *J Clin Pathol.* 1993;46:193–197.

Cooke RA, Stewart B. *Colour Atlas of Anatomical Pathology.* New York, NY: Churchill Livingstone; 1987.

Fazzini E, Weber D, Waldo E. *A Manual for Surgical Pathologists.* Springfield, IL: Charles C Thomas; 1972.

Geller SA, Gerber MA. Guidelines for high risk autopsy. In: Hutchins GM, ed. *Autopsy Performance and Reporting.* Northfield, IL: College of American Pathologists; 1995:94–97.

Hammond ME, Compton CC. Protocols for the examination of tumors of diverse sites: introduction; Cancer Committee of the College of American Pathologists. *Arch Pathol Lab Med.* 2000;124:13–16.

International Union Against Cancer. Hermanek P, Henson DE, Hutter RVP, Sobin LH, eds. *TNM Supplement 1993: A Commentary on Uniform Use.* Berlin: Springer-Verlag; 1993.

International Union Against Cancer. Hermanek P, Sobin LH, eds. *TNM Classification of Malignant Tumours.* 4th ed. (2nd rev.) Berlin: Springer-Verlag; 1992.

International Union Against Cancer. Spiessl B, Beahrs OH, Hermanek P, et al. eds. *TNM Atlas: Illustrated Guide to the TNM/pTNM Classification of Malignant Tumours.* 3rd ed. (2nd rev.). Berlin: Springer-Verlag; 1992.

Lowe DG, Jeffrey IJM. *Surgical Pathology Techniques.* Philadelphia, PA: BC Decker; 1990.

Markel SF, Hirsch SD. Synoptic surgical pathology reporting. *Hum Pathol.* 1991;22:807–810.

Protection of Laboratory Workers From Infectious Disease Transmitted by Blood, Body Fluids, and Tissue. 2nd ed. NCCLS document M29-T2. Villanova, PA: National Committee on Clinical Laboratory Standards; 1991.

Richardson JM, Redford LK, Motton H, James R, Porterfield J. Protective garb. *N Engl J Med.* 1988;318:1333. Letter.

Rosai J, members of the Department of Pathology, Memorial Sloan-Kettering Cancer Center. Standardized reporting of surgical pathology diagnoses for the major tumor types: a proposal. *Am J Clin Pathol.* 1993;100:240–255.

Rosai J, Bonfiglio TA, Corson JM, et al. Standardization of the surgical pathology report. *Mod Pathol.* 1992;5:197–199.

Schmidt WA. *Principles and Techniques in Surgical Pathology.* Reading, Mass: Addison-Wesley; 1983.

Scully C, Samaranayake L, Martin M. HIV: answers to common questions on transmission, disinfection and antisepsis in clinical dentistry. *Br Dent J.* 1993;175:175–179.

A Summary of Major Provisions of the Final Rule Implementing the Occupational Safety and Health Administration Bloodborne Pathogens Regulation and Supplemental Information. Northfield, IL: College of American Pathologists; 1992.

Surgical Pathology/Cytopathology Quality Assurance Manual. Northfield, IL: College of American Pathologists; 1993.

Teloh HA. *Methods in Surgical Pathology.* Springfield, IL: Charles C Thomas; 1957.

Travers H, Davey D, Cleary K, Tazelaar H, Minielly J, eds. *Quality Improvement Manual in Anatomic Pathology.* Northfield, IL: College of American Pathologists; 1993.

Laboratory Techniques

Culling CFA. *Handbook of Histopathological and Histochemical Techniques.* 3rd ed. Boston, Mass: Butterworths; 1974.

Dawson PJ, Deckys MC. Rapid (same day) processing of biopsies using Carnoy's fixative. *Am J Surg Pathol.* 1987;11:82.

Greer CE, Peterson SL, Kiviat NB, Manos MM. PCR amplification from paraffin-embedded tissues. *Am J Clin Pathol.* 1991;95:117–124.

Hopwood D. Fixation and fixatives. In: Bancroft JD, Stevens A, eds. *Theory and Practice of Histological Techniques.* New York, NY: Churchill Livingstone; 1977:16–28.

Kelley DB, Abt AB. An improved method for mounting frozen-section specimens. *Am J Surg Pathol.* 1990;14:186–187.

Kok LP, Boon ME, Suurmeijer AJH. Major improvement in microscopic-image quality of cryostat sections. Combining freezing and microwave-stimulated fixation. *Am J Clin Pathol.* 1987;88:620–623.

Luna LG, ed. *Manual of Histologic Staining Methods of the Armed Forces Institute of Pathology.* 3rd ed. New York, NY: McGraw-Hill; 1968.

Naish SJ, Boenisch T, Farmilo AJ, Stead RH, eds. *Handbook. Immunochemical Staining Methods.* Carpinteria, Calif: DAKO Corp; 1989.

Page DL, Nolen C, Womack JL. Histologic technique. *Am J Surg Pathol.* 1989;13:1072. Letter.

Pearse AGE. *Histochemistry. Theoretical and Applied.* 2nd ed. Boston, Mass: Little, Brown; 1960.

Radivoyevitch MA. Stamping method for frozen section. *Am J Surg Pathol.* 1989;13:244–245.

Rogers C, Klatt EC, Chandrasoma P. Accuracy of frozen-section diagnosis in a teaching hospital. *Arch Pathol Lab Med.* 1987;111:514–517.

Sheehan DC, Hrapchak BB. Fixation. In: Sheehan DC, Hrapchak, BB, eds. *Theory and Practice of Histotechnology.* 2nd ed. St Louis, MO: CV Mosby Co; 1980;40–58.

Shi SR, Cote RJ, Taylor CR. Antigen retrieval immunohistochemistry and molecular morphology in the year 2001. *Appl Immunohistochem Mol Morphol.* 2001;9:107–116.

SooHoo W, Ruebner B, Vogt P, Wiese D. Orientation of small, flat frozen-section specimens. *Am J Surg Pathol.* 1988;12:573–574.

Start RD, Cross SS, Smith JHF. Assessment of specimen fixation in a surgical pathology service. *J Clin Pathol.* 1992;45:546–547.

Therkildsen MH, Pilgaard J. Microwave-assisted frozen section diagnosis: a comparison between conventional cryostat technique and the combination of freezing and microwave-stimulated fixation. *Acta Pathol Microbiol Immunol Scand.* 1990;98:200–202.

Werner M, Chott A, Fabiano A, Battifora H. Effect of formalin tissue fixation and processing on immunohistochemistry. *Am J Surg Pathol.* 2000;24:1016–1019.

Woosley JT. Improved histology from inadequately fixed paraffin-embedded biopsy specimens. *Am J Surg Pathol.* 1989;13:246–247.

Wright JR Jr. The development of the frozen section technique, the evolution of surgical biopsy, and the origins of surgical pathology. *Bull Hist Med.* 1985;59:295–326.

Tissue Collection for Molecular Genetic Studies

Coombs NJ, Gough AC, Primrose JN. Optimisation of DNA and RNA extraction from archival formalin-fixed tissue. *Nucleic Acids Res.* 1999;27(16):e12.

Dei Tos AP, Dal Cin P. The role of cytogenetics in the classification of soft tissue tumours. *Virchows Arch.* 1997;431:83–94.

Florell SR, Coffin CM, Holden JA, et al. Preservation of RNA for functional genomic studies: a multidisciplinary tumor bank protocol. *Mod Pathol.* 2001;14:116–128.

Gillespie JW, Best CJ, Bichsel VE, et al. Evaluation of non-formalin tissue fixation for molecular profiling studies. *Am J Pathol.* 2002;160:449–457.

Lymph Nodes for Metastatic Tumors

Association of Directors of Anatomic and Surgical Pathology. ADASP recommendations for processing and reporting lymph node specimens submitted for evaluation of metastatic disease. *Am J Surg Pathol.* 2001;25:961–963.

Baisden BL, Askin FB, Lange JR, Westra WH. HMB-45 immunohistochemical staining of sentinel lymph nodes: a specific method for enhancing detection of micrometastases in patients with melanoma. *Am J Surg Pathol.* 2000;24:1140–1146.

Fitzgibbons PL, LiVolsi VA. Recommendations for handling radioactive specimens obtained by sentinel lymphadenectomy; Surgical Pathology Committee of the College of American Pathologists, and the Association of Directors of Anatomic and Surgical Pathology. *Am J Surg Pathol.* 2000;24:1549–1551.

Weaver DL. Sentinel lymph node biopsy in breast cancer: creating controversy and defining new standards. *Adv Anat Pathol.* 2001;8:65–73.

Yared MA, Middleton LP, Smith TL, et al. Recommendations for sentinel lymph node processing in breast cancer. *Am J Surg Pathol.* 2002;26:377–382.

Photography

Burgess CA. Gross specimen photography—a survey of lighting and background techniques. *Med Biol Illustr.* 1975;25:159–166.

Cutignola L, Bullough PG. Photographic reproduction of anatomic specimens using ultraviolet illumination. *Am J Surg Pathol.* 1991;15:1096–1099.

Haberlin C. Specimen photography. In: Hansell P, ed. *A Guide to Medical Photography.* London: MTP Press; 1979:77–97.

Vetter JP. The color presentation and photography of gross specimens. *J Audiovis Med.* 1983;6:7–12.

Vetter JP. The color photography of gross specimens. *J Coll Am Pathologist.* 1984;3:155–161.

White W. *Photomacrography, an Introduction.* Boston, Mass: Butterworth; 1987:97–133.

William AR. Closeup photography and photomicrography. In: Morton R, ed. *Photography for the Scientist.* London: Academic Press; 1984:355–391.

Head and Neck General

Barnes L, Johnson JT. Pathologic and clinical considerations in the evaluation of major head and neck specimens resected for cancer. *Pathol Annu.* 1986;21: 173–250.

Batsakis JG. *Tumors of the Head and Neck: Clinical and Pathological Considerations.* 2nd ed. Baltimore, MD: Williams & Wilkins; 1979.

Gnepp DR, ed. *Contemporary Issues in Surgical Pathology: Pathology of the Head and Neck.* New York, NY: Churchill Livingstone; 1988.

Larynx

Association of Directors for Anatomic and Surgical Pathology. Recommendations for the reporting of larynx specimens containing laryngeal neoplasms. *Pathol Int.* 1997;47:809–811.

Association of Directors for Anatomic and Surgical Pathology. Recommendations for the reporting of specimens containing oral cavity and oropharynx neoplasms. *Virchows Arch.* 2000;437:345–347.

Association of Directors for Anatomic and Surgical Pathology. Recommendations for the reporting of specimens containing oral cavity and oropharynx neoplasms. *Am J Clin Pathol.* 2000;114:336–338.

Harwood AR. Cancer of the larynx. *J Otolaryngol.* 1982; 11:2–21.

Hollinger LD, Miller AW. A specimen mount for small laryngeal biopsies. *Laryngoscope.* 1982;92:524–526.

Kashima HK. The characteristics of laryngeal cancer correlating with cervical lymph node metastasis (analysis based on 40 total organ sections). *Can J Otolaryngol.* 1975;4:893–902.

Kirchner JA, Carter D. The larynx. In: Sternberg SS, ed. *Diagnostic Surgical Pathology.* New York, NY: Raven Press; 1994:893–916.

Levendag PC, Veeze-Kuijpers B, Knegt PPM, et al. Cancer of the supraglottic larynx with neck node metastasis treated by radiation therapy only: the revised 1987 URIC classification system as prognostic indicator. *Acta Oncol.* 1990;29:603–609.

McGavran MH, Bauer WC, Ogura JH. The incidence of cervical lymph node metastases from epidermoid carcinoma of the larynx and their relationship to certain characteristics of the primary tumor. *Cancer.* 1961;14:55–66.

Min KW, Houck JR Jr. Protocol for the examination of specimens removed from patients with carcinomas of the upper aerodigestive tract: carcinomas of the oral cavity including lip and tongue, nasal and paranasal sinuses, pharynx, larynx, salivary glands, hypopharynx, oropharynx, and nasopharynx; Cancer Committee, College of American Pathologists. *Arch Pathol Lab Med.* 1998;122:222–230.

Olofsson J. Growth and spread of laryngeal carcinoma. *Can J Otolaryngol.* 3:1974;446–459.

Vermund H. Role of radiotherapy in cancer of the larynx as related to the TNM system of staging: a review. *Cancer.* 1970;25:485–504.

Zarbo RJ, Barnes L, Crissman JD, Gnepp DR, Mills SE. Recommendations for the reporting of specimens containing oral cavity and oropharynx neoplasms; Association of Directors of Anatomic and Surgical Pathology. *Hum Pathol.* 2000;31:1191–1193.

Salivary Glands

Ellis GL, Auclair PL, Gnepp DR, eds. *Surgical Pathology of the Salivary Glands.* Philadelphia, PA: Saunders; 1991.

Min KW, Houck JR Jr. Protocol for the examination of specimens removed from patients with carcinomas of the upper aerodigestive tract: carcinomas of the oral cavity including lip and tongue, nasal and paranasal sinuses, pharynx, larynx, salivary glands, hypopharynx, oropharynx, and nasopharynx; Cancer Committee, College of American Pathologists. *Arch Pathol Lab Med.* 1998;122:222–230.

Radical Neck Dissection

Merlano M, Vittale V, Rosso R, et al. Treatment of advanced squamous-cell carcinoma of the head and neck with alternating chemotherapy and radiotherapy. *N Engl J Med.* 1992;327:1115–1121.

Robbins KT, Medina JE, Wolfe GT, Levine PA, Sessions RB, Pruet CW. Standardizing neck dissection terminology. *Arch Otolaryngol Head Neck Surg.* 1991;117: 601–605.

Vikram B, Strong EW, Shah J, Spiro RH. Elective postoperative radiation therapy in stages III and IV epidermoid carcinoma of the head and neck. *Am J Surg.* 1980;140:580–584.

Digestive System—General

Appelman HD, ed. *Contemporary Issues in Surgical Pathology: Pathology of the Esophagus, Stomach, and Duodenum*. New York, NY: Churchill Livingstone; 1984.

Haggitt RC. Handling of gastrointestinal biopsies in the surgical pathology laboratory. *Lab Med*. 1982;13: 272–278.

Maxilla

Min KW, Houck JR Jr. Protocol for the examination of specimens removed from patients with carcinomas of the upper aerodigestive tract: carcinomas of the oral cavity including lip and tongue, nasal and paranasal sinuses, pharynx, larynx, salivary glands, hypopharynx, oropharynx, and nasopharynx; Cancer Committee, College of American Pathologists. *Arch Pathol Lab Med*. 1998;122:222–230.

Zarbo RJ, Barnes L, Crissman JD, Gnepp DR, Mills SE. Recommendations for the reporting of specimens containing oral cavity and oropharynx neoplasms; Association of Directors of Anatomic and Surgical Pathology. *Hum Pathol*. 2000;31:1191–1193.

Esophagus

Association of Directors for Anatomic and Surgical Pathology. Recommendations for the reporting of resected esophageal carcinomas. *Am J Clin Pathol*. 2000;114:512–514.

Lee RG, Compton CC. Protocol for the examination of specimens removed from patients with esophageal carcinoma: a basis for checklists; The Cancer Committee, College of American Pathologists, and the Task Force on the Examination of Specimens from Patients with Esophageal Cancer. *Arch Pathol Lab Med*. 1997;121:925–929.

Ming S-C. *Tumors of the Esophagus and Stomach*. Washington, DC: Armed Forces Institute of Pathology; 1973.

Stomach

Compton C, Sobin LH. Protocol for examination of specimens removed from patients with gastric carcinoma: a basis for checklists; Members of the Cancer Committee, College of American Pathologists, and the Task Force for Protocols on the Examination of Specimens from Patients with Gastric Cancer. *Arch Pathol Lab Med*. 1998;122:9–14.

Japanese Research Society for Gastric Cancer. The general rules for the gastric study in surgery and pathology. Part I. Clinical classification. *Jpn J Surg*. 1981;11:127–139.

Rotterdam H, Enterline HT, *Pathology of the Stomach and Duodenum*. New York, NY: Springer-Verlag, 1989.

Non-Neoplastic Intestinal Disease

Ming SC, Goldman H, eds. *Pathology of the Gastrointestinal Tract*. Philadelphia, PA: Saunders; 1992.

Norris HT, ed. *Pathology of the Colon, Small Intestine, and Anus*. New York, NY: Churchill Livingstone; 1983.

Neoplastic Intestinal Disease

Association of Directors for Anatomic and Surgical Pathology. Recommendations for the reporting of resected large intestine carcinomas. *Am J Clin Pathol*. 1996;106:12–15.

Compton CC, Henson DE, Hutter RVP, Sobin LH, Bowman HE. Updated protocol for the examination of specimens removed from patients with colorectal carcinoma: a basis for checklists. *Arch Pathol Lab Med*. 1997;121:1247–1254.

Henson DE, Hutter RVP, Sobin LH, Bowman HE. Protocol for the examination of specimens removed from patients with colorectal cancer. *Arch Pathol Lab Med*. 1994;118:122–125.

Hermanek P, Giedl J, Dworak O. Two programmes for examination of regional lymph nodes in colorectal carcinoma with regard to the new pN classification. *Pathol Res Pract*. 1989;185:867–873.

Qizilbash AH. Pathologic studies in colorectal cancer: a guide to the surgical pathology examination of colorectal specimens and review of features of prognostic significance. *Pathol Annu*. 1982;17:1–46.

Rickert RR, Compton CC. Protocol for examination of specimens from patients with carcinomas of the anus and anal canal: a basis for checklists; Cancer Committee of the College of American Pathologists. *Arch Pathol Lab Med*. 2000;124:21–25.

Zarbo RJ. Interinstitutional assessment of colorectal carcinoma surgical pathology report adequacy: a College of American Pathologists Q-probes study of practice patterns from 532 laboratories and 15,940 reports. *Arch Pathol Lab Med*. 1992;116:1113–1119.

Appendix

Gray GF Jr, Wackym PA. Surgical pathology of the vermiform appendix. *Pathol Annu*. 1986;21:111–144.

Liver

Arias IM, Popper H, Shachter D, Shafritz DA. *The Liver: Biology and Pathobiology*. New York: Raven Press; 1982.

Elias H, Sherrick JC. *Morphology of the Liver*. New York, NY: Academic Press; 1969.

Ruby SG. Protocol for the examination of specimens from patients with hepatocellular carcinoma and cholangiocarcinoma, including intrahepatic bile ducts; Cancer Committee of the College of American Pathologists. *Arch Pathol Lab Med*. 2000;124:41–45.

Sherlock S. *Diseases of the Liver and Biliary System*. Philadelphia, PA: Davis; 1968.

Gallbladder and Extrahepatic Biliary System

Albores-Saavedra J, Henson DE. *Atlas of Tumor Pathology: Tumors of the Gallbladder and Extrahepatic Bile Ducts*. Washington, DC: Armed Forces Institute of Pathology; 1986.

Henson DE, Albores-Saavedra J, Compton CC, Members of the Cancer Committee, College of American Pathologists. Protocol for the examination of specimens from patients with carcinomas of the gallbladder, including those showing focal endocrine differentiation: a basis for checklists. *Arch Pathol Lab Med*. 2000; 124:37–40.

Henson DE, Albores-Saavedra J, Compton CC, Members of the Cancer Committee, College of American Pathologists. Protocol for the examination of specimens from patients with carcinomas of the extrahepatic bile ducts, exclusive of sarcomas and carcinoid tumors: a basis for checklists. *Arch Pathol Lab Med*. 2000;124:26–29.

Sobin LH, Wittekind C, eds. *TNM Classification of Malignant Tumours: International Union Against Cancer*. 5th ed. New York, NY: Wiley; 1997.

Pancreas

Albores-Saavedra J, Heffess C, Hruban RH, Klimstra D, Longnecker D. Recommendations for the reporting of pancreatic specimens containing malignant tumors: The Association of Directors of Anatomic and Surgical Pathology. *Am J Clin Pathol*. 1999;111:304–307.

Compton CC, Henson DE. Protocol for the examination of specimens removed from patients with carcinoma of the exocrine pancreas: a basis for checklists; Cancer Committee, College of American Pathologists. *Arch Pathol Lab Med*. 1997;121:1129–1136.

Compton CC. Protocol for the examination of specimens from patients with carcinoma of the ampulla of Vater: a basis for checklists; Cancer Committee, College of American Pathologists. *Arch Pathol Lab Med*. 1997;121:673–677.

Compton CC. Protocol for the examination of specimens from patients with endocrine tumors of the pancreas, including those with mixed endocrine and acinar cell differentiation: a basis for checklists; Cancer Committee of the College of American Pathologists. *Arch Pathol Lab Med*. 2000;124:30–36.

Cruickshank AH. *Pathology of the Pancreas*. Berlin: Springer-Verlag; 1986.

Cubilla AL, Fitzgerald PJ. *Atlas of Tumor Pathology: Tumors of the Exocrine Pancreas*. Washington, DC: Armed Forces Institute of Pathology; 1984.

Klöppel G, Heitz PU, eds. *Pancreatic Pathology*. Edinburgh: Churchill Livingstone; 1984.

Heart Valves and Vessels

Billingham ME, Cary NR, Hammond ME, et al. A working formulation for the standardization of nomenclature in the diagnosis of heart and lung rejection: Heart Rejection Study Group; The International Society for Heart Transplantation. *J Heart Transplant*. 1990;9:587–593.

Hackel DB. Anatomy and pathology of the cardiac conducting system. In: Edwards JE, ed. *The Heart*. Baltimore, MD: Williams & Wilkins; 1974:232–247.

Hutchins GM. Special studies on the heart and lungs. In: Hutchins GM, ed. Autopsy: Performance & Reporting. Northfield, Ill, College of American Pathologists; 1990;108–114.

Morse D, Steiner RM. Cardiac valve identification atlas and guide. In: Morse D, Steiner RM, Fernandez J, eds. *Guide to Prosthetic Cardiac Valves*. New York, NY: Springer-Verlag; 1985.

Schoen FJ, Sutton MSJ. Contemporary issues in the pathology of valvular heart disease. *Hum Pathol*. 1987; 18:568–576.

Schoen FJ. Symposium on cardiovascular pathology. Part II. Surgical pathology of removed natural and prosthetic heart valves. *Hum Pathol*. 1987;18:558–567.

Silver MD. *Cardiovascular Pathology*. New York, NY: Churchill Livingstone, 1983.

Virmani R, Atkinson J, Fenoglio JJ. *Cardiovascular Pathology*. Philadelphia, PA: Saunders; 1991.

Lungs

Association of Directors of Anatomic and Surgical Pathology. Recommendations for the reporting of resected primary lung carcinomas. *Mod Pathol*. 8: 796–798, 1995.

Carter D. Pathologic examination of major pulmonary specimens resected for neoplastic disease. *Pathol Annu*. 1983;18:315–332.

Churg A. An inflation procedure for open lung biopsies. *Am J Surg Pathol*. 1983;7:69–71.

Colby TV, Koss M, Travis WD. *Atlas of Tumors of the Lower Respiratory Tract*. 3rd Series. Washington, DC: Armed Forces Institute of Pathology; 1995.

Dail DH, Hammar SP, eds. *Pulmonary Pathology*. 2nd ed. New York, NY: Springer-Verlag; 1994.

Halbower AC, Mason RJ, Abman SH, Tuder RM. Agarose infiltration improves morphology of cryostat sections of lung. *Lab Invest*. 1994;71:149–153.

Katzenstein A-LA, Askin FB. *Surgical Pathology of Nonneoplastic Lung Disease*. 2nd ed. Philadelphia, PA: Saunders; 1990.

Mark EJ. The second diagnosis: the role of the pathologist in identifying pneumoconioses in lungs excised for tumor. *Hum Pathol*. 1981;12:585–587.

Naruke T, Suemasu K, Ishikawa S. Lymph node mapping and curability at various levels of metastasis in resected lung cancer. *J Thorac Cardiovasc Surg*. 1978;76:832–839.

Thurlbeck WM, ed. *Pathology of the Lung*. New York, NY: Thieme Medical Publishers; 1988.

Transplantation

Banff schema for grading liver allograft rejection: an international consensus document. *Hepatology*. 1997;25:658–663.

Billingham ME, Cary NR, Hammond ME, et al. A working formulation for the standardization of nomenclature in the diagnosis of heart and lung rejection: Heart Rejection Study Group; The International Society for Heart Transplantation. *J Heart Transplant*. 1990;9:587–593.

Racusen LC, Solez K, Colvin RB, et al. The Banff 97 working classification of renal allograft pathology. *Kidney Int*. 1999;55:713–723.

Solez K, Axelsen RA, Benediktsson H, et al. International standardization of criteria for the histologic diagnosis of renal allograft rejection: the Banff working classification of kidney transplant pathology. *Kidney Int*. 1993;44:411–422.

Yousem SA, Berry GJ, Cagle PT, et al. Revision of the 1990 working formulation for the classification of pulmonary allograft rejection: Lung Rejection Study Group. *J Heart Lung Transplant*. 1996;15:1–15.

Bone

Dahlin DC. *Bone Tumors: General Aspects and Data on 6,221 Cases*. 3rd ed. Springfield, IL: Charles C Thomas; 1978.

Fechner RE, Mills SE. *Atlas of Tumor Pathology: Tumors of the Bone and Joints*. 3rd series, fascicle 8. Washington, DC: Armed Forces Institute of Pathology; 1993.

Huvos AG. *Bone Tumors: Diagnosis, Treatment, and Prognosis*. Philadelphia, PA: Saunders; 1991.

Vincic L, Weston S, Riddell RH. Bone core biopsies: plastic or paraffin? *Am J Surg Pathol*. 1989;13:329–334.

Soft Tissue, Nerves, and Muscle

Anthony DC, Crain BJ. Practical topics in neuropathology: nerve biopsy. *Arch Pathol Lab Med*. 1996;120:26–34.

Association of Directors for Anatomic and Surgical Pathology. Recommendations for the reporting of soft tissue sarcomas. *Am J Clin Pathol*. 1999;111:594–598.

Carpenter S, Karpati G. *Pathology of Skeletal Muscle*. New York, NY: Churchill Livingstone; 1984.

Dabowitz V. *Muscle Biopsy: A Practical Approach*. 2nd ed. Philadelphia, PA: Baillière Tindall, 1985.

De la Monte SM. Postmortem evaluation of neuromuscular diseases. In: Hutchins GM, ed. *Autopsy. Performance and Reporting*. Northfield, IL: College of American Pathologists; 1990:99–105.

Enzinger FM, Weiss SW. *Soft Tissue Tumors*. 3rd ed. St Louis, MO: Mosby; 1994.

Pearl G, Ghatak N. Practical topics in neuropathology: muscle biopsy. *Arch Pathol Lab Med*. In press.

Skin

Ackerman AB. *Pathology of Malignant Melanoma*. New York, NY: Masson; 1981.

Elder DE, Murphy GF. *Atlas of Tumor Pathology: Melanocytic Tumors of the Skin*. 3rd series, fascicle 2. Washington, DC: Armed Forces Institute of Pathology; 1991.

Holmes EC, Clark W. Morton DL, Eilber FR, Bochow AJ. Regional lymph node metastases and the level of invasion of primary melanoma. *Cancer*. 1976; 37:199–201.

Mondragon G, Nygaard F. Routine and special procedures for processing biopsy specimens for lesions suspected to be malignant melanomas. *Am J Dermatopathol*. 1981;3:265–272.

Murphy GF, Elder DE. *Atlas of Tumor Pathology: Nonmelanocytic Tumors of the Skin*. 3rd series, fascicle 1. Washington, DC: Armed Forces Institute of Pathology; 1991.

White CR Jr. Laboratory handling of skin biopsy specimens. *Lab Med*. 1982;13:211–217.

Wick MR, Compton C. Protocol for the examination of specimens from patients with carcinomas of the skin, excluding eyelid, vulva, and penis: a basis for checklists; Cancer Committee, College of American Pathologists. *Arch Pathol Lab Med*. 2001;125:1169–1173.

Breast

Abraham SC, Fox K, Fraker D, Solin L, Reynolds C. Sampling of grossly benign breast reexcisions: a multidisciplinary approach to assessing adequacy. *Am J Surg Pathol*. 1999;23:316–322.

Association of Directors of Anatomic and Surgical Pathology. Immediate management of mammographically detected breast lesions. *Am J Surg Pathol.* 1993; 17:850–851.

Association of Directors of Anatomic and Surgical Pathology. Recommendations for the reporting of breast carcinoma. *Hum Pathol.* 1996;27:220–224.

Azzopardi JG, Ahmed A, Millis RR. Problems in breast pathology. In: Bennington JL, ed. *Major Problems in Pathology.* Philadelphia, PA: Saunders; 1979;2:1.

Carey K. Board OKs health reform policy, breast implant protocol. *CAP Today.* 1994;8:26–28.

Henson DE, Oberman HA, Hutter RV. Practice protocol for the examination of specimens removed from patients with cancer of the breast: a publication of the Cancer Committee, College of American Pathologists; Members of the Cancer Committee, College of American Pathologists, and the Task Force for Protocols on the Examination of Specimens from Patients with Breast Cancer. *Arch Pathol Lab Med.* 1997;121:27–33.

Murad TM. What to expect from the pathology report concerning breast tumors. *Ala J Med Sci.* 1975;12: 222–224.

National Cancer Institute. Standardized management of breast specimens. *Am J Clin Pathol.* 1978;60:789–798.

Owings DV, Hann L, Schnitt SJ. How thoroughly should needle localization breast biopsies be sampled for microscopic examination? A prospective mammographic/pathologic correlative study. *Am J Surg Pathol.* 1990;14:578–583.

Schnitt SJ, Connolly JL. Processing and evaluation of breast excision specimens: a clinically oriented approach. *Am J Clin Pathol.* 1992;98:125–137.

Schnitt SJ, Wang HH. Histologic sampling of grossly benign breast biopsies: how much is enough? *Am J Surg Pathol.* 1989;13:505–512.

Gynecologic—General

Fox H, Wells M, eds. *Haines & Taylor Obstetrical and Gynaecological Pathology.* 4th ed. New York, NY: Churchill Livingstone; 1995.

Hoskins WJ, Perez CA, Young RC, eds. *Principles and Practice of Gynecologic Oncology.* 3rd ed. Philadelphia, PA: Lippincott Williams & Wilkins; 2000.

Robboy SJ, Bentley RC, Krigman H, Silverberg SG, Norris HJ, Zaino RJ. Synoptic reports in gynecologic pathology. *Int J Gynecol Pathol.* 1994;13:161–174.

Robboy SJ, Kraus FT, Kurman RJ. Gross description, processing, and reporting of gynecologic and obstetric specimens. In: Kurman RJ, ed. *Blaustein's Pathology of the Female Genital Tract.* 4th ed. New York, NY: Springer-Verlag; 2002.

Rock JA, Thompson JD. *TeLinde's Operative Gynecology.* 8th ed. Philadelphia, PA: Lippincott-Raven; 1997.

Scully RE, Bonfiglio TA, Kurman RJ, Silverberg SG, Wilkinson EJ. *Histologic Typing of Female Genital Tract Tumors.* 2nd ed. Berlin: Springer-Verlag; 1994.

Vulva, Uterus, Cervix, and Vagina

Kurman RJ, Amin MB. Protocol for the examination of specimens from patients with carcinomas of the cervix: a basis for checklists; Cancer Committee of the American College of Pathologists. *Arch Pathol Lab Med.* 1999;123:55–61.

Kurman RJ, Norris HJ, Wilkinson E. *Atlas of Tumor Pathology: Tumors of the Cervix, Vagina, and Vulva.* 3rd series, fascicle 4. Washington, DC: Armed Forces Institute of Pathology; 1992.

Mazur MT, Kurman RJ. *Diagnosis of Endometrial Biopsies and Curettings.* New York, NY: Springer-Verlag; 1994.

Scully RE. Protocol for the examination of specimens from patients with carcinomas of the vagina: a basis for checklists; Cancer Committee of the American College of Pathologists. *Arch Pathol Lab Med.* 1999;123:62–67.

Silverberg SG. Protocol for the examination of specimens from patients with carcinomas of the endometrium: a basis for checklists; Cancer Committee of the American College of Pathologists. *Arch Pathol Lab Med.* 1999;123:28–32.

Silverberg SG, Kurman RJ. *Atlas of Tumor Pathology: Tumors of the Uterine Corpus and Gestational Trophoblastic Disease.* 3rd series, fascicle 3. Washington, DC: Armed Forces Institute of Pathology; 1992.

Wilkinson EJ. Protocol for the examination of specimens from patients with carcinomas and malignant melanomas of the vulva: a basis for checklists; Cancer Committee of the American College of Pathologists. *Arch Pathol Lab Med.* 2000;124:51–56.

Wright TC, Gagnon S, Richart RM, Ferenczy A. Treatment of cervical intraepithelial neoplasia using the loop electro-surgical excision procedure. *Obstet Gynecol.* 1992;79:173–178.

Ovary and Fallopian Tube

Hendrickson MR, ed. *State of the Art Reviews: Surface Epithelial Neoplasms of the Ovary.* Philadelphia, PA: Hanley & Belfus; 1993.

Scully RE, Young RH, Clement PB. *Atlas of Tumor Pathology: Tumors of the Ovary, Maldeveloped Gonads, Fallopian Tube, and Broad Ligament.* 3rd series, fascicle 23. Washington, DC: Armed Forces Institute of Pathology; 1998.

Scully RE, Antman KH. Protocol for the examination of specimens from patients with tumors of the peritoneum: a basis for checklists; Cancer Committee of the American College of Pathologists. *Arch Pathol Lab Med*. 2001;125:1174–1176.

Scully RE, Henson DE, Nielsen ML, Ruby SG. Practice protocol for the examination of specimens removed from patients with ovarian tumors: a basis for checklists; Cancer Committee of the American College of Pathologists. *Arch Pathol Lab Med*. 1995;119:1012–1022.

Scully RE, Henson DE, Nielsen ML, Ruby SG. Protocol for the examination of specimens removed from patients with carcinoma of the fallopian tube: a basis for checklists; Cancer Committee of the American College of Pathologists. *Arch Pathol Lab Med*. 1999;123:33–38.

Products of Conception and Placentas

Benirschke K, Kaufmann P. *Pathology of the Human Placenta*. 4th ed. New York, NY: Springer-Verlag; 2000.

Driscoll SG, Langston C. College of American Pathologists conference XIX on the examination of the placenta: report of the working group on methods for placental examination. *Arch Pathol Lab Med*. 1991;115:704–708.

Lage J. Protocol for the examination of specimens removed from patients with gestational trophoblastic malignancies: a basis for checklists. Cancer Committee of the American College of Pathologists. *Arch Pathol Lab Med*. 1999;123:50–54.

Szulman AE. Examination of the early conceptus. *Arch Pathol Lab Med*. 1991;115:696–700.

Wigglesworth JS, Singer DB, eds. *Textbook of Fetal and Perinatal Pathology*. Boston, Mass: Blackwell Science, 1998.

Penis

Cubilla AL, Barreto J, Caballero C, Ayala G, Riveros M. Pathologic features of epidermoid carcinoma of the penis: a prospective study of 66 cases. *Am J Surg Pathol*. 1993;17:753–763.

Cubilla AL, Piris A, Pfannl R, Rodriguez I, Agüero F, Young RH. Anatomic levels: important landmarks in penectomy specimens: a detailed anatomic and histologic study based on 44 cases. *Am J Surg Pathol*. 2001;25:1091–1094.

Mostofi FK, Price EB. *Tumors of the Male Genital System*. Washington, DC: Armed Forces Institute of Pathology; 1973.

Prostate

Association of Directors of Anatomic and Surgical Pathology. Recommendations for the reporting of resected prostate carcinomas. *Pathol Int*. 1997;47:268–271.

Bova GS, Fox WM III, Epstein JI. Methods of radical prostatectomy specimen processing: a novel technique for harvesting fresh prostate cancer tissue and review of processing techniques. *Mod Pathol*. 1993;6:201–207.

Epstein JI. Evaluation of radical prostatectomy capsular margins of resection: the significance of margins designated as negative, closely approaching, and positive. *Am J Surg Pathol*. 1990;14:626–632.

Epstein JI. Evaluation of radical prostatectomy specimens: therapeutic and prognostic implications. *Pathol Annu*. 1991;26:159–210.

Epstein JI. Pathologic assessment of the surgical specimen. *Urol Clin North Am*. 2001;28:567–594.

Fechner RE. Recommendations for the reporting of resected prostate carcinomas. *Virchows Arch*. 1996;428:203–206.

Hall GS, Kramer CE, Epstein JI. Evaluation of radical prostatectomy specimens: a comparative analysis of sampling methods. *Am J Surg Pathol*. 1992;16:315–324.

Henson DE, Hutter RVP, Farrow G. Practice protocol for the examination of specimens removed from patients with carcinoma of the prostate gland. *Arch Pathol Lab Med*. 1994;118:779–783.

Moore GH, Lawshe B, Murphy J. Diagnosis of adenocarcinoma in transurethral resectates of the prostate gland. *Am J Surg Pathol*. 1986;10:165–169.

Mostofi FK. Prostate sampling. *Am J Surg Pathol*. 1986;10:175. Letter.

Murphy WM, Dean PJ, Brasfield JA, Tatum L. Incidental carcinoma of the prostate: how much sampling is adequate? *Am J Surg Pathol*. 1986;10:170–174.

Randall A. *Surgical Pathology of Prostatic Obstructions*. Baltimore, MD: Williams & Wilkins; 1931.

Ruijter ET, Miller GJ, Aalders TW, et al. Rapid microwave-stimulated fixation of entire prostactectomy specimens: Biomed-II MPC Study Group. *J Pathol*. 1997;183:369–375.

Schmid H-P, McNeal JE. An abbreviated standard procedure for accurate tumor volume estimation in prostate cancer. *Am J Surg Pathol*. 1992;16:184–191.

Yatani R, Furusato M, Sakamoto A, Harada M. Editorial comments regarding the American Association of Directors of Anatomic and Surgical Pathology recommendations for the reporting of resected prostate carcinomas; Committee of the Japanese Pathological Society for the General Rules for Clinical and Pathological Studies on Prostatic Cancer. *Pathol Int*. 1997;47:272–274.

Testis

Association of Directors for Anatomic and Surgical Pathology. Protocol for malignant and potentially malignant neoplasms of the testis and paratestis. *Am J Clin Pathol.* 2000;114:339–342.

Borski AA. Diagnosis, staging and natural history of testicular tumors. *Cancer.* 1973;32:1202–1205.

Collins DH, Pugh RCB. *The Pathology of Testicular Tumors.* Edinburgh: E&S Livingstone; 1964.

Pugh RCB, ed. *Pathology of the Testis.* Oxford, UK: Blackwell Scientific Publications; 1976.

Talerman A, Roth LM, eds. *Contemporary Issues in Surgical Pathology: Pathology of the Testis and Its Adnexa.* New York, NY: Churchill Livingstone; 1986.

Kidney

Association of Directors for Anatomic and Surgical Pathology. Recommendations for the reporting of resected neoplasm of the kidney. *Hum Pathol.* 1996;27:1005–1007.

Holland JM. Cancer of the kidney: natural history and staging. *Cancer.* 1973;32:1030–1042.

Murphy WM, Beckwith JB, Farrow GM. *Atlas of Tumor Pathology: Tumors of the Kidney, Bladder, and Related Structures.* 3rd series, fascicle 11. Washington, DC: Armed Forces Institute of Pathology; 1994.

Bladder

Association of Directors of Anatomic and Surgical Pathology. Recommendations for the reporting of urinary bladder specimens containing bladder neoplasms. *Pathol Int.* 1997;47:329–331.

Friedell GH, Parija GC, Nagy GK, Soto EA. The pathology of human bladder cancer. *Cancer.* 1980;45:1823–1831.

Murphy WM, Beckwith JB, Farrow GM. *Atlas of Tumor Pathology: Tumors of the Kidney, Bladder, and Related Structures.* 3rd series, fascicle 11. Washington, DC: Armed Forces Institute of Pathology; 1994.

Skinner DG. Current state of classification and staging of bladder cancer. *Cancer Res.* 1977;37:2838–2842.

Young RH, ed. *Contemporary Issues in Surgical Pathology: Pathology of the Urinary Bladder.* New York, NY: Churchill Livingstone; 1989.

Eye

Apple DJ, Rabb MF. *Ocular Pathology: Clinical Applications and Self-Assessment.* St Louis, MO: Mosby-Year Book; 1991:1–13.

Beck K, Jensen OA. *External Ocular Tumors. Textbook and Atlas.* Philadelphia, PA: Saunders; 1978.

Doxanas MT, Green WR, Iliff CE. Factors in the successful surgical management of basal cell carcinoma of the eyelids. *Am J Ophthalmol.* 1981;91:726–736.

Duane T. *Clinical Ophthalmology.* New York, NY: Harper & Row; 1976.

Engel H, de la Cruz ZC, Green WR, Michels RG. Cytopreparatory techniques for eye fluid specimens obtained by vitrectomy. *Acta Cytol.* 1982;26:551–560.

Folberg R, Verdick R, Weingeist TA, Montague PR. The gross examination of eyes removed for choroidal and ciliary body melanomas. *Ophthalmology.* 1986;93:1643–1647.

Hogan MJ, Zimmerman LE. *Ophthalmic Pathology. An Atlas and Textbook.* 2nd ed. Philadelphia, PA: Saunders, 1962.

Luna LG. *Manual of Histologic Staining Methods of the Armed Forces Institute of Pathology.* New York, NY: McGraw-Hill; 1968:53–54.

Menocal NG, Ventura DB, Yanoff M. Eye techniques: routine processing of ophthalmic tissue for light microscopy. In: Sheehan DC, Hrapchak BB, eds. *Theory and Practice of Histotechnology.* 2nd ed. St Louis, MO: Mosby; 1980:285–291.

Shields JA, Shields CL, Ehya H, Eagle RC Jr, De Potter P. Fine-needle aspiration biopsy of suspected intraocular tumors. *Ophthalmology.* 1993;100:1677–1684.

Spencer WH, ed. *Ophthalmic Pathology: An Atlas and Textbook.* 3rd ed. Philadelphia, PA: Saunders, 1985.

Torczynski E. Preparation of ocular specimens for histopathologic examination. *Ophthalmology.* 1981;88:1367–1371.

Yanoff M, Fine B. *Ocular Pathology. A Text and Atlas.* New York, NY: Harper & Row; 1975.

Thyroid

LiVolsi VA. *Surgical Pathology of the Thyroid.* Philadelphia, Pa: Saunders; 1990.

Rosai J, Carcangiu ML, DeLellis RA. *Atlas of Tumor Pathology: Tumors of the Thyroid Gland.* 3rd series, fascicle 5. Washington, DC: Armed Forces Institute of Pathology; 1992.

Rosai J, Carcangiu ML, DeLellis RA, Simoes MS. Recommendations for the reporting of thyroid carcinomas; Association of Directors of Anatomic and Surgical Pathology. *Hum Pathol.* 2000;31:1199–1201.

Sneed DC. Protocol for the examination of specimens removed from patients with malignant tumors of the thyroid gland, exclusive of lymphnas: a basis for checklists; Cancer Committee, College of American Pathologists. *Arch Pathol Lab Med.* 1999;123:45–49.

Yamashina M. Follicular neoplasms of the thyroid: total circumferential evaluation of the fibrous capsule. *Am J Surg Pathol.* 1992;16:392–400.

Parathyroid Glands

DeLellis RA. *Atlas of Tumor Pathology: Tumors of the Parathyroid Gland.* 3rd series, fascicle 6. Washington, DC: Armed Forces Institute of Pathology; 1993.

Geelhoed GW, Silverberg SG. Intraoperative imprints for the identification of parathyroid tissue. *Surgery.* 1984;96:1124–1131.

Grimelius L, Åkerström, G, Johansson H, Bergström R. Anatomy and histopathology of human parathyroid glands. *Pathol Annu.* 1981;16:1–24.

LiVolsi VA, Hamilton R. Intraoperative assessment of parathyroid gland pathology: a common view from the surgeon and the pathologist. *Am J Clin Pathol.* 1994;102:365–373.

Adrenal Glands

Association of Directors for Anatomic and Surgical Pathology. Recommendations for the reporting of tumors of the adrenal cortex and medulla. *Am J Clin Pathol.* 1999;112:451–455.

Lack EE, ed. *Contemporary Issues in Surgical Pathology: Pathology of the Adrenal Glands.* New York, NY: Churchill Livingstone; 1990.

Neville AM, O'Hare MJ. *The Human Adrenal Cortex.* New York, NY: Springer-Verlag; 1982.

Page DL, DeLellis RA, Hough AJ Jr. *Atlas of Tumor Pathology: Tumors of the Adrenal.* 2nd series, fascicle 23. Washington, DC: Armed Forces Institute of Pathology; 1985.

Pediatric Tumors

Coffin CM, Dehner LP. Soft tissue neoplasms in childhood: a clinicopathologic overview. In: Finegold M, Bennington JL, eds. *Pathology of Neoplasia in Children and Adolescents.* Philadelphia, PA: Saunders; 1986.

Helwig EB. Malignant melanoma in children. In: *Neoplasms of the Skin and Malignant Melanoma.* Proceedings of the 20th Annual Clinical Conferences on Cancer, Houston, Tex. Chicago, IL: Year Book Medical Publishers; 1975:11–26.

Pochedly C, Miller D, Finklestein JZ. *Wilms' Tumor.* New York, NY: John Wiley; 1976.

Brain and Spinal Cord

Bell JE, Ironside JW. How to tackle a possible Creutzfeldt-Jakob disease necropsy. *J Clin Pathol.* 1993;46: 193–197.

Brown P. Guidelines for high risk autopsy cases: special precautions for Creutzfeldt-Jakob disease. In: Hutchins GM, ed. *Autopsy Performance and Reporting.* Northfield, IL: College of American Pathologists; 1990:68–74.

Burger PC, Scheithauer BW. *Atlas of Tumor Pathology: Tumors of the Central Nervous System.* 3rd series, fascicle 10. Washington, DC: Armed Forces Institute of Pathology; 1994.

Burger PC, Scheithauer BW, Vogel SF. *Surgical Pathology of the Nervous System and Its Coverings.* New York, NY: Churchill Livingstone; 1991.

Scheithauer BW. Surgical pathology of the pituitary: the adenomas. *Pathol Annu.* 1984;19:317–374.

Lymph Nodes

Compton CC, Ferry JA, Ross DW. Protocol for the examination of specimens from patients with Hodgkin's Disease; Cancer Committee, College of American Pathologists. *Arch Pathol Lab Med.* 1999;123: 75–80.

Compton CC, Harris NL, Ross DW. Protocol for the examination of specimens from patients with non-Hodgkin's lymphona; Cancer Committee, College of American Pathologists. *Arch Pathol Lab Med.* 1999;123:68–74.

Compton CC, Sobin LH. Protocol for the examination of specimens removed from patients with gastrointestinal lymphoma: a basis for checklists; Cancer Committee, College of American Pathologists, and the Task Force for Protocols on the Examination of Specimens from Patients with Gastrointestinal Lymphoma. *Arch Pathol Lab Med.* 1997;121:1042–1047.

Crowley KS. Lymph node biopsy. *Pathology.* 1983;15: 137–138.

Durkin K, Haagensen CD. An improved technique for the study of lymph nodes in surgical specimens. *Ann Surg.* 1980;191:419–429.

Jaffee ES. *Surgical Pathology of the Lymph Nodes and Related Organs*, 2nd ed. Philadelphia, PA: Saunders; 1995.

Mufarrij A, Valensi QJ. A method for the dissection of lymph node specimens (anatomic method). *Am J Surg Pathol.* 1981;5:497–500.

Spleen

Burke JS. Surgical pathology of the spleen: an approach to the differential diagnosis of splenic lymphomas and leukemias. Part 1. Diseases of the white pulp. *Am J Surg Pathol.* 1981;5:551–563.

Burke JS. Surgical pathology of the spleen: an approach to the differential diagnosis of splenic lymphomas and leukemias. Part II. Diseases of the red pulp. *Am J Surg Pathol.* 1981;5:681–694.

Thymus

Moran CA, Suster S. On the histologic heterogeneity of thymic epithelial neoplasms: impact of sampling in subtyping and classification of thymomas. *Am J Clin Pathol.* 2000;114:760–766.

Nezelof C. Thymic pathology in primary and secondary immunodeficiencies. *Histopathology*. 1992;21:499–511.

Rosai J, Levine GD. *Tumors of the Thymus*. 2nd series, fascicle 13. Washington, DC: Armed Forces Institute of Pathology; 1976.

Bone Marrow

Arber DA, Rainer P, Helbert B, Rappaport ES. Agar processing of bone marrow aspirate material. *Lab Med*. 1992;23:479–484.

Brunning RD, McKenna RW. *Atlas of Tumor Pathology: Tumors of the Bone Marrow*. 3rd series, fascicle 9. Washington, DC: Armed Forces Institute of Pathology; 1994.

Knowles DM, ed. *Neoplastic Hematopathology*. Baltimore, MD: Williams & Wilkins; 1992.

Common Uncomplicated Specimens

Daftari TK, Levine J, Fischgrund JS, Herkowitz HN. Is pathology examination of disc specimens necessary after routine anterior cervical discectomy and fusion? *Spine*. 1996;21:2156–2159.

Dohar JE, Bonilla JA. Processing of adenoid and tonsil specimens in children: a national survey of standard practices and a five-year review of the experience at the Children's Hospital of Pittsburgh. *Otolaryngol Head Neck Surg*. 1996;115:94–97.

Netser JC, Robinson RA, Smith RJ, Raab SS. Value-based pathology: a cost-benefit analysis of the examination of routine and nonroutine tonsil and adenoid specimens. *Am J Clin Pathol*. 1997;108:158–165.

Partrick DA, Bensard DD, Karrer FM, Ruyle SZ. Is routine pathological evaluation of pediatric hernia sacs justified? *J Pediatr Surg*. 1998;33:1090–1092.

Reddy P, Williams R, Willis B, Nanda A. Pathological evaluation of intervertebral disc tissue specimens after routine cervical and lumbar decompression: a cost-benefit analysis retrospective study. *Surg Neurol*. 2001;56:252–255.

Strong EB, Rubinstein B, Senders CW. Pathologic analysis of routine tonsillectomy and adenoidectomy specimens. *Otolaryngol Head Neck Surg*. 2001;125:473–477.

Wenner WJ Jr, Gutenberg M, Crombleholme T, Flickinger C, Bartlett SP. The pathological evaluation of the pediatric inguinal hernia sac. *J Pediatr Surg*. 1998;33:717–718.

Index

Acid hydrolysis, decalcification with, 19
Adenoids, 236–237
Adrenal glands
  in nephrectomy specimens, 187
  normal appearance of, 208
  sampling from adrenalectomies, 208–210
Amputations
  sampling for gangrene, 238
  sampling for tumors, 119
Anatomic landmarks, 4, 7, 9
  See also specific organ or structure
Anatomic orientation, 4, 9
Ancillary testing, fixation for, 14
Anorchia, 183
Appendix, 74–75
Arteries, 101
Association of Directors of Anatomic and Surgical Pathology (ADASP), ix, xi

B5, fixation with, 15, 16
Barrett's esophagus, 58, 61
Biliary system, 82–87
Biohazardous trash, 2–3
Bioprosthetic heart valves, 100
Bone
  amputation, specimens from, 119
  challenges in dissection of, 114, 116
  decalcifying specimens of, 116
  fragments, specimens from, 114–116
  segmental resections of, 116–118
  specimen radiographs of, 114
Bone marrow
  fluid aspiration of, 232–234
  trephine core biopsies of, 232, 234
Bouin's, fixation with, 15
Bowel, sampling of, 66–69
Brain and spinal cord
  cytologic preparations from, 218
  electron microscopy of tissues from, 220
  frozen sections and permanent sections from, 218–220
  needle biopsy specimens of, 218
  tissues from specific entities in, 220–221
Breast
  additional margins in lumpectomies of, 134, 137
  calcifications, presence of, 133
  core needle biopsies of, 133
  examining and processing fresh tissue of, 132
  lumpectomies of, 134, 135, 136
  mammographic abnormalities, biopsies for, 133–134, 135
  mastectomies of, 134, 138, 139
  reduction mammoplasty, sampling of, 138, 140
  slide index for a modified radical mastectomy, 12
Breast implants, evaluation of, 140

Cardiovascular system. *See* Heart; Heart valves; Transplantation
Carnoy's, fixation with, 16
Cataract specimens, 198–199
Cavitronic Ultrasonic Surgical Aspirator (CUSA), 142
Central nervous system, 218–221
Cervix
  cervical cancer, radical hysterectomy for, 154–155, 156–158
  cone biopsy of, 148, 149
  large loop excision of the transformation zone (LLETZ) of, 146, 148
  loop electrocautery excision procedure (LEEP) of, 146–148
  See also Uterus; Vagina
Children's Oncology Group, The (COG), 212
Cholecystectomies, 82–85
Choledochal cysts, 87
College of American Pathologists (CAP), ix, xi
Complex specimens, basic approach to, 44–47
Conception, products of, 166, 168
Cone biopsy of the cervix, 148, 149
Consistency of specimens, documenting in gross descriptions of, 7
Contamination
  as a "pickup," 4
  of specimens for RNA/DNA examination, 25
  of staining solutions, 21
  See also Laboratory techniques
Cooling sprays, 20
Craniofacial bones, resecting tumors from, 48–53
Creutzfeldt-Jakob disease, 221
Crush preparation, 20
Curettings, 146
Cutting stations, 4

Cystectomies of ovaries, 161–165
Cystic kidneys, 187
Cystic masses in the pancreas, 92
Cystoprostatectomy, 189–190, 192
Cytogenetics, sampling for, 22

Decalcification, process of, 19
Defibrillators, 100
Digestive system, 58–92
Digital images, supplementing gross descriptions with, 8, 29–30
Dissection, fundamentals of
  anatomic orientation of specimens, 4, 9
  dissecting the specimen in, 4–7
  fixing specimens in, 6
  gross description in, 7–8, 9
  inking specimens for, 5, 9
  lymph nodes, sampling of, 11, 13
  margins, sampling of, 9, 10
  normal tissues, sampling of, 11, 13
  opening and sectioning specimens, 5–6, 9
  requisition forms in, 3–4, 11
  small specimens, handling of, 4–5
  specimen orientations in, 3–4, 9
  storing specimens for, 6–7
  surgical pathology report in, 11
Distal pancreatectomies, 89–92
DNA. *See* Molecular genetic analysis, tissue collection for
Documentation of findings, 7–8, 10, 11–12, 23
See also specific organ or structure

Ectopic pregnancy, sampling of, 160
Electrolysis, decalcification with, 19
Electron microscopy, 14, 23, 220
En bloc resections, specimens from, 192
Endocervical curettings, 146
Endocrine system, 202–210
Endometrial curettings, 146
Esophagus, 58–61
Ethmoid sinus, 50
Ethyl alcohol, fixation with, 14, 16
Explanted heart, examination of, 94–96, 97
Extrahepatic biliary system, 82–87
Eye
  cataract specimens from, 198–199
  enucleation specimens of, 194–198
  fixation of ocular tissue of, 194–195
  landmarks for examination of, 195, 196, 198
  sectioning of, 196, 197, 198
  techniques for processing tissue from, 198, 199–200
Eyelid excisions, specimens from, 199

Fallopian tubes, sampling of, 160–162
Fetal parts, 166
Fixation, 6
  with acetic acid, 14, 16
  with aldehydes, 14, 15
  with ethyl alcohol, 14, 16
  group classification of, 14
  handling of small specimens with, 5
  with mercury-based fixatives, 14, 15
  with methyl alcohol, 14, 16
  of ocular tissue, 194–195
  with oxidizing agents, 14, 15
  with picric acid, 14, 15, 16
  with protein-denaturing agents, 14, 16
See also specific organ or structure
Flow cytometry, sampling for, 22, 23, 225
Foreskin, 172
Formaldehyde, fixation with, 14, 15
Fresh frozen tissue banks, 23, 25
Frontal sinus, 49
Frozen section, method of, 20–21

Gallbladder
  calculi in, 83, 85
  cholecystectomies, sampling of, 82–83, 85
  extrahepatic biliary tree excisions, sampling of, 84, 85–87
Gangrene, sampling amputations for, 238
Gastrectomies, sampling of, 62–65
Gastroesophageal junction (GEJ), 58, 62, 64
Genetic analysis, tissue collection for, 22–25
Genitourinary system
  female, 142–170, 188–192
  male, 172–192
Genomic studies, tissue collection for, 6, 22–25
Gestation, verification of, 166–168
Gliomas, 219, 220
Glottic cancers, 42
Glutaraldehyde, fixation with, 14, 15
Gram Weigert's (GW), staining with, 17, 18
Gross clearance, 64
Gross descriptions
  distributing tissues, documentation of, 8
  goals and features of, 7–8, 9
  as a legal document, 8
  role in slide indexes, 7–8, 12
  supplementing with photographic images, 8, 26–32

Heart
  arteries and veins, sampling of, 101
  cardiac tumors in, 97
  conduction system, examination of, 96
  endomyocardial biopsy of, 96–97
  evaluating transplants of, 94–96, 97, 110–111
  left ventricular devices in, 100
  pacemakers and defibrillators in, 100
  pericardium in, 97–98
Heart valves
  bioprosthetic heart valves in, 100
  mechanical heart valves in, 98–101
  native heart valves in, 98
Helicobacter pylori, 65, 227
Helly's fluid, fixation with, 15
Hematopoietic tumors, genetic profiling of, 22
Hematoxylin and eosin (H&E), staining with, 17
Hepatectomies, partial or total, 76–81

Hernia sacs, 237
Histofreeze, 20
Histology
   handling small and delicate specimens for, 5
   inking specimens for, 5, 9
   See also specific organ or structure
Human Genome Project, 22

Immunohistochemical staining, 14, 19
Impression smears, 19–20
Inflammatory bowel disease, 66–69
Inking specimens, 5, 9
   See also specific organ or structure
In situ hybridization, 14
Instruments, safe handling of, 2–3
Interface zones, sampling of, 8–10, 13
Internal Review Board (IRB), 25
International Society for Heart and Lung
   Transplantation (ISHLT), 110–111
Intersex syndromes, 183
Intervertebral disk material, 237–238
Intestinal disease, non-neoplastic or neoplastic, 66–73
Intraoperative consultation
   crush preparations, method of, 20
   cytologic slides, preparation of, 19–20
   frozen section, method of, 20–21
   with impression smears, 19–20
   scrapings, method of, 20
   with touch preparations, 20
Intrauterine pregnancy. *See* Placentas; Products of conception

Kidneys
   biopsies of, 184
   cystic kidneys, sections of, 187
   evaluating transplants of, 111
   nephrectomies for neoplastic disease, sampling of, 184–187
   nephrectomies for non-neoplastic disease, 186, 187
   partial nephrectomies, sampling of, 187
   pediatric renal neoplasms, 213–215

Laboratory techniques
   approaches to complex specimens, 44–47
   decalcification, methods of, 19
   fixation, 14–17
   immunohistochemical staining in, 19
   intraoperative consultation in, 19–21
   special staining in, 17–19
Large loop excision of the transformation zone (LLETZ), 146, 148
Larynx
   anatomy and landmarks of, 38–39, 40
   subtotal laryngectomies, specimens from, 42
   supraglottic, glottic, or subglottic cancers in, 42
   total laryngectomy, sampling of, 39, 41–42
Left ventricular devices, 100
Lesions, localizing of, 6, 9
Liver
   biopsies of, 76
   evaluating transplants of, 111
   explants, sampling of, 79–81
   hepatectomies, sampling from, 76–79
Loop electrocautery excision procedure (LEEP), 146–147
Lumpectomies of breast tissue, 134, 135, 136, 137
Lungs
   components of, 102
   evaluating transplants of, 111
   limited pulmonary resections, sampling of, 102–104
   lobectomies and pneumonectomies, 104–105, 107
   pleural resections for malignant mesotheliomas in, 105–109
   wedge resections of, 102–104
Lymph nodes
   in adrenalectomy specimens, 210
   biopsy of sentinel lymph nodes, 3, 34–36
   in esophagectomy specimens, 59
   evaluating for metastatic disease, 34–36
   extranodal specimens with, 226–227
   finding and sampling of, 11, 13
   pelvic lymph dissection of, 179
   in radical neck dissections, 54
   rapid handling specimens of, 224–226
   within thyroidectomies, 204
   tissues to submit, 224–226
   See also specific organ or structure
Lymphomas, 220–221

Malignant mesothelioma, 105, 109
Margins
   additional margins in lumpectomies of, 134, 137
   sampling of, 9, 10, 13
Mastectomies, 134, 138, 139
Maxilla, 48–53
Medical devices
   evaluation of heart valves and assistive devices, 98–101
   storing specimens of, 7
Melanomas, 128–129
Meningiomas, 220
Mercuric chlorides, fixation with, 14, 15
Metastatic disease, evaluating lymph nodes for, 34–36
Modified neck dissections, 54–56
Modified radical mastectomy, 12
Moh's micrographic surgery of skin, 128
Molecular genetic analysis, tissue collection for, 22–25
Muscles, biopsies of, 122–123

Nasal cavity and sinuses, 48–53
Neck dissections, 54–56
Needle biopsy
   of brain and spinal cord, 218
   of breast tissue, 133
   of the liver, 76

Neoplastic intestinal disease
  polypectomy, sampling of, 70–71
  resected intestinal neoplasms, specimens from, 72–73
Nephrectomies, sampling of, 184–187
Nerves, biopsies of, 122–123
Non-neoplastic intestinal disease
  sampling for inflammatory bowel disease, 66–69
  small and large intestine resections, sampling of, 66–69

Oil red O (ORO), staining with, 17
Oligodendrogliomas, 220
Omentectomies, sampling of, 165
Oophorectomies, 161–165
Open enucleation of the prostate, 176
Opening and sectioning specimens, fundamentals of, 5–6, 9
Orchiectomies, 180–183
Organic chelation, decalcification with, 19
Orientation of specimens, 3–4, 9
Osmium tetroxide, fixation with, 14
Ovary
  biopsies and wedge resections of, 160
  ovarian cystectomies and oophorectomies of, 161–165
  specimens for tumor staging, 165

Pacemakers, 100
Pancreas
  ampulla of Vater, sampling of, 92
  cystic tumors in, 92
  distal pancreatectomies, sampling of, 89, 90, 92
  pancreaticoduodenectomies, specimens of, 88–89, 91
  Whipple procedure, sampling of, 88–89, 91
Papanicolaou (PAP), staining with, 17, 18–19
Parallel section, sampling of margins with, 9, 10, 13
Paranasal sinuses, 48–53
Parathyroid glands, 7, 206–207
Parotid glands, 43
Pediatric tumors
  general guidelines for, 212
  pediatric renal neoplasms, 213–215
  small blue cell tumors of childhood, 212–213
  tissue for biologic studies and classification, 212
Pelvic exenterations, 157, 158–159
Penectomies, 172–174
Penis
  components of, 172
  foreskin, sampling of, 172
  penectomies, sampling of, 172–174
Peptic ulcer disease, 62, 63
Periodic acid-Schiff (PAS), staining with, 17–18
Perpendicular section, sampling of margins with, 9, 10, 13
Photographing specimens
  backgrounds and lighting for, 26–28
  camera stands and lens selection for, 26
  determining standardized exposure times, 28–29
  digital photography in, 29–30
  managing shapes and other features of specimens, 30–31
  placing scales in, 29
  setting up a system, 26–30
  steps of, 30
  supplementing gross descriptions with, 8
  troubleshooting and maintaining system of, 31–32
  using 35-mm slides, 28
"Pickup," cancer fragments in, 4
Picric acid, fixation with, 14, 15, 16
Pituitary adenomas, 221
Placentas, 167–170
Pneumonectomies, 104–105
Polymerase chain reaction (PCR)-based molecular testing, 16, 25
Polypectomies, 70–71
Potassium dichromate, fixation with, 14, 15
Potassium permanganate, fixation with, 14
Primitive tumors, genetic profiling of, 22
Products of conception, 166, 167
Prostate
  biopsies of, 176
  pelvic lymph dissection with, 179
  prostate chips, 176
  radical prostatectomies, 176–179
  transurethral resections and open enucleations of, 176
  See also Cystoprostatectomy
Prosthetic Cardiac Valves, Guide to, 100
Prosthetic devices
  breast implants in, 140
  in the heart, 98–101
  storing specimens of, 7
Pulmonary resections, 102–109
Punch biopsies of skin, 127–128

Radical neck dissections, 54–56
Radical orchiectomies, 180–182
Radical prostatectomies, 176–179
Radioactive specimens, 3, 35
Rectum, 67, 72
Reduction mammoplasty, sampling of, 138, 140
Requisitions forms, 3–4, 11
Resected intestinal neoplasms, 72–73
Respiratory system. See Lungs
RNA. See Molecular genetic analysis, tissue collection for
RNAlater™, 23, 25
Roswell Park Memorial Institute (RPMI), medium of, 22, 23, 25, 224

Safety in the pathology laboratory
  disposal of instruments and trash, 2–3
  handling radioactive specimens, 3, 35
  preventing needle sticks or knife cuts, 239
  protective gear for, 2
  storage of specimens in, 2–3
  universal precautions for, 2

Salivary glands, 43
Salpingectomies, 160–162
Salpingo-oophorectomy, 161–165
Scrapings, method of, 20
Sectioning, artifacts in, 20
Segmental resections of bone, 116–118
Seizures, temporal lobe specimens for, 221
Selective neck dissections, 54–56
Selective sampling, 8, 13
Sentinel lymph nodes
   biopsy and examination of, 34–36
   handling radioactive specimens of, 3, 35
Shape of specimens, documenting in gross
     descriptions of, 7, 9
Shave specimens, 10, 13
Size of specimens, documenting in gross
     descriptions of, 7, 9
Skin
   biopsies of, 124–127
   elliptical and round specimens of, 124–127
   examining nontraditional specimens of, 128
   punch biopsies of, 127–128
   specimens from Moh's micrographic surgery, 128
Slide index
   documenting method of sampling margins in, 10
   function of gross description with, 7–8, 12
Small blue cell tumors of childhood, 212–213
Soft tissue
   dissection and sampling of, 120–122
   sampling gangrene from amputations, 238
Specimens, sampling of
   goals of, 8–11, 13
   selective sampling in, 8, 13
Spinal cord. *See* Brain and spinal cord
Spleen
   processing specimens from, 228–229
   red or white pulp of, 228–229
Staging neoplasms, 7, 11
Staining
   with Gram Weigert's (GW), 17, 18
   with hematoxylin and eosin (H&E), 17
   immunohistochemical stains in, 19
   with oil red O (ORO), 17
   with periodic acid-Schiff (PAS), 17–18
   with Ziehl-Neelsen, 17, 18
Stomach
   anatomic regions of, 62–64
   gastrectomies, sampling of, 62–65
   See also Neoplastic or Non-neoplastic intestinal
     disease
Storing specimens, 6–7
Subglottic cancers, 42
Subtotal laryngectomies, 42
Supraglottic tumors, 42
Surgical pathology reports, 11

Tags or sutures, role in anatomical orientation,
   4, 7, 9
Teeth, handling of, 49, 50, 51
Temporal artery, biopsy of, 101

Testis
   anorchia and intersex syndromes in, 183
   bilateral orchiectomies for prostate cancer of,
     182–183
   biopsies of, 180
   radical orchiectomy of, 180–182
   testicular neoplasms, sampling of, 182
   torsion, infarction, or infectious disease in, 183
   undescended testis, processing of, 182
Thymus, 231
Thyroid, 202–205
Tissue
   dissecting soft tissues, 120–122
   documenting distribution of, 8, 23
   documenting surgical removal of structures, 11, 13
   handling of, 4–5
Tissue banks, 23, 25
Tonsils and adenoids, 236–237
Torsion of testis, 183
Total colectomies, 68
Total cystectomies, sampling of, 188–192
Total laryngectomy, sampling of, 39, 41–42
Touch imprints, distributing tissue for, 23
Touch preparation, 20
Transplantation
   biopsies from transplant recipients, 110
   complications of, 110
   hearts, sampling of, 94–96, 97, 110–111
   kidneys, evaluating transplants of, 111
   liver, sampling of, 79–81, 111
   lungs, evaluating transplants of, 111
Transurethral resection of the prostate, 176
Tumors
   classification by genetic profiling of, 22, 25
   gross descriptions of, 7
   multidisciplinary tumor bank protocol with, 23
   pediatric tumors, processing of, 212–215
   periphery, sampling from, 8, 10, 13
   sampling of, 8, 10
   staging of, 7, 11
   See also specific organs or structure

Undescended testis, 182
Universal precautions, 2
Urachal tract, 189–192
Urinary bladder
   biopsies of, 188
   cystectomies, sampling of, 188–190
   cystoprostatectomy, sampling of, 189–190, 192
   en bloc resections, specimens from, 192
Uterus
   evaluating appearance of, 148–150
   hysterectomy for endometrial cancer, 152–154
   hysterectomy for nonmalignant disease of,
     150–152
   pelvic exenterations and vaginectomies of, 157,
     158–159
   radical hysterectomy for cervical cancer, 154–155,
     156–158
   See also Cervix; Vagina

Vagina
  biopsies of, 146
  vaginectomies, sampling of, 158–159
  See also Cervix; Uterus
Veins, sampling of, 101
Vulva
  Cavitronic Ultrasonic Surgical Aspirator (CUSA) biopsies of, 142
  components of, 142
  excisional biopsies of, 142, 144
  small biopsies of, 142
  vulvectomies, specimens from, 143, 144–145

Vulvar intraepithelial neoplasia (VIN), 142, 144, 145

Wedge biopsy
  of the liver, 76
  of lungs, 102–104
  of ovaries, 160
Weight of specimens, documenting in gross descriptions of, 7, 9
Whipple procedure, 88–89, 91

Zenker's, fixation with, 15
Ziehl-Neelsen, staining with, 17, 18